FOCUS Psychiatry Review:
400 Self-Assessment Questions

FOCUS Psychiatry Review: 400 Self-Assessment Questions

A workbook with questions covering the
ABPN outline of topics for recertification:

Anxiety Disorders
Bipolar Disorder
Child and Adolescent Psychiatry
Clinical Neuroscience and Genetics
Forensic and Ethical Issues in Psychiatry
Gender, Race, and Culture
Geriatric Psychiatry
Major Depressive Disorders
Personality Disorders
Posttraumatic Stress Disorder
Psychopharmacology
Psychosomatic Medicine
Psychotherapy
Schizophrenia
Sleep, Sex, and Eating Disorders
Substance-Related Disorders

Editors

Deborah J. Hales, M.D.

Mark Hyman Rapaport, M.D.

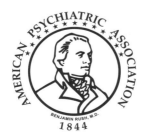

Manufactured in the United States of America on acid-free paper

American Psychiatric Association
1000 Wilson Boulevard
Arlington, VA 22209-3901
www.psych.org

ISBN-13: 978-**0-89042-297-7**

Contents

Introduction

In today's world it is hard to keep up with the explosive growth in knowledge. Psychiatric practice is rapidly improving thanks to developments in evidence-based practice and advances in neuroscience research. The editors of *FOCUS* developed the *FOCUS Psychiatry Review* as an aid for psychiatrists in lifelong learning in the field. This workbook contains 400 board-type multiple-choice questions from *FOCUS*'s annual Self-Assessment Examinations that can help psychiatrists prepare for examinations and identify areas for further study. The questions, developed by the *FOCUS* self-assessment board, are consistent in form and process with the questions used by high-stakes examinations. They cover important clinical areas of psychiatric practice and closely follow the American Board of Psychiatry and Neurology (ABPN) outline of topics for the recertification examination in psychiatry.

The *FOCUS Psychiatry Review* is designed to test current knowledge and its clinical application. The workbook is flexible in format, allowing readers to use the educational approach that works best for them. Readers can review resource materials prior to answering questions, or they can use the workbook to review the references listed in the critiques after scoring test sections.

The workbook will be useful for anyone committed to lifelong learning in the field—psychiatric residents, practicing psychiatrists, and psychiatrists preparing for examinations.

- The *FOCUS Psychiatry Review* contains 400 clinical questions that can be used to identify areas of strength and weakness.
- It provides up-to-date critiques and current references to facilitate further study.
- It is a complementary component to a larger overall program of lifelong learning for the psychiatrist who wants to keep current in the field.

This edition covers the following topics:

Anxiety Disorders

Bipolar Disorder

Child and Adolescent Psychiatry

Clinical Neuroscience and Genetics

Forensic and Ethical Issues in Psychiatry

Gender, Race, and Culture

Geriatric Psychiatry

Major Depressive Disorders

Personality Disorders

Posttraumatic Stress Disorder

Psychopharmacology

Psychosomatic Medicine

Psychotherapy

Schizophrenia

Sleep, Sex, and Eating Disorders

Substance-Related Disorders

The *FOCUS Psychiatry Review* provides up to 50 hours of Continuing Medical Education Credit.

APA is accredited by ACCME to provide continuing medical education for physicians.
APA designates this educational activity for a maximum of 50 AMA PRA Category 1 credits. Physicians should claim credit commensurate with the extent of their participation in the activity.

Educational Objectives

At the completion of the activity, participants will
1) have an increased understanding of new developments in psychiatric diagnosis and treatment;
2) be aware of resources available for learning more about these developments; and
3) recognize areas of strength and areas where more study is needed.

To obtain Continuing Medical Education Credit, complete and send this page to:

American Psychiatric Association
Department of CME
1000 Wilson Blvd., Suite 1825
Arlington, VA 22209
Fax: 703-907-7849
plee@psych.org

Begin date: July 2006
End date: July 2009

AMERICAN PSYCHIATRIC ASSOCIATION
FOCUS Psychiatry Review:
400 Self-Assessment Questions

I have participated for _____ hours (up to 50) in completion of this CME activity.

Name (please print): _____

Address: _____

Address: _____

City/State/Zip: _____

E-mail_____   Fax _____

Please send my certificate by: Mail _____   Fax _____   E-mail _____

1. The quality of the *FOCUS Psychiatry Review* workbook was excellent.
   Strongly agree   Agree   Disagree   Strongly disagree

2. The *FOCUS Psychiatry Review* workbook was useful to me in preparing for examinations.
   Strongly agree   Agree   Disagree   Strongly disagree

3. The workbook was useful in helping me understand my areas of strength and weakness.
   Strongly agree   Agree   Disagree   Strongly disagree

4. The workbook will be helpful to me in my clinical practice.
   Strongly agree   Agree   Disagree   Strongly disagree

5. The material in the *FOCUS Psychiatry Review* was presented without bias.
   Strongly agree   Agree   Disagree   Strongly disagree

6. The questions were: too hard ___, just right ___, too easy ___.

Comments:

_____

_____

_____

Section 1: Self-Assessment Questions

1

A clinician is considering combination therapy for treatment-resistant depression. Which of the following combinations has the most potential for serious adverse reactions?

(A) Bupropion and fluoxetine
(B) Buspirone and nortriptyline
(C) Paroxetine and desipramine
(D) Phenelzine and lithium carbonate
(E) Venlafaxine and tranylcypromine

2

Which of the following conditions is most commonly comorbid with prepubertal bipolar disorder?

(A) Attention deficit hyperactivity disorder (ADHD)
(B) Autistic disorder
(C) Separation anxiety disorder
(D) Tourette's disorder

3

A 39-year-old actuary for an insurance company is offered a substantial promotion that will require her to move to another city. Her new office will be on the 23rd floor of a high-rise building. She informs her psychiatrist that she is "terrified" of riding in an elevator and terrified of heights, but desperately wants the new job. Which of the interventions listed below is most likely to be successful for her?

(A) Cognitive therapy
(B) Hypnotherapy
(C) Insight-oriented psychotherapy
(D) Selective serotonin reuptake inhibitors
(E) Systematic desensitization

4

During resettlement, a refugee takes on the values and attitudes of the new culture and does not retain his original cultural values. Which of the following best describes this process?

(A) Integration
(B) Assimilation
(C) Separation
(D) Marginalization

5

Parasomnias can be differentiated from dyssomnias because parasomnias involve abnormalities in which of the following aspects of sleep?

(A) Amount of sleep
(B) Initiation of sleep
(C) Physiological systems that occur during sleep
(D) Quality of sleep
(E) Timing of sleep

6

A 27-year-old male patient with an initial episode of schizophrenia is treated with risperidone at an initial dose of 2 mg daily, and after 1 week of treatment he no longer experiences agitation. By the third week of treatment, with gradual titration of risperidone to 6 mg daily, his delusions and hallucinations are significantly improved. At week 4, he describes some trouble sleeping at night because of restlessness but reports that he is much less fearful and no longer hears voices. When seen for a scheduled appointment at week 6, however, he is noticeably drooling and is in constant motion, rocking back and forth and fidgeting in his chair. The side effect of treatment that he is most likely experiencing is:

(A) akathisia.
(B) neuroleptic malignant syndrome.
(C) restless leg syndrome.
(D) serotonin syndrome.
(E) tardive dyskinesia.

7

A patient takes a medication for bipolar I disorder throughout pregnancy and delivery. The newborn is noted to be cyanotic and in respiratory distress. An echocardiogram reveals significant displacement of two leaflets of the tricuspid valve into the ventricle and a large atrial septal defect consistent with Ebstein's anomaly. Of the following medications, which was the woman most likely taking during her pregnancy?

(A) Carbamazepine
(B) Gabapentin
(C) Lithium
(D) Topiramate
(E) Valproate

8

A forensic psychiatric evaluation differs from a general psychiatric evaluation in that a forensic evaluation:

(A) typically includes a mental status examination.
(B) does not have a doctor-patient relationship.
(C) requires a completed written report.
(D) requires the presence of a lawyer during the evaluation.

9

A 30-year-old man reports that he is unable to sleep and hears noises and voices at night even though he lives alone. The symptoms started abruptly on the day preceding the visit. During the interview, he repeatedly brushes off his arms, muttering about bugs. The information that would be most helpful in determining initial interventions would be the history of:

(A) family disorders.
(B) medical problems.
(C) psychiatric hospitalization.
(D) recent stresses.

10

The practice of obtaining informed consent from an individual prior to initiating any treatment fulfills which of the following ethical principles?

(A) Nonmaleficence
(B) Autonomy
(C) Justice
(D) Competence

11

Which of the following psychotherapies has the best documented effectiveness in the treatment of major depressive disorder?

(A) Supportive
(B) Psychodynamic
(C) Interpersonal
(D) Psychoeducational
(E) Family

12

Which of the following antidepressants would be the best choice for a patient concerned about erectile dysfunction?

(A) Bupropion
(B) Fluoxetine
(C) Nortriptyline
(D) Imipramine
(E) Venlafaxine

13

The National Comorbidity Survey identified a number of gender differences in exposure and in the development of posttraumatic stress disorder (PTSD). Compared with females, males have:

(A) higher trauma exposure, and higher prevalence of PTSD.
(B) lower trauma exposure, and lower prevalence of PTSD.
(C) higher trauma exposure, and lower prevalence of PTSD.
(D) lower trauma exposure, and higher prevalence of PTSD.
(E) the same trauma exposure, and the same prevalence of PTSD.

14

A cancer patient with significant nausea requires an antidepressant. Which of the following medications would be the best choice?

(A) Bupropion
(B) Duloxetine
(C) Mirtazapine
(D) Paroxetine
(E) Venlafaxine

15

When non-substance abusing men and women drink the same amount of alcohol, the women are likely to have higher alcohol blood levels than the men. The best explanation for this is that compared with men, women:

(A) have a larger volume of distribution.
(B) have lower excretion rates.
(C) only metabolize by first-order kinetics.
(D) metabolize less alcohol in the gut.
(E) are deficient in acetaldehyde dehydrogenase.

16

Which of the following situations best describes when weight considerations should determine hospitalization for anorexia nervosa in children and young adolescents?

(A) Weight is less than 20% of recommended healthy body weight.
(B) Weight is less than 25% of ideal body weight.
(C) Weight is being rapidly lost and outpatient efforts are ineffective, regardless of actual weight.
(D) The family asks for hospitalization.
(E) Weight is fluctuating unpredictably over 2–3 months.

17

Which of the following antipsychotic drugs is most likely to be associated with hyperprolactinemia?

(A) Aripiprazole
(B) Clozapine
(C) Olanzapine
(D) Quetiapine
(E) Risperidone

18

Which of the following atypical antipsychotic drugs is a D$_2$ receptor partial agonist?

(A) Aripiprazole
(B) Olanzapine
(C) Quetiapine
(D) Risperidone
(E) Ziprasidone

19

A 33-year-old man started twice-weekly psychodynamic psychotherapy 6 months ago with the goal of exploring issues stemming from his distant relationship with his father and his inability to form adequate mentoring relationships in his work as a research chemist. He reports an increasing preoccupation with his therapist's unwillingness to see him more frequently. The patient has been speaking in therapy of his wish that the therapist see him on Sunday. He believes that the therapist refuses to have extra sessions because he prefers other patients. Which of the following best explains the patient's behavior?

(A) Transference neurosis
(B) Delusional system
(C) Obsessional diathesis
(D) Erotomania
(E) Psychotic distortion

20

Which of the following disorders has the highest relative risk for first-degree relatives?

(A) Alcoholism
(B) Anorexia
(C) Bipolar disorder
(D) Panic disorder
(E) Somatization disorder

21

A 68-year-old man has a grand mal seizure that is attributed to an abrupt hyponatremia, with a serum sodium concentration of 110 mmol/L. Which of the following medications is the most likely cause?

(A) Gabapentin
(B) Lithium
(C) Oxcarbazepine
(D) Topiramate
(E) Valproate

22

Social rhythm therapy, which is designed specifically for bipolar disorder, is based on which of the following models?

(A) Psychoeducation
(B) Object relations and self psychology theory
(C) Circadian regulation and interpersonal psychotherapy
(D) Cognitive therapy techniques to address social dysfunction
(E) Supportive psychotherapy

23

Rapid cycling in bipolar I or II disorder is associated with:

(A) menopause.
(B) antidepressant use.
(C) cocaine abuse.
(D) early onset.
(E) alcohol abuse.

24

A 65-year-old woman has a history of a left frontal lobe stroke. Which of the following psychiatric symptoms is most commonly associated with a stroke in this area of the brain?

(A) Panic
(B) Mania
(C) Depression
(D) Obsessions
(E) Anxiety

25

Genetic studies of obsessive-compulsive disorder have revealed linkages to which of the following disorders?

(A) Alcohol dependence
(B) Schizophrenia
(C) Shared psychotic disorder
(D) Somatoform disorder
(E) Tourette's syndrome

26

A psychiatrist proposes to use an FDA-approved drug not previously used for the treatment of mania because it has biochemical properties similar to known antimanic agents. The psychiatrist has also read several articles describing open-label studies suggesting efficacy of the drug. The patient in question has not responded to any agent thus far. The psychiatrist must do which of the following?

(A) Get an institutional review board approval, since what is proposed is clinical research.
(B) Notify the FDA, since the drug is being used for a non-FDA-approved purpose.
(C) Obtain informed consent from the patient or from an appropriate proxy agent.
(D) Wait until there is higher-quality data to support this use of the drug.

27

A 75-year-old retired physicist who is suffering from metastatic cancer is referred to a psychiatrist by the primary care physician because the patient wants to die and has requested assistance in suicide. On evaluation, the psychiatrist finds that the patient's cognition is intact. The most appropriate next step for the psychiatrist is to:

(A) be as persuasive as possible so that the patient accepts the cancer treatment.
(B) find out whether there are areas of suffering that can be addressed by available palliative care measures.
(C) tell the referring physician that the patient can be given assistance in suicide because the patient is a competent adult.
(D) tell the referring physician that even though the patient's cognition appears intact, the patient is probably incapacitated by virtue of the unreasonable choice that is being made.

28

Of the following ethnic groups, which is at lowest risk of completed suicide?

(A) African Americans
(B) Asian Americans
(C) Caucasian Americans
(D) Hispanic Americans
(E) Native Americans

29

A 15-year-old boy is referred for psychiatric evaluation after taking an overdose of an over-the-counter cold medication. The patient denies that this was a suicide attempt. The patient acknowledges that he has been having difficulties for about a year, since the separation of his parents. He often feels angry and irritable, has difficulty sleeping, has little appetite, has lost weight, has little interest in his usual activities, and often wishes he was dead. His grades have dropped to the point that he is failing his courses. Over the past year, he has been smoking 1–2 packs of cigarettes a day, drinking to the point of intoxication on the weekends, and taking over-the-counter cold medication to enhance the effects of the alcohol. His past psychiatric history is significant for attention deficit hyperactivity disorder (ADHD), for which he has a prescription for a stimulant medication. He has not taken his medication as prescribed. Instead, he hoards the medication and then takes large quantities to experience a euphoric effect. Which of the following medications would be the most efficacious in addressing this patient's symptom constellation?

(A) Bupropion
(B) Citalopram
(C) Desipramine
(D) Trazodone
(E) Venlafaxine

30

A psychiatrist attends a dinner lecture sponsored by a major pharmaceutical company, the maker of a newly approved drug for major depression. The company's representative approaches the psychiatrist after the lecture and says, "I hope we can count on you to prescribe our medication. This is a great medication!" The psychiatrist does not know what to say and later feels troubled by this encounter. Which of the following statements reflects the psychiatrist's ethical obligation in this situation?

(A) The psychiatrist can accept dinners and "repay" the company with favorable prescribing practices if the psychiatrist chooses to do so.
(B) The psychiatrist should report the pharmaceutical representative's behavior to the local APA branch's ethics committee.
(C) The psychiatrist should be aware that "strings attached" industry-sponsored activities are unethical.
(D) The psychiatrist must repay the representative for the cost of the dinner, since there are apparent, though unstated, ethical conflicts.

31

More severe and prolonged forms of conduct disorder are most often associated with which of the following comorbid disorders?

(A) Anxiety disorders
(B) Attention deficit hyperactivity disorder
(C) Depression
(D) Eating disorder
(E) Tic disorder

32

A 62-year-old man is taking desipramine for depression. He presents with marked sedation, tachycardia, and postural hypotension about 10 days after the addition of a second antidepressant. Which of the following medications is most likely responsible?

(A) Venlafaxine
(B) Mirtazapine
(C) Citalopram
(D) Sertraline
(E) Fluoxetine

33

Which of the following diseases associated with dementia characteristically has early changes in personality and a late decline in memory?

(A) HIV infection
(B) Creutzfeldt-Jakob disease
(C) Parkinson's disease
(D) Lewy body dementia
(E) Pick's disease

34

Which of the following features best distinguishes anorexia nervosa from bulimia nervosa?

(A) Amenorrhea
(B) Decreased body weight
(C) Calluses on the dorsum of the hand
(D) Dental enamel erosion
(E) Enlarged parotid glands

35

Which of the following aspects of cognitive performance is most likely to decline in the course of normal aging?

(A) Short-term memory
(B) Speed of performance
(C) Store of knowledge
(D) Syntax
(E) Vocabulary

36

Disorders with significant psychiatric symptoms that can be linked to a single gene include:

(A) attention deficit hyperactivity disorder.
(B) bipolar disorder.
(C) fragile X syndrome.
(D) major depression.
(E) schizophrenia.

37

The rule of confidentiality is waived in a psychiatrist-patient interaction when the treatment or evaluation includes:

(A) a minor.
(B) a forensic consultation.
(C) an impaired physician.
(D) a patient who reveals a past felony.

38

The highest percentage of persons with mental retardation have an intelligence quotient of:

(A) <20.
(B) 20 to 35.
(C) 35 to 50.
(D) 50 to 70.
(E) 70 to 90.

39

A 4-year-old girl who has been cared for in seven different foster homes since the age of 6 months, now exhibits excessive familiarity with strangers. Her current foster parents, with whom she has lived for the past 5 months, state that she does not seem to be particularly close to them. The girl's biological mother is reported to have used alcohol in a binge pattern during her pregnancy. Which of the following is the most likely diagnosis?

(A) Attention deficit hyperactivity disorder
(B) Fetal alcohol syndrome
(C) Oppositional defiant disorder
(D) Pervasive developmental disorder
(E) Reactive attachment disorder

40

An 8-year-old girl insists on keeping a rigid routine when dressing, will wear only certain clothes, insists on recopying her homework if there are any mistakes, and has temper tantrums when the items on her desk are moved. During a discussion of the diagnosis and treatment options, her parents express reluctance to use medication and want to explore other options. The first recommendation would be:

(A) cognitive behavior therapy.
(B) family therapy.
(C) interpersonal psychotherapy.
(D) parent training.
(E) supportive psychotherapy.

41

Which of the following are common hyperarousal symptoms in posttraumatic stress disorder (PTSD)?

(A) Intense psychological distress at exposure to external cues resembling the trauma
(B) Difficulty falling or staying asleep
(C) Intrusive images of the event
(D) Feelings of estrangement from others

42

Which of the following medications is considered first-line monotherapy for posttraumatic stress disorder?

(A) Clonazepam
(B) Sertraline
(C) Olanzapine
(D) Valproate
(E) Propranolol

43

A 50-year-old woman has a long history of difficulty with driving because she worries that she might hit a car or a person accidentally. She also worries excessively about her son getting hurt or attacked when he goes out. Her husband can often reassure her. Which of the following diagnoses is most appropriate?

(A) Agoraphobia
(B) Delusional disorder
(C) Generalized anxiety disorder
(D) Obsessive-compulsive disorder
(E) Panic disorder

44

A 40-year-old woman with chronic headaches has undergone trials with several narcotic and nonnarcotic agents with variable success. Her physician elects to try her on a newer antidepressant medication. Which of the following medications is most likely to be effective?

(A) Bupropion
(B) Mirtazapine
(C) Nefazodone
(D) Sertraline
(E) Venlafaxine

45

Echolalia and echopraxia are most likely manifestations of which of the following disorders?

(A) Hypochondriasis
(B) Bipolar disorder, mixed episode
(C) Depression with catatonic features
(D) Lewy body dementia
(E) Frontotemporal dementia

46

An adolescent female took an unknown drug at an all-night dance party. She was brought to the emergency department for evaluation of altered mental status and marked hyperthermia. Which of the following was most likely the drug that was ingested?

    (A) Ketamine
    (B) Methylenedioxymethamphetamine (MDMA)
    (C) Flunitrazepam
    (D) Gamma-hydroxybutyrate (GHB)
    (E) Phencyclidine (PCP)

47

A 23-year-old man who is hospitalized for psychosis displays prominent, excessive, and purposeless motor activity together with peculiar voluntary movements. On one occasion, he stands in the middle of the ward immobile and mute. He demonstrates waxy flexibility. The appropriate medical intervention is:

    (A) benztropine.
    (B) clonidine.
    (C) lorazepam.
    (D) propranolol.
    (E) ziprasidone.

48

A 49-year-old woman is referred for treatment of chronic, severe major depression. Which of the following treatment approaches is most likely to be associated with sustained improvement in her symptoms?

    (A) Antidepressant medication plus psychotherapy
    (B) Psychotherapy alone
    (C) Antidepressant medication alone
    (D) ECT alone
    (E) ECT plus psychotherapy

49

In people with typical left-brain dominance, the ability to interpret the emotional tone of speech is a function of the:

    (A) left premotor cortex (Broca's area).
    (B) right premotor cortex.
    (C) left parietotemporal cortex (Wernicke's area).
    (D) right parietotemporal cortex.
    (E) anterior cingulate gyrus.

50

Which of the following psychotherapies has the greatest body of evidence demonstrating efficacy for social phobia?

    (A) Insight-oriented psychotherapy
    (B) Interpersonal psychotherapy
    (C) Brief psychodynamic psychotherapy
    (D) Cognitive behavior psychotherapy
    (E) Supportive psychotherapy

51

A patient who is completely deaf arrives with an interpreter at the outpatient clinic for an evaluation of depressed mood. You wish to know about the patient's sleep quality. Of the following, which is the most appropriate way to work with the interpreter and the patient?

    (A) Ask the interpreter, "How is she sleeping?"
    (B) Ask the interpreter, "Please ask her how she is sleeping."
    (C) Look at the patient and ask, "How are you sleeping?"
    (D) Loudly enunciate "How are you sleeping?" to the patient.
    (E) Write out "How are you sleeping?" and give it to the patient.

52

An internist consults a psychiatrist because of his frustration with an elderly patient who has a diagnosis of hypochondriasis. Medical tests are negative, but the patient is unable to accept that he is not ill. The psychiatrist confirms the diagnosis of hypochondriasis. Which of the following is the best management strategy for a patient with hypochondriasis?

    (A) Refer the patient to a more psychologically minded internist colleague.
    (B) Have regularly scheduled appointments with limited reassurance.
    (C) See the patient as needed, but for a limited time.
    (D) Instruct the patient to call only for urgent matters.
    (E) Refer the patient for psychotherapy.

53

A 29-year-old woman presents for an initial evaluation. She describes periods of mood lability and unstable interpersonal relationships, particularly with men. During periods of stress, she reports feeling angry and "empty" and sometimes scratches herself with sharp items. Sleep is often a problem, and alprazolam has been helpful. In developing a treatment plan, which of the following principles would be most appropriate?

(A) Restrict pharmacotherapy to antidepressants and mood stabilizers
(B) Treat with multiple classes of medications for potential future symptoms
(C) Target specific symptoms that are currently causing disruption
(D) Refuse to prescribe a benzodiazepine
(E) Withhold medications if the patient engages in acting out behavior

54

A 45-year-old woman with bipolar disorder who has been successfully maintained on lithium presents at the clinic with the complaint of swelling in her ankles. Examination reveals 2+ pitting edema. Her serum lithium level is 0.8 mEq/L. The physician prescribes a thiazide diuretic. Four days later the patient presents at the emergency department with confusion, a coarse tremor in her extremities, and ataxia. Her serum lithium level is now 2.6 mEq/L. Urinalysis reveals a slightly elevated specific gravity and an absence of blood, ketones, and protein. Which of the following best explains the patient's lithium toxicity?

(A) Acute nephrogenic diabetes insipidus
(B) Increased reabsorption in the proximal tubules
(C) Decreased glomerular filtration rate
(D) Glomerulonephritis
(E) Tubulointerstitial nephropathy

55

A random community sample contains 100 individuals who meet diagnostic criteria for borderline personality disorder. Which of the following is the best estimate of the gender ratio of the sample?

(A) 50% men and 50% women
(B) 40% men and 60% women
(C) 25% men and 75% women
(D) 10% men and 90% women

56

The Child Behavior Checklist is a commonly used instrument completed by parents about their children's behaviors. In a study comparing the results from subject groups obtained from multiple cultures, girls scored higher than boys across all cultures on which behavior scale?

(A) Aggression
(B) Anxious/depressed
(C) Attention problems
(D) Delinquency
(E) Thought problems

57

Characteristic cognitive processes in persons with obsessive-compulsive disorder include:

(A) above average spatial recognition.
(B) better memory for pleasant events.
(C) decreased capacity for selective attention.
(D) impaired reality testing.
(E) normal confidence in one's own memory.

58

In family studies of patients with schizophrenia, the personality disorder that has been found to occur most frequently in first-degree relatives is:

(A) borderline.
(B) histrionic.
(C) paranoid.
(D) schizoid.
(E) schizotypal.

The following vignette applies to questions 59 and 60.

A 25-year-old woman presents to the emergency department with the chief complaint, "I think I'm having a heart attack." She reports that while grocery shopping she suddenly felt "scared to death." Her heart was racing, she felt short of breath and dizzy, and she was nauseated and broke out in a sweat. Her fingers and hands and the area around her mouth felt numb. The episode lasted about 10 minutes and dissipated on its own. She managed to drive herself to the emergency department. Physical examination and laboratory studies, including a chest X-ray, blood chemistries, cardiac enzymes, and electrocardiogram, are normal.

59

In the lab, which of the following substances would be most likely to induce an episode with these symptoms?

(A) Carbon monoxide
(B) Sodium lactate
(C) Physostigmine
(D) Propranolol
(E) Sodium pyruvate

60

The medication that is most likely to be effective in the long-term treatment of her condition with the best tolerance of side effects is:

(A) alprazolam.
(B) buspirone.
(C) paroxetine.
(D) propranolol.
(E) imipramine.

61

A 38-year-old man with migraine headaches had successfully obtained relief by taking codeine. Recently his physician started him on a trial of paroxetine for suspected depression. The patient notes improvement in his symptoms of depression and now has headaches less frequently, but when he does have one, he must take twice the amount of codeine for pain relief. Which of the following best describes this drug interaction?

(A) Cytochrome P450 enzymes: inhibition
(B) Cytochrome P450 enzymes: induction
(C) Increased protein binding
(D) Decreased absorption
(E) Increased excretion

62

Which of the following antidepressants is most likely to be associated with substantial weight gain?

(A) Bupropion
(B) Fluoxetine
(C) Sertraline
(D) Venlafaxine
(E) Mirtazapine

63

Expert consensus suggests that the length of time for a pharmacological trial in obsessive-compulsive disorder should be at least:

(A) 3 weeks.
(B) 6 weeks.
(C) 9 weeks.
(D) 12 weeks.

64

A 35-year-old man presents with a 4-week history of low mood, crying spells, poor sleep with early morning awakening, poor appetite with a 12-pound weight loss, and difficulty in concentrating at work. At age 27 he had been hospitalized with an episode of mania, but shortly thereafter he decided not to continue in outpatient follow-up treatment. He has no medical problems and takes no medications. As initial pharmacotherapeutic treatment, which of the following is most appropriate?

(A) Lamotrigine
(B) Nortriptyline
(C) Sertraline
(D) Valproate
(E) Venlafaxine

65

A patient with borderline personality disorder is in dialectical behavior therapy. She has left messages on the therapist's voice-mail while he is on vacation despite an agreement that she would not call him at all during his vacation and would go to the emergency department if she became suicidal. The best approach in dialectical behavior therapy is for the therapist to:

(A) explain that a treatment boundary has been violated and therapy will have to end.
(B) wait for the patient to bring up the issue before discussing the implications for therapy.
(C) explain to the patient that the treatment plan will have to change if she cannot keep the agreement.
(D) make an exception since there is a history of serious attempts and safety is an issue.

66

A patient being treated with interferon for hepatitis C complains of depression, anxiety, and irritability. Which of the following pharmacological agents has the most evidence for efficacy in treating those symptoms?

(A) Trazodone
(B) Haloperidol
(C) Risperidone
(D) Nefazodone
(E) Sertraline

67

An 11-year-old girl is referred for an evaluation of school problems. Her teachers and parents describe her as argumentative, hostile, disrespectful, and difficult. The girl often refuses to listen, will not obey instructions, does not do her work, has temper tantrums, and insists on having her own way. She has been this way since preschool. The most likely diagnosis is:

(A) antisocial personality disorder.
(B) attention deficit hyperactivity disorder.
(C) conduct disorder.
(D) intermittent explosive disorder.
(E) oppositional defiant disorder.

68

Patients with end-stage renal disease who are on hemodialysis are most likely to present with which of the following psychiatric symptoms?

(A) Major depression
(B) Delirium
(C) Psychosis
(D) Panic attacks
(E) Generalized anxiety

69

A 27-year-old woman has had five hospitalizations over the 3-year period since she was initially diagnosed with schizophrenia. On each occasion, recurrent psychotic symptoms have been associated with treatment nonadherence. Which of the following strategies is supported by the greatest body of research evidence as the most likely to improve medication adherence for this patient?

(A) Cognitive-motivational interventions
(B) Insight-oriented psychotherapy
(C) Psychoeducational interventions
(D) Family therapy
(E) Supportive group psychotherapy

70

Which of the following is the most likely symptom in cocaine intoxication?

(A) Paranoid delusions
(B) Hypotension
(C) Bradycardia
(D) Depersonalization

71

A consultation-liaison psychiatrist, on arriving on the internal medicine hospital unit, learns that the patient's nurse requested the consultation and that the attending internist does not want the consultation. Of the following, the best action for the psychiatrist would be to:

(A) talk briefly with the nurse about why he or she considered the consultation important.
(B) apologize to the attending internist and leave the unit.
(C) talk with the nurse's supervisor about the correct way to request a consultation.
(D) proceed with the consultation and make treatment recommendations.
(E) ask to have a case conference about the patient with the physician and nursing staff.

72

Which of the following accurately describes the major quality that fundamentally distinguishes brief dynamic psychotherapy from long-term dynamic psychotherapy? Brief therapy has:

(A) no more than five sessions.
(B) limited focus and goals.
(C) less demonstrated efficacy.
(D) no transference or countertransference phenomena.
(E) fewer demands on the therapist.

73

A 68-year-old man with bipolar I disorder has been adequately maintained on lithium. His most recent serum lithium level was 0.8 mEq/L. He has a variety of medical problems for which he takes several medications. He now presents with pressured speech, racing thoughts, increased energy, and little sleep. His serum lithium level is 0.3 mEq/L. His wife reports that the patient has been adherent to his medication regimen, but she began to notice a change 2 weeks after his primary care physician started him on a new medication. What was the most likely class of medication added to his regimen?

(A) Angiotensin-converting enzyme inhibitors
(B) Beta-blockers
(C) Nonsteroidal anti-inflammatory drugs
(D) Thiazide diuretics
(E) Xanthine bronchodilators

74

A patient with an alcohol problem is ambivalent about starting acamprosate. The psychiatrist explores the patient's thoughts about the advantages and disadvantages of taking and not taking the medication, attempting to tip the patient's decisional balance in favor of taking the medication. Which of the following techniques is the physician using?

(A) Cognitive reframing
(B) Contingency management
(C) Motivational enhancement
(D) Pessimistic anticipation
(E) Rational emotion

75

Which of the following differentiates Lewy body dementia from dementia of the Alzheimer's type?

(A) Apraxia
(B) Choreiform movements
(C) Executive dysfunction
(D) Gradual progression of deficits
(E) Recurrent visual hallucinations

76

The symptom of "flashbacks" is a manifestation of which of the following psychological states?

(A) Psychosis
(B) Fugue
(C) Hyperarousal
(D) Dissociation

77

Response prevention is a useful psychotherapeutic technique for which of the following disorders?

(A) Generalized anxiety disorder
(B) Intermittent explosive disorder
(C) Obsessive-compulsive disorder
(D) Pedophilia
(E) Schizophrenia

78

A patient with alcoholism wants a psychiatrist to bill the patient's insurance company under another diagnosis because the patient is afraid of the stigma attached to the diagnosis. The psychiatrist should:

(A) tell the patient that this would be lying and refuse to comply.
(B) comply with the request because stigmas are inherently unfair to patients.
(C) comply with the request provided the patient's fears are adequately addressed.
(D) explore the reasons behind the request and explain why this is something the psychiatrist is reluctant to do.

79

In a patient experiencing bereavement, which of the following suggests the diagnosis of major depression?

(A) A poor appetite
(B) Initial insomnia
(C) A feeling of worthlessness
(D) Hallucinations of the deceased
(E) Sadness

80

Which CNS structure is most responsible for arousal and sleep-wake cycles?

(A) Amygdala
(B) Hippocampus
(C) Hypothalamus
(D) Reticular activating system
(E) Ventral striatum

81

A 38-year-old patient provides a 12-year history of obsessive concerns about dirt, germs, and contamination and spends more than 3 hours a day with washing and cleaning rituals. Which of the following would be preferred as an initial medication treatment?

(A) Desipramine
(B) Duloxetine
(C) Paroxetine
(D) Phenelzine
(E) Venlafaxine

82

A 59-year-old woman is seen for an initial outpatient psychiatric assessment. Her husband says that increasingly over the past 2 years she has seemed less like her usual outgoing self. She has been increasingly apathetic and uninterested in her usual activities, and more recently she has behaved inappropriately in social interactions, making unusual comments and returning home with items that do not belong to her. Recently, her husband has had to begin helping her dress in the morning, and he notes that she is occasionally incontinent of urine. On mental status examination, her affect is blunted and her speech is sparse, although she does not report specific psychotic symptoms or changes in mood. She knows the year and the season but not the month or date, and she has particular difficulty in naming objects. MRI shows prominent frontal and some temporal atrophy with relative sparing of other cortical regions. Which of the following diagnoses is most likely in this patient?

(A) Dementia of the Alzheimer's type
(B) Creutzfeldt-Jakob disease
(C) Dementia associated with Huntington's disease
(D) Dementia associated with Parkinson's disease
(E) Pick's disease

83

A psychiatrist decides that a patient with alcohol dependence would benefit from regular laboratory monitoring. Which of the following single tests would best provide information about heavy alcohol use over the preceding 7 to 10 days?

(A) Aspartate aminotransferase (AST)
(B) Carbohydrate-deficient transferrin (CDT)
(C) Exhaled ethanol concentration (e.g., Breathalyzer)
(D) Mean corpuscular volume (MCV)

84

A patient with major depression shows no improvement after an adequate trial (in dose and duration) of an antidepressant. The best next step is to:

(A) augment the antidepressant with thyroid hormone.
(B) augment with lithium.
(C) augment with both thyroid hormone and lithium.
(D) switch to a different class of antidepressant.
(E) conduct a "washout" by stopping all medication for 4 weeks, and then reassess.

85

Of the following, which is the most common reason psychiatrists are sued for malpractice?

(A) Sexual improprieties with patients
(B) Suicide
(C) Failure to obtain informed consent
(D) Tardive dyskinesia
(E) Unnecessary commitment

86

Anorexia nervosa is most commonly comorbid with which of the following personality disorders?

(A) Dependent
(B) Paranoid
(C) Schizotypal
(D) Obsessive-compulsive
(E) Histrionic

87

The use of which of the following has been associated with hyperparathyroidism?

(A) Lamotrigine
(B) Divalproex
(C) Lithium
(D) Topiramate

88

Narcolepsy is characterized by which of the following signs and symptoms?

(A) Daytime nonrefreshing sleep episodes
(B) Bouts of urinary incontinence
(C) Early morning awakening
(D) Sleepwalking
(E) Sudden episodes of muscle tone loss

89

The four major components of a psychodynamic view of personality disorders are a biologically based temperament, a set of internalized object relations, an enduring sense of self, and:

(A) an assessment of reality testing.
(B) a punitive superego.
(C) an intact ego ideal.
(D) a specific constellation of defense mechanisms.

90

The antidepressant duloxetine may simultaneously improve mood and:

(A) panic attacks.
(B) chronic pain.
(C) flashbacks.
(D) psychotic symptoms.
(E) night terrors.

91

A 48-year-old man with a medical history of gastro-esophageal reflux disease (GERD) is referred for a psychiatric evaluation of his anxiety. For the past month, since the patient's initial evaluation and treatment for GERD, he complains of an increasing sense of unease, nervousness, restlessness, and inability to sit and read the paper. His medications include 20 mg/day of esomeprazole, 10 mg of metoclopramide q.i.d., and 0.5 mg of lorazepam t.i.d. orally or as needed. He is very concerned about his condition because a sibling who had a similar problem died from esophageal carcinoma. Other than being noticeably fidgety, his mental status exam is unremarkable. What is the most likely explanation?

(A) Development of generalized anxiety disorder
(B) Adjustment disorder with anxious features
(C) Somatoform disorder not otherwise specified (i.e., "sympathy symptoms" with deceased sibling)
(D) Akathisia from metoclopramide
(E) Benzodiazepine withdrawal

92

A 30-year-old patient with no prior history of mental health treatment presents with a major depressive episode. Which of the following elements would be the most important in choosing a medication for treatment?

(A) Co-occurring diagnosis of alcohol dependence in full sustained remission
(B) Good antidepressant response to fluoxetine in a first-degree relative
(C) History of a hypomanic episode
(D) Inactive hepatitis C infection
(E) Suicide attempt by aspirin overdose at age 16

93

A 32-year-old woman with bipolar I disorder has been adequately maintained on lamotrigine. Recently she has experienced an exacerbation of her manic symptoms, and her physician elects to add a second mood stabilizer. Instead of improving, the patient's symptoms worsen. Her serum lamotrigine levels are nearly undetectable. What was the most likely mood stabilizer that was added?

(A) Olanzapine
(B) Carbamazepine
(C) Valproate
(D) Topiramate
(E) Lithium

94

Obsessive-compulsive disorder is hypothesized to involve a neural circuit connecting the cortex and striatum with the:

(A) amygdala.
(B) hippocampus.
(C) hypothalamus.
(D) mammillary body.
(E) thalamus.

95

Which of the following psychiatric disorders occurs most commonly as a comorbid disorder with anorexia nervosa?

(A) Somatization disorder
(B) Generalized anxiety disorder
(C) Major depressive disorder
(D) Obsessive-compulsive disorder
(E) Social phobia

96

Which of the following is the LEAST problematic for the psychiatrist according to ethical principles?

(A) A psychiatrist in a metropolitan area agrees to treat her financial adviser's child.
(B) A psychiatrist in a remote area with no other psychiatrists is involved in a romantic relationship with a patient's adult grandchild.
(C) A psychiatrist hires a current patient to perform clerical work in the psychiatrist's office.
(D) A psychiatrist convinces a patient who was sexually abused by a former clinician to file a suit against that former clinician and serves as the forensic expert for the patient.

97

In the initial assessment, a psychiatrist is consulted by a lesbian couple seeking help for some problems in their long-standing committed relationship. Which of the following is the best approach for the psychiatrist to take in assessing the possibility of domestic violence within the couple?

(A) Ask about it only when material is presented that suggests the problem.
(B) Ask routine questions about battering while taking the history.
(C) Obtain information from collateral sources.
(D) The topic need not be raised because domestic violence is low in lesbian couples.
(E) Wait until the therapy is well established before asking about it.

98

A patient is being treated for a cat phobia. The therapist encourages the patient to pass by a pet store that has cats in the window. From which of the following psychotherapy approaches does this strategy derive?

(A) Cognitive behavior
(B) Insight oriented
(C) Interpersonal
(D) Short-term anxiety-regulating
(E) Supportive

99

Which of the following cognitive functions is most likely to remain stable with normal aging?

(A) Language syntax
(B) Recent memory
(C) Speed of information processing
(D) Topographic orientation
(E) Working memory

100

A consultation is requested for a 22-year-old man because of a gradual onset of behavioral symptoms that include irritability, aggression, and personality change. Associated findings include mild jaundice, dysarthria, and choreiform movements. The consultation-liaison psychiatrist also notices a golden-brown discoloration of the cornea. The most likely diagnosis is:

(A) Huntington's disease.
(B) Wilson's disease.
(C) Parkinson's disease.
(D) progressive supranuclear palsy.
(E) adrenoleukodystrophy.

101

According to DSM-IV-TR, a patient with recurrent hypomanic episodes without intercurrent depressive features would receive which of the following diagnoses?

(A) Bipolar I disorder
(B) Bipolar II disorder
(C) Cyclothymic disorder
(D) Bipolar disorder, not otherwise specified

102

The ventral tegmentum, the nucleus accumbens, and the prefrontal cortex are brain structures or regions most involved in the neurobiology of:

(A) alcohol dependence.
(B) anorexia nervosa.
(C) bipolar disorder.
(D) panic disorder.
(E) schizophrenia.

103

A 32-year-old man with panic disorder treated with lorazepam for several years begins combination therapy (which includes ritonavir) for HIV infection. Two weeks later, his panic attacks increase in frequency. What is the most likely explanation?

(A) An HIV-related brainstem lesion
(B) An HIV-related lung infection
(C) A direct side effect of one of his HIV medications
(D) Ritonavir is decreasing blood lorazepam levels
(E) Failure to take lorazepam as directed

104

A 24-year-old man who lives with his parents is being treated for schizophrenia in a continuing day treatment program. Since the onset of his illness at age 20, he has had three hospitalizations for recurrent psychosis. He is currently on quetiapine 300 mg b.i.d., and his auditory hallucinations have resolved, but he still has some concerns that a government conspiracy may be operating and spying on him. Apart from his family and the day treatment program, he has few interactions with others and no outside interests. If family therapy were instituted with this patient's parents, which of the following outcomes would be most likely to be observed?

(A) Improved employability
(B) Improved social functioning
(C) Reduced likelihood of psychotic relapse and rehospitalization
(D) Reduced number and severity of negative symptoms
(E) Reduced number and severity of positive symptoms

105

Biological relatives of individuals with antisocial personality disorder have an increased risk of having antisocial personality disorder and substance-related disorders. These relatives, especially if they are female, are also at greater risk of:

(A) autism.
(B) narcissistic personality disorder.
(C) bipolar disorder.
(D) schizophrenia.
(E) somatization disorder.

106

Compared with younger adults, the elderly require lower doses of lithium to achieve a given serum lithium concentration because of:

(A) impaired hepatic metabolism.
(B) more complete absorption.
(C) reduced fat storage.
(D) reduced renal excretion.
(E) reduced serum protein binding.

107

Which of the following is the best description of the therapist's empathy?

(A) Envisioning what it would be like for the therapist to be in the patient's situation
(B) Mirroring the patient's presentations of a vulnerable self
(C) Understanding the patient's inner experience from the patient's perspective
(D) Maintaining an attitude of compassion and sympathy
(E) Avoiding making the patient anxious or uncomfortable

108

A 39-year-old secretary must do everything meticulously. Her work area is extremely neat and organized. However, she is not very productive, because she will restart any project if she makes an error. She typically works through lunch and rarely socializes with her coworkers. At home, she is in constant conflict with her children about the tidiness of their rooms, the neatness of their schoolwork, and the need to be frugal. Her children and coworkers tell her that her behaviors "drive them nuts." She does not believe she has a problem and in fact thinks her habits represent "strong moral values." Which term best describes the woman's lack of distress about her problems?

(A) Ambivalence
(B) Denial
(C) Ego-syntonic
(D) La belle indifference
(E) Projection

109

An 18-year-old female patient who is being evaluated for depression reveals that she worries excessively about her weight. She states that she is unable to diet and consumes large quantities of food about once a month. She appears to have normal weight for her height. What is the most likely diagnosis?

(A) Anorexia nervosa
(B) Body dysmorphic disorder
(C) Bulimia nervosa
(D) Eating disorder not otherwise specified
(E) Factitious disorder

110

Patients with bulimia nervosa who engage in binge/purge behaviors are at risk for which of the following medical disorders?

(A) Hyperkalemia
(B) Decreased serum amylase
(C) Cardiomyopathy
(D) Hypothyroidism
(E) Osteopenia

111

A 76-year-old woman presents with weakness, fatigue, somnolence, and depression. Her husband has also noticed that there has been some cognitive slowing and her voice is hoarse. Which of the following endocrine disorders is the most likely diagnosis?

(A) Cushing's disease
(B) Hyperparathyroidism
(C) Hypoparathyroidism
(D) Hypothyroidism
(E) Pheochromocytoma

112

Early-onset Alzheimer's dementia due to mutations in the amyloid precursor protein genes, presenilin-1 and presenilin-2, are transmitted by what mode of inheritance?

(A) Autosomal dominant
(B) Autosomal recessive
(C) X-linked
(D) Trinucleotide repeat
(E) Polygenic

113

A 27-year-old man has a long-standing history of marked discomfort in social situations and avoids group discussions, parties, dating, and speaking at meetings. He also has a history of binge alcohol use, particularly when he has to engage in social activities. The class of medication preferred for treatment of this patient would be:

(A) benzodiazepines.
(B) beta-blockers.
(C) tricyclics.
(D) second-generation antipsychotics.
(E) selective serotonin reuptake inhibitors.

114

The consultation-liaison psychiatrist is called to the emergency department to evaluate a 17-year-old patient who is highly agitated and floridly psychotic with findings of ataxia, nystagmus, dysarthria, miosis, and elevated blood pressure. Intoxication with which of the following substances best explains this presentation?

(A) Heroin
(B) Psilocybin
(C) Cannabis
(D) LSD
(E) Phencyclidine

115

A 35-year-old nurse is admitted to the medical service with numerous ecchymoses on her body and a complaint of tarry stools. Her prothrombin time was 4 INR (international normalized prothrombin ratio) units (normal, 0.78–1.22). Several days after admission her prothrombin time was normal. A medical workup failed to identify the cause of her abnormal clotting time. Her stool was weakly positive for blood. Four days after admission, more ecchymoses appeared and her prothrombin time was again elevated. The patient expressed concern that she might have leukemia and inquired if she would need a bone marrow biopsy. On the fifth day of admission, a warfarin pill was found beneath her bed. The patient signed out of the hospital that evening. Which of the following is the most likely diagnosis?

(A) Somatization disorder
(B) Malingering
(C) Hypochondriasis
(D) Factitious disorder
(E) Body dysmorphic disorder

116

Patients who suffer from depression after a myocardial infarction should be treated with which of the following antidepressants?

(A) A monoamine oxidase inhibitor
(B) Bupropion
(C) Trazodone
(D) A tricyclic antidepressant
(E) An SSRI

117

Cocaine-induced euphoria is most highly associated with which of the following neurotransmitters?

(A) Serotonin
(B) Dopamine
(C) Norepinephrine
(D) Gamma-aminobutyric acid
(E) Acetylcholine

118

Which of the following is an example of an instrumental activity of daily living that becomes impaired in the mild to moderate stages of dementia?

(A) Ambulating
(B) Dressing
(C) Feeding oneself
(D) Remembering appointments
(E) Toileting

119

A 66-year-old patient who is being treated for bipolar disorder presents comatose with a serum sodium concentration of 112 mmol/L. Which of the following is most likely to be the cause of the sodium imbalance?

(A) Divalproex
(B) Carbamazepine
(C) Lithium
(D) Olanzapine

120

Which of the following features differentiates delirium from dementia of the Alzheimer's type?

(A) Acuity of onset and level of consciousness
(B) Level of consciousness and orientation
(C) Acuity of onset and orientation
(D) Visual hallucinations and memory
(E) Memory and level of consciousness

121

Which of the following sleep disorders is more common in males than females during childhood?

(A) Breathing-related sleep disorder
(B) Nightmare disorder
(C) Primary insomnia
(D) Sleep terror disorder
(E) Sleepwalking disorder

122

A physician elects to treat a depressed patient with imipramine. Four days after the start of treatment, the physician receives a call from the emergency department reporting that the patient has fallen. The staff report that the patient stood up quickly after being in bed overnight, felt dizzy, and then lost consciousness, falling to the floor. Examination reveals a pulse of 76 bpm; blood pressure is 136/82 mm Hg lying and 84/46 mm Hg standing. An electrocardiogram is unremarkable. Which of the following best explains the patient's symptoms?

(A) α-Adrenergic receptor blockade
(B) Cholinergic receptor blockade
(C) Histamine receptor blockade
(D) First-degree atrioventricular block
(E) Prolongation of the QTc interval

123

Soon after ECT, a patient is most likely to have problems with which of the following items on the Mini-Mental State Examination?

(A) Reporting the date
(B) Spelling "WORLD" backwards
(C) Repeating "no ifs ands or buts"
(D) Following a three-step command
(E) Writing a sentence

124

Imaging genetics is a form of:

(A) association study.
(B) double-blind study.
(C) linkage study.
(D) randomized study.

125

Which of the following is the most appropriate indication for ECT in a patient with borderline personality disorder?

(A) Comorbid major depression
(B) Severe mood instability
(C) Poor response to valproate
(D) Noncompliance with medications
(E) Recurrent transient psychotic episodes

126

A 70-year-old woman presents with a depression that has not responded to treatment with sertraline, paroxetine, or escitalopram. She has said that she would like to die, and she has a history of an overdose in the past 3 months. Although abdominal computerized tomography shows no abnormalities, she is convinced that a hole in her liver is causing her to lose weight. Mental status examination is also significant for severe psychomotor retardation, and physical examination shows evidence of dehydration. She is currently being treated with 150 mg/day of venlafaxine. Which of the following recommendations is most appropriate at the present time?

(A) Increase the dose of venlafaxine
(B) Recommend ECT
(C) Change to mirtazapine
(D) Add lamotrigine
(E) Obtain a liver scan to assess for evidence of carcinoma

127

A 29-year-old unmarried woman is admitted to an acute inpatient unit after police spotted her wandering along a busy highway gesturing and muttering to herself. On admission, she was disheveled and bizarrely clothed. Her speech was tangential, and she reported auditory hallucinations commenting on her behavior and telling her that "criminal elements" were watching her. She had recently been residing with her parents and gave permission for staff to contact them. Her parents report that her first hospitalization was at age 25, just after she began working on her thesis for a Ph.D. in mathematics. She responded rapidly to treatment with risperidone 3 mg daily, and several months later, with the support of her adviser, she was able to resume work on her thesis. Over the past 6 months, after she decided to stop her medication, her symptoms have returned. In responding to the parents' questions about her prognosis, which of the following factors would be the best predictor of a good prognosis for this patient?

(A) Age at onset of illness
(B) Initial response to medication
(C) Marital status
(D) Number and duration of remissions between psychotic episodes
(E) Premorbid cognitive functioning

128

A patient with a history of "manic and major depressive episodes" who has persistent delusions or hallucinations even when prominent mood symptoms are absent, would have which of the following diagnoses?

(A) Bipolar I disorder
(B) Delusional disorder, grandiose type
(C) Schizoaffective disorder
(D) Schizophrenia, disorganized type

129

A patient with borderline personality disorder reports prominent lability, sensitivity to rejection, anger, outbursts, and "mood crashes." As an initial approach to pharmacotherapy, which of the following would be most appropriate?

(A) Gabapentin
(B) Sertraline
(C) Quetiapine
(D) Phenelzine
(E) Valproic acid

130

Which of the following schools of therapy has its base in the idea that family problems are due to structural imbalances in family relationships and symptoms are communications?

(A) Cognitive behavior
(B) Insight oriented
(C) Psychoeducational
(D) Solution focused
(E) Strategic

131

Compared with depressed elderly individuals who had a first episode of depression in young adulthood, individuals with a first episode of depression in late life are more likely to have:

(A) brain imaging findings suggesting dementia.
(B) comorbid personality disorder.
(C) first-degree relatives with depression.
(D) good response to treatment.
(E) suicidal ideation.

132

A 10-year-old boy has a well-documented episode of moderately severe non-bipolar major depression. Which of the following medications is FDA-approved for use in this patient?

(A) Bupropion
(B) Duloxetine
(C) Fluoxetine
(D) Sertraline
(E) Venlafaxine

133

A 35-year-old man has a 10-year history of schizophrenia and poor adherence with outpatient treatment. He has been stabilized on 20 mg of olanzapine in the hospital, and he has previously done well on 10 mg of oral haloperidol. He has agreed to switch to haloperidol decanoate injections once a month. He is given an initial injection of 50 mg. Which of the following is the most likely amount of time he will need to continue taking the oral olanzapine?

(A) Two days
(B) Two weeks
(C) One month
(D) Three months
(E) One year

134

A 51-year-old woman presents to her physician with the chief complaint of feeling depressed over the past month. She has no energy, is disinterested in her children, and has lost 25 pounds. She is unable to fall asleep until the early morning hours. She has begun to feel that she is unworthy of her family. With the onset of these symptoms, she is quite certain that she has developed a degenerative nerve condition, although all investigations have been negative. The most appropriate first step in treating this patient is to start her on:

(A) a serotonin reuptake inhibitor alone.
(B) a serotonin-norepinephrine reuptake inhibitor alone.
(C) a serotonin reuptake inhibitor and an antipsychotic.
(D) a serotonin-norepinephrine reuptake inhibitor and a benzodiazepine.

135

Which of the following is NOT a predisposing risk factor for the development of posttraumatic stress disorder (PTSD) after a traumatic event?

(A) Recent life stressors
(B) Female gender
(C) Internal locus of control
(D) Past history of depression

136

A patient with schizophrenia, paranoid type, and methamphetamine dependence receives mental health care through a community mental health clinic (CMHC). The patient has appeared to clinically deteriorate over a period of 6 weeks and is hospitalized with a psychotic decompensation. A drug screen on admission shows methamphetamine and amphetamine in the patient's urine. After a 3-day hospital stay, the patient is ready for discharge. The outpatient psychiatrist should do which of the following?

(A) Resume psychiatric care through the CMHC, deferring substance dependence treatment unless the patient resumes methamphetamine use.
(B) Resume psychiatric care at the CMHC, with increased emphasis on the provision of substance dependence treatment by the mental health team.
(C) Enroll the patient in a separate program specifically for substance dependence and continue to provide psychiatric care through the CMHC.
(D) Enroll the patient in a separate program specifically for substance dependence and resume psychiatric care at the CMHC once a period of sobriety is achieved.

137

Which of the following is the most accurate way to diagnose early-stage dementia of the Alzheimer's type?

(A) Apolipoprotein E genotyping
(B) Brain MRI
(C) History of stepwise memory decline
(D) Neuropsychological testing
(E) Patient self-report of memory difficulties

138

A man reports that he avoids public urinals even when he has great urgency to urinate. This type of chief complaint is most consistent with a diagnosis of:

(A) body dysmorphic disorder.
(B) obsessive-compulsive disorder.
(C) panic disorder with agoraphobia.
(D) social phobia.
(E) posttraumatic stress disorder.

139

A patient with mild dementia of the Alzheimer's type is brought in by his wife, who is also his primary caregiver, for follow-up evaluation. She brings along a list of his medications. The patient is taking donepezil, hydrochlorothiazide, and warfarin. The use of which of the following herbal or over-the-counter products by this patient would be of the most concern?

(A) Ginkgo biloba
(B) Ginseng
(C) Hawthorn
(D) Vitamin C
(E) Vitamin E

140

What diagnostic specifier would be most appropriate for a depressed patient who complains of a sense of leaden paralysis and difficulty being around other people but is able to enjoy himself when good things happen?

(A) With atypical features
(B) With catatonic features
(C) With melancholic features
(D) With psychotic features

141

A 34-year-old woman with two previous episodes of major depressive disorder is treated with 100 mg/day of sertraline. Her most recent episode occurred 9 months ago. At that time sertraline was initiated, with the dose titrated up to 150 mg/day over a 2-week period. Her symptoms remitted after 6 weeks, but she experienced significant sexual side effects that resolved with a decrease in the sertraline dose to 100 mg/day. Over the past 7 months she has remained free of depressive symptoms and now inquires about decreasing her dose of medication. Which of the following recommendations is most appropriate?

(A) Continue sertraline at 100 mg/day.
(B) Decrease sertraline to 50 mg/day and continue at that dose.
(C) Discontinue sertraline after tapering the dose.
(D) Initiate psychotherapy and then decrease sertraline to 50 mg/day.
(E) Initiate psychotherapy and then gradually discontinue sertraline.

142

Which of the following antipsychotic drugs has the greatest effect on prolonging the QT interval on the electrocardiogram?

(A) Aripiprazole
(B) Haloperidol
(C) Olanzapine
(D) Thioridazine
(E) Ziprasidone

143

The therapeutic benefit of acamprosate is best established for which of the following conditions?

(A) Alcohol dependence
(B) Barbiturate dependence
(C) Cocaine withdrawal
(D) Heroin addiction
(E) Methamphetamine abuse

144

A 25-year-old woman with bipolar disorder is about to be started on lamotrigine for maintenance therapy. She should receive one-half of the usual starting dose if she is taking which of the following medications?

(A) Carbamazepine
(B) Lithium
(C) Oral contraceptive
(D) Phenytoin

145

Of the following, which is the most important factor in determining whether a patient is suited to brief psychodynamic psychotherapy?

(A) Ability to recognize and discuss feelings
(B) Existence of multiple conflicts
(C) Compliance with medication
(D) Lack of meaningful relationships
(E) Failure of long-term psychodynamic psychotherapy

146

Compared with men, women with schizophrenia taking equivalent doses per weight of antipsychotics are less likely to have which of the following?

(A) Acute dystonia
(B) Drug-drug interactions
(C) Lower serum drug levels
(D) Sedation

147

A 22-year-old man presents at the emergency department with agitated, guarded behavior, paranoid delusional thoughts, and a 7-month history consistent with a diagnosis of schizophrenia, paranoid type. Understanding the man's cultural background would be most helpful for:

(A) choosing his acute and maintenance medications.
(B) determining the cause of his disorder.
(C) determining safety issues and the need for hospitalization.
(D) understanding the content of the delusions and hallucinations.

148

Hypertension is most associated with which of the following medications?

(A) Bupropion
(B) Fluvoxamine
(C) Mirtazapine
(D) Paroxetine
(E) Venlafaxine

149

A patient reports regularly taking a drug bought on the street. Its effect is pleasurable, but it sometimes causes nausea, restlessness, and teeth grinding. The drug is most likely:

(A) methamphetamine.
(B) flunitrazepam (Rohypnol).
(C) methylenedioxymethamphetamine (MDMA).
(D) cocaine.

150

Indications of caffeine withdrawal:

(A) are evident following an average intake of 50 mg/day.
(B) include symptoms that typically last 3 weeks.
(C) include a flushed face and diuresis.
(D) include headache.

151

A 23-year-old college student from Ethiopia is admitted to the hospital for a psychotic disorder. His symptoms include paranoid ideation, hallucinations, and disorganized thinking. He is initially started on 0.5 mg of risperidone twice daily, which is rapidly titrated to 4 mg/day. Despite this treatment, there is no improvement in his symptoms. No detectable plasma levels of the parent compound are noted. What is the most likely explanation for these results?

(A) Binding of the drug to fatty tissue
(B) First-pass effect
(C) Impaired absorption of the drug
(D) Increased excretion
(E) Ultrarapid metabolism of the drug

152

The preferred initial pharmacological treatment for a 26-year-old woman who was violently assaulted 3 years ago and suffers from recurrent nightmares about the event, hypervigilance, difficulty concentrating, and constricted range of affect would be:

(A) alprazolam.
(B) clomipramine.
(C) clonidine.
(D) valproate.
(E) sertraline.

153

In the initial assessment of a depressed patient, what is the most critical decision that the psychiatrist must make?

(A) Type of psychotherapy
(B) Choice of medication
(C) Level of care
(D) Medical workup
(E) Involvement of family

154

A 27-year-old patient announces that she is pregnant despite having taken an oral contraceptive for 4 years. Which of the following medications might account for the failure of her oral contraceptive?

(A) Lithium
(B) Divalproex
(C) Carbamazepine
(D) Lamotrigine
(E) Gabapentin

155

Screening for hepatitis C (HCV) infection is LEAST important in patients with:

(A) methamphetamine dependence.
(B) marijuana dependence.
(C) heroin dependence.
(D) history of blood transfusion (before 1992).
(E) hemodialysis.

156

Which of the following is best characterized as a degenerative dementia?

(A) Systemic lupus erythematosus
(B) Korsakoff's syndrome
(C) Parkinson's disease
(D) HIV disease
(E) Cerebrovascular accident

157

In a urine test for phencyclidine, a false positive test result can occur if a person has ingested:

(A) dextromethorphan.
(B) ibuprofen.
(C) tonic water.
(D) phenylephrine.
(E) diphenhydramine.

158

A 48-year-old man is admitted to the hospital with cholecystitis, and after diagnosis he consents to and undergoes a cholecystectomy. On the third hospital day he becomes angry at the nursing staff and wishes to leave the hospital against medical advice. In assessing this patient's capacity to refuse further medical care, which of the following questions would be most useful for the psychiatrist to ask?

(A) Have you discussed with your family your decision to leave?
(B) What is the danger of your going home at this time?
(C) Have you been troubled by depression?
(D) Are you able to name all of your medications?
(E) When did you first become ill, and do you remember your symptoms?

159

Which of the following disorders has been shown to have genetic or familial links?

(A) Autistic disorder
(B) Dissociative amnesia
(C) Factitious disorder
(D) Hypoactive sexual desire disorder
(E) Pyromania

160

A 45-year-old man and his monozygotic twin have been diagnosed as having the same personality disorder. Which of the following diagnoses is most likely?

(A) Histrionic personality disorder
(B) Obsessive-compulsive personality disorder
(C) Narcissistic personality disorder
(D) Antisocial personality disorder
(E) Avoidant personality disorder

161

Which of the following medication classes is the preferred treatment for obsessive-compulsive disorder?

(A) Atypical antipsychotics
(B) Anticonvulsants
(C) Mood stabilizers
(D) SSRIs
(E) Benzodiazepines

162

Which of the following interventions is the best first step in the management of agitation in the elderly patient?

(A) Haloperidol, 5 mg twice a day, whatever the cause of the agitation
(B) Physical restraints
(C) Evaluation of the patient's surroundings and daily schedule
(D) Diazepam, 5 mg every 6 hours, or until the patient is asleep
(E) Seclusion until the behavior ceases

163

Which of the following will double the blood level of lamotrigine?

(A) Carbamazepine
(B) Divalproex
(C) Phenytoin
(D) Phenobarbital

164

Buspirone has been found to be most consistently effective in the treatment of which of the following anxiety disorders?

(A) Generalized anxiety disorder
(B) Obsessive-compulsive disorder
(C) Panic disorder with agoraphobia
(D) Panic disorder without agoraphobia
(E) Social phobia

165

Which of the following parental transmissions of the fragile X trinucleotide repeat is most likely to result in an affected child?

(A) Mother-to-daughter
(B) Mother-to-son
(C) Father-to-daughter
(D) Father-to-son
(E) No parental gender difference

166

Which of the following is NOT a relative contraindication for the use of disulfiram as an adjunct in the treatment of alcohol dependence?

(A) Impulsive behavior
(B) Psychotic symptoms
(C) Suicidal thoughts
(D) A family history of alcoholism
(E) Impaired judgment

167

Which of the following signs and symptoms is more likely to occur in females than in males at first presentation of psychosis?

(A) Amotivation
(B) Cognitive impairment
(C) Dysphoric mood state
(D) Paranoid ideation
(E) Social isolation

168

A 45-year-old woman complains of blurred vision, ocular pain, and headache and was noted to have increased intraocular pressure. Which of the recently started medications is the most likely cause?

(A) Lamotrigine
(B) Oxcarbazepine
(C) Tiagabine
(D) Topiramate
(E) Valproate

169

A married 50-year-old woman is admitted to the hospital with an acute myocardial infarction. It is recommended that she have a cardiac catheterization with a possible procedure based on the findings. The patient refuses. Which of the following would be a reasonable approach to the patient at this time?

(A) Discharge the patient to home so that she can make up her mind.
(B) Call for a family meeting with her husband and adult children to discuss the options.
(C) Tell her that there is no guarantee that she wouldn't die if she leaves the hospital without treatment.
(D) Consider treatment for depression since she does not seem to want to live.
(E) Recommend treatment against her will because of the seriousness of the condition.

170

Which of the following treatments is most effective for patients with bulimia nervosa and major depressive disorder?

(A) Cognitive behavior therapy
(B) Fluoxetine
(C) Imipramine
(D) Bupropion
(E) Combined cognitive behavior therapy and fluoxetine

171

Which of the following describes the American Academy of Pediatrics statement regarding maternal lithium use during breast-feeding?

(A) Associated with significant side effects in some nursing infants; use with caution
(B) Unknown effects on nursing infants; may be of concern
(C) Absolutely contraindicated
(D) Usually compatible

172

Treatment with which of the following cytokines has been linked to suicidal behavior?

(A) Erythropoietin
(B) Granulocyte colony-stimulating factor
(C) Interferon-α
(D) Interleukin-1 receptor agonist
(E) Anti-tumor-necrosis-factor antibodies

173

The amygdala is most specifically involved in which of the following brain functions?

(A) Determining social behavior
(B) Emotional coding of sensory cues
(C) Generating normal sleep patterns
(D) Recalling previously learned material
(E) Signaling reward by exogenous substances

174

A 22-year-old woman wants to take an antidepressant for treatment of her major depression but is concerned about possible sexual side effects. Which of the following medications is the best choice for her?

(A) Bupropion
(B) Clomipramine
(C) Escitalopram
(D) Sertraline
(E) Venlafaxine

175

Which of the following factors is UNRELATED to a positive treatment outcome for cocaine dependence?

(A) Counseling rapport
(B) Treatment retention
(C) Patient choice of program type
(D) Comorbid depressive symptoms

176

Weight gain is most likely to occur with which of the following antipsychotic drugs?

(A) Aripiprazole
(B) Clozapine
(C) Haloperidol
(D) Ziprasidone
(E) Risperidone

177

A 16-year-old female patient is admitted to the hospital for gastric rupture. On interview, she reports that in the past 2 months, whenever she has felt anxious, angry, or sad, she has eaten unusually large quantities of cookies, candy, crackers, "or whatever I can get my hands on like I'm a maniac, totally out of control." She reports that after gorging, she feels better emotionally but is afraid that she will "get fat." She gags herself to induce vomiting, and recently she has begun drinking ipecac as an emetic after such episodes. This morning, after an episode of self-induced vomiting, she developed severe abdominal pain and was brought to the emergency department by her parents. On physical examination, her height is 5'6" and her weight is 120 pounds. The psychotherapy that has been found to be most effective in treating her eating disorder is:

(A) cognitive behavior therapy.
(B) family therapy.
(C) group therapy.
(D) psychodynamically oriented individual therapy.

178

Despite intensive psychosocial treatment for alcohol dependence, a patient continues to drink alcohol. The psychiatrist decides to recommend adjunctive medication. Which of the following medications would NOT be an acceptable treatment?

(A) Disulfiram
(B) Bromocriptine
(C) Naltrexone
(D) Ondansetron
(E) Acamprosate

179

The anxiety disorder that includes a dissociation-like phenomenon in its criteria is:

(A) generalized anxiety disorder.
(B) obsessive-compulsive disorder.
(C) panic disorder.
(D) posttraumatic stress disorder.
(E) social phobia.

180

Patients with which of the following personality disorders would be expected to benefit most from adjunctive pharmacotherapy?

(A) Borderline
(B) Schizoid
(C) Antisocial
(D) Obsessive-compulsive
(E) Dependent

181

When assessing a patient's suitability for short-term psychodynamic psychotherapy, of the following factors, which is the most important?

(A) The DSM-IV-TR diagnosis
(B) Family psychiatric history
(C) Level of education
(D) An identifiable focus
(E) Need for psychoactive medication

182

A psychiatrist is treating an 8-year-old child of a divorced single parent who is the child's custodial parent. The noncustodial parent wishes to be informed of the child's source of problems and progress of treatment. The psychiatrist should share clinical information with the noncustodial parent:

(A) without consent of the custodial parent or the child.
(B) only with the informed consent of the custodial parent and the child.
(C) only with informed consent of the custodial parent.
(D) only with the informed consent of the child.

183

Cerebral ventricular enlargement, one of the most consistent structural brain findings in patients with schizophrenia, is most closely associated with:

(A) prominent negative symptoms.
(B) rapid onset of the disorder.
(C) improved response rates to atypical antipsychotics.
(D) retained memory- and language-processing capabilities.
(E) increased risk of developing tardive dyskinesia.

184

A patient with heroin dependence purchases a drug on the street. The patient feels a mild opiate high but then, despite continued injection of a sizable volume of drug, feels opiate withdrawal coming on. The drug injected is most likely:

(A) buprenorphine.
(B) heroin.
(C) methadone.
(D) naloxone.

185

Which of the following would be the most important consideration when evaluating an individual for a personality disorder?

(A) Culture
(B) Intelligence
(C) Gender
(D) Socioeconomic status
(E) Education

186

Treatments shown to be effective for smoking cessation include all of the following EXCEPT:

(A) bupropion.
(B) brief advice intervention.
(C) 12-step programs.
(D) nicotine replacement therapy.

187

Based on the mental status examination, the psychiatrist believes that a patient is delirious. The examination reveals disorientation, changing levels of consciousness, and visual illusions. Which of the following tests has the greatest evidence supporting its use in confirming a diagnosis of delirium?

(A) Positron emission tomography
(B) Magnetic resonance imaging
(C) Computerized tomography
(D) EEG

188

The diagnosis of shared psychotic disorder is most commonly found in which of the following groups?

(A) Couple relationships
(B) Groups larger than two people
(C) Groups of men, rather than women
(D) Family blood relations
(E) Children and adolescents

189

A colleague who is a cardiac surgeon asks for a psychiatrist's help in raising funds for a new wing of the local hospital. The cardiac surgeon asks the psychiatrist to solicit patients for charitable contributions. The psychiatrist's ethical response should be to agree to solicit funds from:

(A) only former patients, because there is no longer a doctor-patient relationship.
(B) only wealthy patients who have the means to contribute.
(C) no patients, because of the nature of the psychiatrist-patient relationship.
(D) both current and former patients, since patients can make autonomous decisions.

190

A managed care organization (MCO) is refusing to pay for additional treatment days for a patient in an inpatient psychiatric facility. The attending psychiatrist believes that the additional treatment days may be needed to ensure the patient's safety. Which of the following statements is correct regarding this situation?

(A) The psychiatrist is legally responsible to abide by the MCO's decision.
(B) The psychiatrist is responsible for making provisions for continuity of needed care even if additional days are not covered by the MCO.
(C) As long as the psychiatrist documents that the MCO will not pay, the psychiatrist may discharge the patient.
(D) The psychiatrist may inform the patient of his or her right to appeal the MCO's decision only if there are no "gag clauses" that limit what the psychiatrist is allowed to say.

191

The parents of a 14-year-old boy bring him to a clinic because he has been refusing to go to school. In elementary and middle school, he was in a special education class for mildly mentally retarded students. When he has been at school, he ruminates about "something really bad" happening to his mother or father. Recently, he has been awakening with nightmares that his parents have been killed. His parents have had to stay with their son in order for him to get back to sleep. His medical history is significant for strabismus and scoliosis. Physical examination reveals a long face with prominent ears and jaw, a high arched palate, hyperextensible finger joints, macroorchidism, and flat feet. This boy's overall presentation is most consistent with:

(A) Angelman syndrome.
(B) fragile X syndrome.
(C) Prader-Willi syndrome.
(D) Sturge-Weber syndrome.
(E) Williams syndrome.

192

Which of the following therapies explicitly gives the patient permission to be in the sick role?

(A) Brief psychotherapy
(B) Cognitive behavior therapy
(C) Insight-oriented therapy
(D) Interpersonal psychotherapy
(E) Rational-emotional therapy

193

A 29-year-old woman presents to the emergency department complaining of migraine headache. A review of her medical file reveals one brief admission for a transient psychotic episode and depression within the past 3 years. She is noted to be dressed in odd clothing. She insists that she is clairvoyant and telepathic. Her speech is noted to be metaphorical, overelaborate, and stereotyped. She says she has no close friends or confidants other than her mother and father, and that this has been the case since she was a teenager. She is not particularly bothered about her lack of companionship because she has fears of being harmed in relationships. Her presentation is most consistent with which of the following personality disorders?

(A) Avoidant
(B) Histrionic
(C) Paranoid
(D) Schizoid
(E) Schizotypal

194

Which of the following would be most appropriate as initial pharmacotherapy for a patient with borderline personality disorder who is exhibiting impulsivity and behavioral dyscontrol?

(A) Sertraline
(B) Clozapine
(C) Haloperidol
(D) Naltrexone
(E) Alprazolam

195

A 30-year-old man with schizophrenia has made several significant suicide attempts over the past 10 years in response to auditory command hallucinations. Which of the following has been shown in studies to be most likely to reduce his risk for further suicidal behaviors?

(A) Aripiprazole
(B) Clozapine
(C) Lithium
(D) Olanzapine
(E) Risperidone

196

A 23-year-old patient with chronic schizophrenia complains of a milky discharge from her nipples. Medication-induced antagonism of which of the following receptors is responsible?

(A) Acetylcholine
(B) Dopamine
(C) GABA
(D) Norepinephrine
(E) Serotonin

197

Which of the following statements is most accurate regarding the current status of gene therapy for the clinical treatment of psychiatric disorders?

(A) Gene therapy will be clinically applicable within the next 2 years.
(B) Finding vectors to transfer genes into the nervous system is a challenge.
(C) Neurons are among the easiest cells into which to insert new genes.
(D) Target genes for gene therapy have been clearly defined.
(E) Viral vectors quickly spread novel genes throughout the nervous system.

198

Which of the following agents would be most appropriate for a geriatric patient who has Parkinson's disease and agitation?

(A) Risperidone
(B) Diazepam
(C) Quetiapine
(D) Haloperidol
(E) Lithium

199

A 32-year-old man is brought to the emergency department by his family, who notes that he has been spending a lot of time sitting motionless in his room and appears to be losing weight. In the past, he had been fearful that family members were poisoning his food, but his parents state that he has not expressed those concerns recently. On examination, he is disheveled and poorly groomed, and he sits quietly in his chair except for intermittent grimacing. He has minimally spontaneous speech but will occasionally repeat the last few words of a question posed by the interviewer. His affect is generally restricted in range, and he does not answer questions about his mood, hallucinations, delusions, and suicidal or homicidal ideation. Which of the following subtypes of schizophrenia would best describe this patient's current presentation?

(A) Catatonic
(B) Disorganized
(C) Paranoid
(D) Residual
(E) Undifferentiated

200

Which of the following is most predictive of a favorable response to lithium in bipolar disorder?

(A) Comorbid substance abuse
(B) Depression-mania-euthymia course
(C) Euphoric mania
(D) Psychotic features

201

A female patient reveals during a psychotherapy session that she does not enjoy sexual intercourse. She states that she is aroused by her partner but has sharp pains throughout intercourse. She cannot relax and enjoy sex and has begun to avoid sex because of the anticipation of the pain. What is the most likely diagnosis?

(A) Dyspareunia
(B) Female orgasmic disorder
(C) Sexual masochism
(D) Sexual sadism
(E) Sexual aversion disorder

202

A 25-year-old woman presents with severe anxiety after finding out that her biological mother was recently diagnosed with Huntington's disease. There is no family history of the disease on her father's side. She wishes to know if she is affected. The probability that she is affected is:

(A) 0%.
(B) 25%.
(C) 50%.
(D) 75%.
(E) 100%.

203

A 9-year-old boy is referred for evaluation because he is having "temper tantrums" in school. He cannot sit still, constantly disrupts the class, runs out in the hall without permission and refuses to obey directives from the teacher. He frequently fights with his peers, and if he does not get what he wants, he yells, screams, throws objects, and flails about on the floor. Educational testing reveals borderline intellectual functioning and significant delays in reading, writing, spelling, and mathematics. On physical examination, the boy is noted to be in the fifth percentile for head circumference. He has short palpebral fissures, a thin upper lip, and a smooth philtrum. The boy was most likely exposed to which of the following drugs in utero?

(A) Alcohol
(B) Cocaine
(C) Marijuana
(D) Nicotine
(E) Opiates

204

Which of the following is the most accurate statement regarding psychotherapy for posttraumatic stress disorder (PTSD)?

(A) The therapist should be as nondirective as possible for the psychotherapy to be effective.
(B) Multiple modalities of psychotherapy have proven effective for PTSD.
(C) Psychotherapy must be combined with pharmacotherapy to be effective.
(D) Cognitive behavioral therapy (CBT) is of little value for patients with PTSD.

205

A husband and wife present for treatment because the wife is concerned. Her husband recently told her that he believes he was born a woman. He states that he has always felt this way but can't fight it anymore. He has started wearing dresses around the house after he arrives home from work at the end of the day. He says that he loves his wife and kids but that he needs to be happy as well. What is the most likely diagnosis?

(A) Exhibitionism
(B) Gender identity disorder
(C) Sexual arousal disorder
(D) Transvestic fetishism
(E) Voyeurism

206

Which of the following describes the pharmacokinetics of children younger than 12 years old?

(A) Children have a smaller volume of distribution than adults.
(B) Children have more efficient renal function than adults.
(C) Children metabolize through hepatic pathways more slowly than adults.
(D) Children absorb medications more slowly than adults.

207

A 32-year-old woman develops anorgasmia while taking paroxetine. Switching to which of the following medications is most likely to resolve this problem?

(A) Citalopram
(B) Venlafaxine
(C) Sertraline
(D) Bupropion
(E) Fluoxetine

208

A 4-year-old boy is brought to the clinic by his parents with the chief complaint that "he keeps having nightmares." His parents report that for the past month, during the first one-third of the night, the boy awakens from his sleep with a startled scream. When they enter the room, they find that he has broken out in a sweat, is difficult to awaken, and looks "scared to death." The next morning he has no recall of the event. These episodes are most likely occurring during which stage of sleep?

(A) REM
(B) Stage 0 — non-REM
(C) Stage 1 — non-REM
(D) Stage 2 — non-REM
(E) Stage 3 or 4 — non-REM

209

A 25-year-old male with a history of schizophrenia is hospitalized and treated with haloperidol and benztropine. The patient becomes distressed, has a temperature of 103°F and has labile blood pressure. Physical examination reveals hypertonicity, diaphoresis, and tachycardia. Laboratory studies reveal a creatine kinase of 55,000 IU/L. What is the most likely diagnosis?

(A) Anticholinergic syndrome
(B) CNS infection
(C) Malignant hyperthermia
(D) Neuroleptic malignant syndrome
(E) Serotonin syndrome

210

A previously well 24-year-old woman presented with a 4-week history of progressively worsening expansive irritable mood, pressured speech, racing thoughts, grandiosity, and distractibility. More recently she heard the voice of God proclaiming her to be a special messenger. Which of the following is the most likely diagnosis?

(A) Brief psychotic disorder without marked stressor
(B) Bipolar disorder with psychotic features
(C) Schizoaffective disorder, bipolar type
(D) Schizophrenia, catatonic subtype
(E) Schizophreniform disorder

211

According to the principles of dialectical behavior therapy, the core deficit in borderline personality disorder is in:

(A) regulation of affect.
(B) capacity for attachment.
(C) object constancy.
(D) self-integration.
(E) impulsive aggression.

212

According to the American Psychiatric Association guidelines, which of the following is true regarding a psychiatrist engaging in a sexual relationship with a former patient?

(A) Acceptable provided at least 2 years have passed since the termination of the doctor-patient relationship
(B) Acceptable provided at least 5 years have passed since the termination of the doctor-patient relationship
(C) Acceptable provided the former patient initiates the relationship and it is clear to both parties that no exploitation is taking place
(D) Unethical no matter how long it has been since the termination of the doctor-patient relationship

213

A patient with schizophrenia begins treatment with clozapine. The baseline white blood cell count (WBC) is 8100 (normal=4500–11,000/mm³). The absolute neutrophil count (ANC) is 6200 (normal=1500–8000/mm³). The tests remain normal in weekly monitoring. After 3 months, the patient has had significant clinical improvement, but the WBC drops to 3200, the ANC drops to 2100, and immature cell forms are present on peripheral blood smear. Repeat tests show a WBC of 3100, an ANC of 1900, and no immature cell forms. The physical examination is normal, with no fever, sore throat, or other sign of infection. What would be the best next step in the management of this patient?

(A) Continue current dosage of clozapine and begin twice-weekly monitoring of the WBC and differential.
(B) Immediately and permanently discontinue clozapine.
(C) Interrupt clozapine therapy until the WBC is normal, and then resume treatment.
(D) Reduce the dose of clozapine and begin weekly monitoring of the WBC and differential.
(E) Routinely monitor the WBC and differential unless the patient develops signs and symptoms of infection.

214

According to DSM-IV-TR, which personality disorder cannot be diagnosed in children and adolescents?

(A) Paranoid
(B) Dependent
(C) Schizotypal
(D) Borderline
(E) Antisocial

215

The first-line treatment of choice (determined by expert consensus) for acute posttraumatic stress disorder (PTSD) milder severity is:

(A) low-dose venlafaxine.
(B) psychotherapy.
(C) combination of a mood stabilizer and psychotherapy.
(D) any selective serotonin reuptake inhibitor (SSRI).

216

A 54-year-old woman is hospitalized with hyperthermia, myoclonus, delirium, and autonomic instability. Which of the following medication combinations would be most likely to cause this clinical presentation?

(A) Bupropion and venlafaxine
(B) Desipramine and escitalopram
(C) Duloxetine and fluoxetine
(D) Paroxetine and phenelzine
(E) Sertraline and buspirone

217

In addition to lithium, which of the following is recommended as a first-line monotherapy for bipolar I disorder, depressed mood, in the revised *APA Practice Guideline for the Treatment of Patients With Bipolar Disorder* (2002)?

(A) Lamotrigine
(B) Divalproex
(C) Gabapentin
(D) Bupropion

218

A 15-year-old African American male high school freshman is referred to a psychiatrist because of increasing oppositional behavior at school. In middle school he was an honor roll student, played soccer, and was on student council, all of which he continued in his first 9 weeks of high school. On the weekends, he volunteers at a local Boys and Girls Club and plays the keyboard at his church. After a couple of sessions, he finally admits that he needed to "prove myself to my boys because they said I was 'acting white'." Which of the following is the most likely reason for his peers' denigration?

(A) Being on student council
(B) Doing volunteer work
(C) Having honor roll grades
(D) Playing soccer
(E) Playing the keyboard

219

A 55-year-old man presents with depressed mood, poor concentration, poor appetite, feelings of worthlessness, and insomnia 4 weeks after alcohol cessation. There is no history of mania. Which of the following is the best next step?

(A) Begin an antidepressant.
(B) Begin a sleep aid.
(C) Begin an anticonvulsant.
(D) Begin to phase-advance sleep onset.
(E) Wait 7–10 days, then reassess.

220

A 16-year-old girl with depression has suicidal ideation. Which of the following characteristics is the most strongly associated with a greater risk of completed suicide?

(A) Limited cognitive abilities
(B) Perfectionist characteristics
(C) Previous suicide attempt
(D) Strong religious beliefs
(E) Superficial cutting of forearms

221

A psychiatrist routinely receives free golf outings, concert tickets, and dinners as gifts from a local pharmaceutical representative. Which of the following statements most adequately describes the ethics of this practice?

(A) It is ethical if no single gift is worth more than $250.
(B) Self-monitoring and self-regulation are the most effective ways of minimizing harm from conflicts of interest.
(C) There is no evidence that pharmaceutical company marketing to physicians influences physicians' behavior.
(D) This is a conflict of interest for the psychiatrist.

222

The process of gene mapping, performed to determine whether or not a particular allele occurs more frequently than by chance in affected individuals, is known as which type of study?

(A) Twin
(B) Linkage
(C) Association
(D) Family
(E) Segregation analysis

223

Which of the following is the most common psychiatric disturbance among adolescents who die by suicide?

(A) Schizophrenia
(B) Depressive disorders
(C) Antisocial behavior/conduct disorder
(D) Anxiety disorders
(E) Alcohol dependence

224

Which of the following is the best medication treatment for premature ejaculation?

(A) Bupropion
(B) Lorazepam
(C) Paroxetine
(D) Risperidone
(E) Trazodone

225

The highest rates of posttraumatic stress disorder (PTSD) have been reported to be induced by:

(A) combat.
(B) sexual assault.
(C) natural disasters.
(D) motor vehicle accidents.

226

Which of the following laboratory test results is elevated in some patients with anorexia nervosa?

(A) Amylase
(B) Magnesium
(C) Phosphate
(D) Potassium
(E) Zinc

227

Which of the following is the most common side effect of cholinesterase inhibitors?

(A) Anorexia
(B) Muscle cramps
(C) Nausea
(D) Somnolence
(E) Syncope

228

There is accumulating evidence suggesting that all of the following psychotherapies are beneficial in bipolar I disorder EXCEPT:

(A) interpersonal and social rhythm therapy.
(B) cognitive behavioral therapy.
(C) family therapy.
(D) psychoanalysis.

229

A 45-year-old patient with heroin dependence is admitted to the infectious disease service for intravenous antibiotic treatment of bacterial endocarditis. An HIV test is negative. There is no other past psychiatric history. Opiate withdrawal is adequately controlled with oral methadone. On hospital day 3, the patient becomes acutely anxious, has moderate tachycardia, and asks to be discharged from the hospital. A low-grade fever develops, but blood cultures are negative and a complete blood count shows no significant increase or shift in leukocytes. The most likely explanation for the change in the patient's condition is:

(A) an occult infection.
(B) alcohol or sedative-hypnotic withdrawal.
(C) an undiagnosed anxiety disorder.
(D) a medication reaction, most likely to the antibiotic.

230

Long-term treatment with which of the following medications has been demonstrated to reduce suicide risk in bipolar disorder?

(A) Carbamazepine
(B) Divalproex
(C) Lithium
(D) Olanzapine

231

A psychiatric referral is requested to evaluate a 25-year-old woman who wishes to undergo a second rhinoplasty because, she states, "the first one left my nose too big." In tears, the patient states that her discomfort about the appearance of her nose prevents her from having an active social life. She pleads with the psychiatrist to render an opinion that will permit the surgery. The patient does not appear psychotic. She does not express any other obsessional thoughts. In the psychiatrist's opinion, the patient's nose is unremarkable. Which of the following disorders is the most likely diagnosis for this patient?

(A) Delusional disorder, somatic type
(B) Obsessive-compulsive disorder
(C) Body dysmorphic disorder
(D) Hypochondriasis
(E) Somatization disorder

232

A 50-year-old man is treated with several trials of single antidepressants. His unipolar depression has been only partially responsive. Which of the following agents has the best evidence from randomized controlled trials to support its use in augmenting his antidepressant?

(A) Bupropion
(B) Buspirone
(C) Lithium
(D) Methylphenidate
(E) Triiodothyronine (T$_3$)

233

A 65-year-old man seen in the emergency department is agitated, tachycardic, hypertensive, and tremulous. He sees fish swimming on the wall: "It's just like watching television." The most likely diagnosis is:

(A) delirium.
(B) delusional disorder.
(C) depression.
(D) obsessive-compulsive disorder.
(E) schizophrenia.

234

A 42-year-old morbidly obese man is seen for chronic fatigue. Findings on polysomnography indicate obstructive sleep apnea. If the sleep apnea is left untreated over a prolonged period, which of the following conditions is most likely to develop?

(A) Cataplexy
(B) Catalepsy
(C) Pulmonary hypertension
(D) Obstructive pulmonary disease
(E) Sleep paralysis

235

A patient in psychotherapy believes that her therapist wants to help her, she characteristically trusts him with very private material, and she has at times expressed her feeling that they have many things in common and that in many ways she views him as a role model. This patient's alliance is best characterized as:

(A) erotic.
(B) idealized.
(C) positive.
(D) primitive.
(E) mirroring.

236

For which of the anxiety disorders does clonazepam have an FDA indication?

(A) Generalized anxiety disorder
(B) Obsessive-compulsive disorder
(C) Panic disorder
(D) Posttraumatic stress disorder
(E) Social phobia

237

A 22-year-old female presents with symptoms of depression. She is always thinking that the worst will occur in her relationships and employment, and she feels powerless to alter or control these events. She is seeking treatment with a therapist who provides cognitive behavior therapy. What is the most likely focus of the therapy for this patient?

(A) Anger turned inward
(B) Early deprivation
(C) Difficulties in relationships
(D) Self-image
(E) Maladaptive thought patterns

238

A 36-year-old female graduate student presents with atypical depression that has not responded to selective serotonin reuptake inhibitors (SSRIs). Which of the following medications has the most evidence for efficacy in this situation?

(A) Bupropion
(B) Phenelzine
(C) Valproic acid
(D) Trazodone
(E) Imipramine

239

"*Guevodoces*," which translates as "penis at 12," refers to Dominican children with a female appearance at birth, reared as girls, who at puberty develop male secondary sexual characteristics and male-typical sexual urges and behaviors. The genetic condition they have is called:

(A) androgen insensitivity syndrome.
(B) cloacal extrophy.
(C) congenital adrenal hyperplasia.
(D) Klinefelter syndrome.
(E) 5-α reductase deficiency.

240

Rapid cycling is LEAST likely to respond to:

(A) divalproex.
(B) carbamazepine.
(C) haloperidol.
(D) lithium.

241

During an office follow-up visit, a 19-year-old woman with schizophrenia reports no improvement in her symptoms despite being on an appropriate dose of an antipsychotic medication for 3 weeks. The most reasonable initial approach would be to:

(A) add an anticonvulsant medication.
(B) add another antipsychotic medication.
(C) change to another antipsychotic medication.
(D) explore potential nonadherence.
(E) increase the dose of the patient's current medication.

242

A small-town newspaper's reporter calls a psychiatrist to get "a professional's opinion" on the publicized misbehavior of the district's elected representative, who may or may not have bipolar disorder. The reporter asks the psychiatrist, who has never met the representative, "Why do you think the representative misbehaved, doctor?" The psychiatrist's ethical obligations would lead to which of the following responses?

(A) Inform the public about the representative's bipolar disorder, since this person is a public figure.
(B) Comment on the representative's condition only if the representative has not been a patient.
(C) Comment on either childhood dynamic origins or brain abnormality as the possible cause of the representative's problems, if public records contain information that is consistent with such possibilities.
(D) Comment on the general nature of psychiatric illnesses.

243

In psychodynamic psychotherapy, a boundary crossing—unlike a boundary violation—is:

(A) discussed with the patient.
(B) an exploitative break in the therapeutic frame.
(C) generally not examined in the therapy.
(D) harmful to the therapy.
(E) a repeated occurrence.

244

A male psychiatrist has been conducting weekly psychotherapy for the last 4 months with a female patient. The patient has serious financial problems due to overspending. One day, the patient brings in a gift-wrapped box to the session and, handing the box to the psychiatrist, blurts out, "It's a $100 tie ... I couldn't help myself, it just looked like something you'd wear and I'm so grateful for all of your help. Please accept it!" Which of the following is an appropriate response for the psychiatrist to give to this patient?

(A) Accept the gift but donate it to charity without telling the patient.
(B) Accept the gift but make it clear that the psychiatrist is uncomfortable doing so, given the patient's financial difficulties.
(C) Acknowledge the patient's gratitude, discuss the implications, but state that as a general policy the psychiatrist does not accept gifts from patients.
(D) Decline the gift without further explanation.

245

A consultation is requested for a 16-year-old male who has been in detention for the past 2 months on charges of possession of cocaine. The detention center staff describe the youth as hyperactive, inattentive, impulsive, and easily distracted. A review of his educational history indicates that the youth has been in special education classes since the first grade because of attention deficit hyperactivity disorder and a mixed expressive-receptive language disorder. On examination, there is no evidence of a mood or anxiety disorder or current substance abuse. Which of the following medications would be most appropriate for this patient?

(A) Atomoxetine
(B) Clonidine
(C) Desipramine
(D) Mixed salts of amphetamines
(E) Pemoline

246

A 78-year-old patient with major depressive disorder is being treated with atorvastatin and metoprolol for cardiovascular disease. Which of the following antidepressants is best used with these two other medications?

(A) Bupropion
(B) Escitalopram
(C) Fluoxetine
(D) Nefazodone
(E) Paroxetine

247

A 23-year-old woman presents to the clinic with a chief complaint of having sexual problems. She reports that she gets aroused and enjoys intercourse but is unable to have an orgasm. She believes the problem started about a month ago, when her physician prescribed a medication for her "anxiety attacks." The medication was most likely:

(A) bupropion.
(B) buspirone.
(C) citalopram.
(D) mirtazapine.
(E) trazodone.

248

Methylphenidate has its greatest action on which of the following neurotransmitter systems?

(A) Acetylcholine
(B) Dopamine
(C) Gamma-aminobutyric acid
(D) Glutamate
(E) Serotonin

249

Which mental disorder is the most frequent cause of first-onset psychosis after age 60?

(A) Dementia of the Alzheimer's type
(B) Bipolar disorder
(C) Delusional disorder
(D) Major depression
(E) Very late onset schizophrenia

250

Psychotic features do NOT occur during which of the following?

(A) Manic episode
(B) Mixed episode
(C) Hypomanic episode
(D) Major depressive episode

251

The parents of a 7-year-old boy express concern about his bed-wetting. The boy seems well adjusted, and the family has developed a nonstigmatizing system to care for his bed and personal hygiene. He has no medical problems. After explaining the natural history of enuresis, the most reasonable initial approach would be to:

(A) start desmopressin.
(B) start imipramine.
(C) provide observation and follow-up.
(D) order a bell and pad.
(E) start psychotherapy.

252

A psychiatrist repeatedly and increasingly fantasizes about a sexual relationship with a patient in psychotherapy whom the psychiatrist finds very attractive. The psychiatrist is considering the possibility that the prohibition of sex with patients may not apply in this case because of some extenuating circumstances. Which of the following options would be the most ethical behavior on the part of the psychiatrist?

(A) Keep a diary of the sexual fantasies in order to contain them.
(B) Increase the frequency of therapy sessions in order to make the best use of the intensity of the transference that is developing.
(C) Transfer the patient's care to another psychiatrist.
(D) Because there are important psychodynamic therapeutic implications for the patient, share the fantasies with the patient if the benefits seem to outweigh the risks.

253

Which of the following statements about a defendant's competency to stand trial for a criminal offense is NOT correct?

(A) The defendant must be able to remember what he or she was doing at the time of the offense.
(B) The defendant must be able to communicate with attorneys.
(C) The defendant must be able to understand basic courtroom procedure.
(D) The defendant must be able to understand the nature of various possible pleas and their consequences.

254

A 34-year-old Puerto Rican woman presents in distress at the outpatient clinic. She reports that her grandfather recently died, and since then she has been afflicted by several bouts of *ataque de nervios*. She has these spells only when she is upset. A detailed history should be obtained to distinguish *ataque* from which other axis I diagnosis?

(A) Bipolar disorder
(B) Histrionic personality disorder
(C) Obsessive-compulsive disorder
(D) Panic disorder
(E) Schizophrenia

255

Which of the following signs or symptoms alone would be sufficient to meet criterion A for the active phase of schizophrenia?

(A) Bizarre delusions
(B) Catatonic behavior
(C) Incoherent speech
(D) Negative symptoms
(E) Tactile hallucinations

256

A 32-year-old woman was unexpectedly terminated from her job. Two months later she presents tearfully with depressed mood and occasional feelings of hopelessness; she still feels stressed by the loss of her job. She has no prior history of depression, is not suicidal, has not had changes in appetite, weight, sleep, or energy level, and still gets pleasure from family and hobbies. Which of the following diagnoses would be the most appropriate?

(A) Major depressive disorder
(B) Bipolar II disorder
(C) Bereavement
(D) Adjustment disorder
(E) Dysthymic disorder

257

Which of the following has been approved by the FDA for the treatment of alcohol dependence?

(A) Buprenorphine
(B) Levo-alpha-acetylmethadol (LAAM)
(C) Naloxone
(D) Naltrexone

258

A psychiatrist maintains private therapy progress notes, in addition to medical record notes, that contain extremely sensitive clinical information. This practice is:

(A) an acceptable means of enhancing patient confidentiality.
(B) an acceptable way of preventing court-mandated access to sensitive clinical information.
(C) not acceptable, because all clinical material should be included in patients' medical records.
(D) not acceptable, because the risks to the patient outweigh the benefits.

259

Which of the following psychosocial treatments is most likely to be effective in the treatment of obsessive-compulsive disorder?

(A) Cognitive therapy
(B) Supportive psychotherapy
(C) Interpersonal therapy
(D) Behavioral therapy
(E) Group therapy

260

A 7-year-old boy presents to a clinic on referral from the school with a number of behavior problems, including impaired attention, hyperactivity, and impulsivity. His parents have described him as a "whirling dervish" for years. At age five, he was evaluated by his primary care physician and started on methylphenidate, which produced significant improvement in his behavior. However, he then developed jerky, irregular muscle movements around the eyes and mouth that persisted when he was off the medication. The medication that could address all of his symptoms is:

(A) clonidine.
(B) d,l-amphetamine.
(C) haloperidol.
(D) magnesium pemoline.
(E) pimozide.

261

A 16-year-old girl has been blinking her eyes and clearing her throat on an intermittent basis for years. She has no control of the symptoms and has never been free of them for more than a few days, and they cause significant problems. What medication may be helpful for treating this problem?

(A) Pimozide
(B) Nortriptyline
(C) Paroxetine
(D) Lorazepam
(E) Methylphenidate

262

Blocking craving for opiates with subsequent reduction in associated drug use generally requires which of the following daily doses of methadone?

(A) 5 mg
(B) 10 mg
(C) 20 mg
(D) 40 mg
(E) 80 mg

263

Which of the following is the most important consideration for the treatment plan when performing an initial evaluation of a patient with borderline personality disorder in suicidal crisis?

(A) Safety
(B) Goals
(C) Type
(D) Frame
(E) Outcome

264

The best documented treatment for posttraumatic stress disorder (PTSD) precipitated by a violent rape includes:

(A) event recall.
(B) martial arts instruction.
(C) prosecution of the rapist.
(D) cognitive-based therapy.

265

A 40-year-old female comes to the mental health center for the first time. After a thorough assessment, she is told that the best treatment would be a course of brief psychotherapy. She looks concerned and asks if she can be transferred to a doctor of her own race. The appropriate step to take would be to:

(A) attempt to convince her that any doctor is capable.
(B) explore why she feels this is necessary.
(C) grant her request and transfer her.
(D) help her find another clinic that will suit her.
(E) switch to medication management only.

266

DSM-IV-TR cultural formulation for a patient from a culture different than the psychiatrist's requires:

(A) a history of the patient's education and occupational training.
(B) independent information from a cultural consultant.
(C) an understanding of the neurobiology of the patient's disorder.
(D) an understanding of the effect of the psychiatrist's own culture on treatment variables.
(E) use of an interpreter from or assimilated in the patient's culture.

267

A 20-year-old male college student presents in the emergency department with confusion and agitation. He is distracted and talks in a rambling manner. During the interview, he reports seeing an angel who is telling him about his mission. His roommate states that the student has been having problems for months, with worsening grades, not sleeping, and withdrawal from friends. In establishing a diagnosis and preparing to initiate treatment, the most appropriate laboratory test to obtain at this point would be:

(A) a complete blood count, including a platelet count.
(B) an electrocardiogram.
(C) hepatic function tests.
(D) thyroid function tests.
(E) a toxicology screen.

268

A 60-year-old woman presents with daytime fatigue, morning headache, and poor memory. Findings from her physical examination and blood studies are all within normal limits, and she reports that her mood is normal. On further questioning she reports that her husband sleeps in a separate room because of her snoring and thrashing. The most effective treatment for this condition is:

(A) fluoxetine.
(B) continuous positive airway pressure.
(C) lorazepam.
(D) methylphenidate.
(E) relaxation therapy.

269

Which of the following best describes a characteristic of the assertive community treatment (ACT) model for management of schizophrenia?

(A) Clinic-based services
(B) Focus on symptom resolution
(C) Hospital-based services
(D) Psychiatrist-led treatment team
(E) 24-hour availability of services

270

The strong association between physical illness and suicide has been demonstrated for which of the following conditions?

(A) Amyotrophic lateral sclerosis
(B) Blindness
(C) Epilepsy
(D) Hypertension
(E) Diabetes mellitus

271

A 32-year-old man sees his primary care physician because of a recurrent productive cough. The physician recommends blood work and a chest X-ray. When the patient enters the phlebotomy suite, his heart begins to race, he perspires, and his muscles tense. When he sits in the phlebotomy chair and a tourniquet is applied, his symptoms worsen. In addition, he becomes short of breath, begins to hyperventilate, and feels numbness and tingling in his hands and feet and around his mouth. When the phlebotomist uncaps the needle, the patient passes out. He awakens shortly after an ammonia capsule is broken under his nose. He apologizes for his behavior and says, "I always get this way when I see a needle." This presentation is most consistent with:

(A) agoraphobia.
(B) generalized anxiety disorder.
(C) panic disorder.
(D) social phobia.
(E) specific phobia.

272

Which of the following symptoms is significantly more likely to be associated with posttraumatic stress disorder (PTSD) than with normal bereavement?

(A) Initial shock
(B) Depressive symptoms
(C) Numbing
(D) Avoidance of reminders
(E) Sleep disturbance

273

A patient with schizophrenia is in the midst of a severe exacerbation but refuses treatment. The patient is able to paraphrase what the psychiatrist has said about the diagnosis, the prognosis, and the reasons for the proposed treatment with medications. Which of the following statements by the patient is the clearest example of an impaired ability to "appreciate or understand"?

(A) "I have tried all those antipsychotics before. None of them work that well for me so why try again."
(B) "Your office is bugged, but the reason why I do not want to take the medication is that I am really afraid of gaining more weight."
(C) "The space aliens living in my stomach would be injured if I took those pills."
(D) "I am a Christian Scientist and I do not believe that I have a disease."

274

A 42-year-old woman with generalized anxiety disorder has responded favorably to 60 mg/day of buspirone. To avoid substantially increasing the blood level of the medication and producing side effects, you caution her to avoid regular consumption of which of the following beverages?

(A) Apple juice
(B) Coffee
(C) Grapefruit juice
(D) Milk
(E) Red wine

275

Which of the following therapies has the best evidence for effectiveness in the treatment of posttraumatic stress disorder?

(A) Present-centered group therapy
(B) Psychological debriefings
(C) Single-session techniques
(D) Cognitive behavior therapy
(E) Trauma-focused group therapy

276

Linkage analysis can be defined as:

(A) a test to identify which of several genes in a chromosomal region is involved in the disorder in question.
(B) a test to determine the chromosomal region where a disorder resides by searching for co-segregation of a genetic marker with the disorder locus.
(C) a study that requires the cause of the disorder to be a common risk variant.
(D) an analysis that is not sensitive to a genetic model.

277

Which of the following is true regarding adolescents with attention deficit hyperactivity disorder (ADHD) who are treated with methylphenidate?

(A) Significantly reduced risk of substance abuse in later life
(B) Higher level of all substance abuse in adulthood
(C) Increased alcohol abuse in adulthood
(D) Increased cannabis abuse in adulthood

278

Elements of an individual's ability to make decisions about undergoing treatment or participating in research include all of the following EXCEPT:

(A) understanding the information provided.
(B) reasoning with the information or weighing options.
(C) repeating the outlined risks and benefits without prompting.
(D) appreciating the significance of the information for the individual's own situation.

279

A school guidance counselor refers a 5-year-old girl who will not speak. The girl has been enrolled in school for 3 months. During this time, she has been noted to make hand gestures or nod in response to her teacher or peers. The guidance counselor has been meeting with the girl regularly, and recently the child has begun to whisper. However, she will not use a normal voice. The girl's parents report that the child has no problems speaking at home. The girl plays with her peers, makes appropriate eye contact when spoken to, seems interested in others, and has no unusual movements. There have been no delays or abnormalities in development. As an adult, this child is at high risk of developing:

(A) major depressive disorder.
(B) obsessive-compulsive disorder.
(C) posttraumatic stress disorder.
(D) schizophrenia.
(E) social phobia.

280

A 10-year-old boy is brought for consultation for "bed-wetting." His parents report that he began using the toilet and staying dry during the day when he was 3 years old. However, he has never consistently been able to control his bladder during sleep. Physical examination and laboratory studies have demonstrated no abnormalities. His father reports that he also wet the bed as a child but stopped when he was about 12 years old. The intervention that is most likely to have long-term effectiveness with this boy is:

(A) hypnotherapy.
(B) low-dose tricyclic antidepressants.
(C) oral desmopressin.
(D) psychotherapy.
(E) urine alarm (bell and pad).

281

A 58-year-old man has a history of ingesting 1 to 2 pints of vodka on a daily basis over the past 20 years. He presents to the emergency department after a minor motor vehicle accident and appears disorganized. A computerized tomography scan of his head is most likely to show which of the following?

(A) Acoustic neuroma
(B) Caudate calcification
(C) Cerebellar degeneration
(D) Frontal lobe tumor
(E) Prolactinoma

282

Symptoms of obsessive-compulsive disorder respond best to which of the following tricyclic antidepressants?

(A) Imipramine
(B) Amitriptyline
(C) Doxepin
(D) Clomipramine
(E) Desipramine

283

A 23-year-old woman presented with a 2-week history of difficulty sleeping, hearing voices, and problems with thinking. She was fearful and suspicious, and talked about evil alien forces out in the world. Some of her relatives have had "nervous breakdowns" requiring hospitalization. Further evaluation revealed that the woman had been raped about 3 weeks earlier. However, she has no recollection of the event. One week after initial presentation, her symptoms have disappeared and she has returned to normal functioning. The most likely diagnosis at this time is:

(A) acute stress disorder.
(B) brief psychotic disorder.
(C) schizoaffective disorder.
(D) posttraumatic stress disorder.
(E) schizophreniform disorder.

284

Which of the following medications is most likely to be associated with polycystic ovary syndrome?

(A) Carbamazepine
(B) Gabapentin
(C) Lithium
(D) Topiramate
(E) Valproate

285

In the National Institute of Mental Health's Epidemiologic Catchment Area study, the ethnic differences in the 1-month prevalence of mental health disorders dropped after which of the following factors was controlled for?

(A) Age
(B) Education
(C) Gender
(D) Literacy rate
(E) Socioeconomic status

286

A patient has not responded to phenelzine after 10 weeks of treatment, and a switch to fluoxetine is planned. What is the recommended minimum interval between stopping phenelzine and starting fluoxetine?

(A) 1 week
(B) 2 weeks
(C) 4 weeks
(D) 6 weeks
(E) 8 weeks

287

The single most effective treatment for major depression in elderly patients is:

(A) bupropion.
(B) citalopram.
(C) ECT.
(D) nortriptyline.
(E) venlafaxine.

288

A 30-year-old athletic man presents for evaluation of several syncopal episodes over the past month. He has been treated for hypertension during the past year and has responded nicely to 50 mg/day of metoprolol XR and 25 mg/day of hydrochlorothiazide. Three months ago his primary care physician started him on 20 mg/day of fluoxetine and 0.5 mg/day of lorazepam t.i.d. for mixed anxiety and depression. On examination the patient seems mildly anxious and demonstrates orthostatic hypotension. His ECG is unremarkable except for mild sinus bradycardia. What is the most likely explanation?

(A) Transient ischemic attacks
(B) Fluoxetine–metoprolol interaction
(C) Overdiuresis
(D) Benzodiazepine intoxication
(E) Psychogenic syncope

289

Attention deficit hyperactivity disorder (ADHD) appears to be most strongly associated with prenatal exposure to:

(A) caffeine.
(B) lithium.
(C) nicotine.
(D) SSRIs.
(E) valproic acid.

290

Compared with Caucasian Americans, African Americans are more likely to receive a diagnosis of:

(A) bipolar disorder, depressed.
(B) bipolar disorder, manic.
(C) major depression.
(D) schizophrenia.
(E) substance-induced psychosis.

291

The clinical sign that best differentiates delirium from dementia is:

(A) agitation.
(B) confusion.
(C) fluctuating consciousness.
(D) poor attention span.
(E) psychosis.

292

Gabapentin has FDA approval as an indication for which of the following?

(A) Postmenopausal hot flashes
(B) Posttraumatic stress disorder (PTSD)
(C) Postherpetic neuralgia
(D) Cocaine dependence

293

A patient with a first episode of a nonpsychotic major depression has responded well to the acute phase medication treatment. What is the typical duration of the continuation phase?

(A) 3 months
(B) 4 to 9 months
(C) 10 to 15 months
(D) 2 years
(E) Lifelong

294

A 40-year-old woman consults a psychiatrist with a chief complaint of anxiety, insomnia with nightmares, loss of appetite, and chest pain. Tearfully, the patient reports that 2 weeks ago her husband left her for another woman. The husband told the patient, "I need someone more adventuresome." She suspected that her husband was having an affair, but she was unprepared for his leaving. She avoids walking by his office in their home because when she sees his litter, still on the desk, she feels chest pain. She reports fear of being alone. She continually daydreams about their life together. She can "barely function" in her job as a hospital administrator. The most likely preliminary diagnosis is:

(A) acute stress disorder.
(B) adjustment disorder with anxiety.
(C) pathological bereavement.
(D) posttraumatic stress disorder.
(E) social phobia.

295

A 74-year-old man falls on an ice patch and bumps his head. During the next 4 weeks, his wife notices that he seems more forgetful and that at night he is disoriented. He also develops a persistent headache. Which of the following diagnoses is most likely to be causing this presentation?

(A) Cerebellar tumor
(B) Multi-infarct dementia
(C) Occipital tumor
(D) Subdural hematoma
(E) Wernicke's encephalopathy

296

What proportion of people with dysthymic disorder experience an episode of major depression in their lifetime?

(A) 5%–10%
(B) 20%–30%
(C) 40%–50%
(D) 70%–80%
(E) 100%

297

Currently, the efficacy of a psychotherapy for treatment of a particular disorder is best judged by:

(A) cohort study.
(B) individual case outcomes.
(C) number needed to treat to number needed to harm ratio.
(D) relative risk reduction measure.
(E) systematic review of controlled studies.

298

A 25-year-old woman is diagnosed with bipolar I disorder. She has a previous history of several suicide attempts. Of the following medications, which would be the most likely to decrease her risk for suicide if administered on a long-term basis?

(A) Carbamazepine
(B) Lamotrigine
(C) Lithium
(D) Risperidone
(E) Verapamil

299

A 29-year-old man has severe panic attacks cued by public speaking. He has developed marked avoidance of such situations, which has greatly compromised his career development. Which of the following is the most appropriate diagnosis?

(A) Agoraphobia without panic disorder
(B) Acute stress disorder
(C) Panic disorder with agoraphobia
(D) Social phobia
(E) Specific phobia

300

A patient whose depression has responded well to an SSRI now reports symptoms of erectile dysfunction associated with the SSRI antidepressant therapy. This dysfunction has persisted for more than a month. The best initial approach would be to:

(A) add bupropion.
(B) take a drug holiday.
(C) reduce the dose of the antidepressant.
(D) switch to a different SSRI.
(E) continue treatment until the patient develops tolerance to the side effect.

301

A patient with a 10-year history of alcohol dependence requests outpatient detoxification. In determining whether outpatient detoxification is an appropriate treatment setting for this patient, the most important variable is:

(A) length of history of alcohol dependence.
(B) support of spouse or significant other.
(C) type of alcohol consumed.
(D) prior history of delirium tremens.

302

During the sexual history, a married 35-year-old male reveals that he considers himself to be "on the down low." Regarding his sexual orientation and partners, he would most likely consider himself to be:

(A) bisexual, and has sex equally with men and women.
(B) heterosexual, and exclusively has sex with women.
(C) heterosexual, but also secretly has sex with men.
(D) homosexual, but also has sex with women.
(E) homosexual, and exclusively has sex with men.

303

In order for a patient to meet the diagnostic criteria for substance abuse, which of the following must be present?

(A) Physiologic tolerance to the substance
(B) Physiologic withdrawal from the substance
(C) Failure to attend to expected cultural role as a result of the substance
(D) Positron emission tomography findings of mesolimbic tract hyperactivity
(E) Family history of addiction

304

Among patients with major depressive disorder, women have which of the following characteristics compared with men?

(A) Earlier age at onset
(B) Shorter episode duration
(C) Higher rates of comorbid drug abuse
(D) Lower rates of comorbid generalized anxiety
(E) Fewer suicide attempts

305

In order to determine the genomic location of a susceptibility gene for panic disorder, which of the following approaches would be most appropriate?

(A) Family risk studies
(B) Genetic epidemiology
(C) Gene finding
(D) Molecular genetics
(E) Twin studies

306

During treatment, a female patient reports sexual encounters with a prior therapist in a state that mandates the reporting of sexual abuse by therapists. In the interest of preserving the confidentiality of the doctor-patient relationship, which of the following is the best response of the therapist?

(A) Refer the patient to another physician for consultation, specifically for the role of advocacy.
(B) Request court immunity from the statute to protect the doctor-patient relationship.
(C) Convince the patient to report the matter herself.
(D) Explore the allegation with the patient to determine whether it actually occurred.

307

Which of the following medications has been shown to be most effective in reducing suicidal behaviors in patients with schizophrenia or schizoaffective disorder?

(A) Clozapine
(B) Haloperidol
(C) Lithium
(D) Olanzapine
(E) Ziprasidone

308

Which of the following diagnostic criteria most clearly distinguishes paranoid personality disorder from paranoid schizophrenia, delusional disorder, and mood disorder with psychotic features?

(A) Absence of positive psychotic symptoms
(B) Age at onset
(C) Degree of impairment in interpersonal relationships
(D) Duration of symptoms
(E) Pervasive nature of symptoms

309

A 19-year-old exchange student from Malaysia is brought to the emergency department by his host parents after he became violent at home and threatened to kill them. The parents report that he seemed fine until they commented to him that he had left the faucet running in the bathroom. Initially, he went to his room and seemed sullen. He then began "ranting and raving" about how he is not an irresponsible person, accused the host parents of spying on him, threatened them, threw objects about, and collapsed on the floor in exhaustion. In the emergency department, the student is calm and cooperative. Mental status examination is unremarkable. The student denies any recall of the episode. This presentation is most consistent with which culture-bound syndrome?

(A) Amok
(B) Dhat
(C) Koro
(D) Locura
(E) Rootwork

310

What is the most common comorbid condition in children with autistic disorder?

(A) Attention deficit hyperactivity disorder
(B) Major depression
(C) Mental retardation
(D) Schizophrenia
(E) Social phobia

311

A 65-year-old patient is admitted to the surgical inpatient service for a hernia repair. The family reported that over the past few months the patient has had episodes of confusion. While on the ward, the patient began to have prominent visual hallucinations. The staff administered 1 mg of haloperidol orally. A second dose was given 3 hours later. Soon after receiving the second dose of haloperidol, the patient had a severe extrapyramidal response. Which of the following is the most likely diagnosis?

(A) Delirium with preexisting dementia
(B) Parkinson's dementia
(C) Lewy body dementia
(D) Major depressive disorder with psychosis
(E) Alcohol withdrawal

312

Which of the following is most likely to be preserved in the early stages of frontotemporal dementia?

(A) Judgment
(B) Personality
(C) Verbal output
(D) Visuospatial skills
(E) Sociability or social involvement

313

Of the following disorders, which has the greatest genetic contribution or heritability?

(A) Major depressive disorder
(B) Alcoholism
(C) Obsessive-compulsive disorder
(D) Schizophrenia
(E) Panic disorder

314

A 25-year-old man collects women's bras and underpants from public laundries and uses the objects to become sexually aroused. This description is most consistent with which of the following DSM-IV-TR diagnoses?

(A) Exhibitionism
(B) Fetishism
(C) Frotteurism
(D) Sexual masochism
(E) Kleptomania

315

A 24-year-old man comes for an evaluation because he cannot relax. He reports that he constantly is thinking about whether his car will break down, his bills will get paid, and if his school performance is adequate. For over a year, he often is tired, irritable, and on edge. Upon reflection, the student is unable to identify any aspect of his life that is going so well that it does not generate concern. The most likely diagnosis is:

(A) depressive disorder not otherwise specified.
(B) generalized anxiety disorder.
(C) obsessive-compulsive disorder.
(D) panic disorder.
(E) social phobia.

316

The side effect of pancreatitis is linked most closely to which of the following?

(A) Divalproex
(B) Oxcarbazepine
(C) Lamotrigine
(D) Topiramate

317

Which of the following is a technique of supportive dynamic psychotherapy?

(A) Transference interpretation
(B) Promoting therapeutic regression
(C) Extreme passivity of therapist
(D) Problem-solving focus
(E) Frequent genetic reconstruction

318

The most effective behavior therapy technique used in the treatment of compulsions of obsessive-compulsive disorder is:

(A) exposure and response prevention.
(B) negative reinforcement.
(C) positive reinforcement.
(D) punishment.
(E) systematic desensitization.

319

A man who is receiving cognitive behavior therapy for depression feels guilty for massive layoffs at his workplace, even though he was not involved in the management decision. Which of the following types of cognitive error is most consistent with this patient's feeling?

(A) Arbitrary inference
(B) Absolutist thinking
(C) Catastrophic thinking
(D) Magnification and minimization
(E) Personalization

320

An actor has received repeated complaints from colleagues about his behavior in professional situations. He has just started rehearsals for a play. The problematic behavior consists of excessive demands for special treatment and outbursts when special treatment is not granted. He is diagnosed as having narcissistic personality disorder. He has been in treatment for several months; treatment has been going well, and there have been fewer demands and outbursts at work. Which of the following is the patient most likely to do next?

(A) Generalize this behavior to his home environment
(B) Demand new concessions from the play's director
(C) Show a new understanding of his behavior
(D) Continue to show appropriate behavior at work
(E) Discuss his feelings about the therapist

321

Of the following, which is the best definition of ethnicity? Human groups that:

(A) share a sociopolitical designation.
(B) share common values, beliefs, history, and customs.
(C) have common identities, ancestries, and histories.
(D) share distinct identifying phenotypic characteristics.
(E) are living together in the same location.

322

Which of the following psychotherapeutic approaches provides the primary framework for dialectical behavior therapy for borderline personality disorder?

(A) Cognitive behavior therapy
(B) Interpersonal psychotherapy
(C) Psychodynamic psychotherapy
(D) Family systems therapy
(E) Supportive psychotherapy

323

The most common DSM-IV-TR axis II personality disorder demonstrated among persons with substance use disorders is:

(A) borderline personality disorder.
(B) narcissistic personality disorder.
(C) dependent personality disorder.
(D) antisocial personality disorder.

324

A 72-year-old woman is hospitalized with findings of dementia, ataxia, and macrocytic anemia. The most likely diagnosis is:

(A) dementia of the Alzheimer's type.
(B) vascular dementia.
(C) vitamin B_{12} deficiency.
(D) Huntington's disease.
(E) pellagra.

325

A 20-year-old woman describes a 6-month history of frequent binge eating followed by self-induced vomiting and laxative use to maintain normal body weight. Which of the following medications is FDA-approved for her disorder?

(A) Bupropion
(B) Citalopram
(C) Escitalopram
(D) Fluoxetine
(E) Venlafaxine

326

A psychiatrist who is grieving from a recent sudden loss of a spouse shares those feelings with a psychotherapy patient. What is the most ethical interpretation of the psychiatrist's actions?

(A) It may be ethically problematic if the psychiatrist was driven by personal needs rather than by serving the patient's needs.
(B) It is always ethically unacceptable because a psychiatrist should never reveal personal information to a patient.
(C) It is problematic to reveal any information other than the psychiatrist's professional training.
(D) It is not ethically problematic because sharing the psychiatrist's authentic feelings with patients is therapeutic for the patient.

327

Which of the following will cause the greatest increase in serum lithium levels?

(A) Theophylline
(B) Ziprasidone
(C) Hydrochlorothiazide
(D) Celecoxib

328

While reviewing the treatment plan for a patient with methamphetamine dependence, the psychiatrist thinks about how best to help the patient progress from the contemplation phase to the preparation phase. The psychiatrist's approach to treatment in this case is based on the principles of:

(A) 12-step facilitation therapy.
(B) cognitive behavior therapy (CBT).
(C) contingency management therapy.
(D) motivational enhancement therapy (MET).

329

Which of the following is the most effective treatment for catatonic features associated with a manic episode?

(A) Lithium
(B) Electroconvulsive therapy
(C) Divalproex
(D) Clozapine

330

The cornerstone of relapse prevention as a modality of treatment for substance-dependent patients is:

(A) psychodynamic technique.
(B) 12-step group attendance.
(C) motivational enhancement.
(D) skills training.

331

Which of the following is the most common sexual disorder in men?

(A) Hypoactive sexual desire disorder
(B) Male erectile disorder
(C) Premature ejaculation
(D) Male orgasmic disorder
(E) Dyspareunia

332

An adult female patient consumes an average of 14 glasses of wine per week, never consuming more than four glasses on any one occasion. Based solely on this drinking pattern, her physician should do which of the following?

(A) Refer her to an addiction specialist for further evaluation.
(B) Recommend that she begin attending AA meetings.
(C) Inform her that she is drinking at a safe level.
(D) Recommend that she reduce her drinking by about 50%.

The following four questions (333–336) form a serial vignette.

333

Mr. B, a high school teacher in his mid-30s, was recently separated from his wife and two children. An intelligent and verbally facile man with a particular talent in the arts, Mr. B was plagued by his conviction that he was unacceptable to other people unless he complied with their expectations and gratified their needs. This was a pleasant, agreeable, and compliant facade that hid his feelings of weakness and stupidity. He constantly sought approval from his superiors, but underneath he felt resentment and rebelliousness about others' expecting him to accommodate to their needs and wishes.

Mr. B's mother was an embittered, burdened woman, contemptuous of men and preoccupied with her own needs and interests. His father, while somewhat approachable, had often been away from home trying to make a living to support the family. Mr. B remembered his father as erratic and moody and given to temper outbursts, which, he recalls, would lead to beatings with a leather strap. The middle of three children, the patient felt that his father favored his older sister and that his mother favored his younger brother, and he saw himself as the neglected outsider.

What is the most likely defense mechanism utilized by this patient when first meeting the psychiatrist?

(A) Regression
(B) Altruism
(C) Undoing projection
(D) Intellectualization rationalization
(E) Dissociation

334

Because of an emergency, Mr. B's psychiatrist was 20 minutes late to the second interview. Mr. B makes an offhand and somewhat negative comment about "doctors being too busy these days." In all likelihood, this is an example of:

(A) reaction formation.
(B) transference.
(C) idealization.
(D) splitting.
(E) suppression.

335

On hearing the irritation in the patient's voice, the clinician begins to explain in detail the reasons for his tardiness and apologizes profusely. He assures the patient that he will not be late for future meetings. This is an example of:

(A) denial.
(B) regression.
(C) countertransference.
(D) deidealization.
(E) dissociation.

336

In beginning a brief therapy with Mr. B, the most important challenge for this psychiatrist is to:

(A) prescribe an antidepressant.
(B) prescribe an antianxiety agent.
(C) contact the patient's wife for additional history.
(D) establish a therapeutic or working alliance.
(E) set clear limits on the patient's behavior.

337

Which of the following psychiatric disorders is considered to be predominantly culture specific?

(A) Bulimia nervosa
(B) Generalized anxiety disorder
(C) Major depressive disorder
(D) Posttraumatic stress disorder
(E) Schizophrenia

338

A 73-year-old man with moderate congestive heart failure and degenerative arthritis in his right knee visits his physician for a scheduled outpatient appointment. Although his physical examination findings from the previous visit are unchanged, the physician notes that the patient appears tired and less interactive than usual. Concerned that the patient may be experiencing a major depressive episode, the physician wishes to gather more information. The presence of which of the following would be most helpful in making a diagnosis of major depressive disorder?

(A) Complaints of pain
(B) Decreased concentration
(C) Loss of appetite
(D) Poor energy
(E) The wish to die

339

A 46-year-old woman presents to her primary care physician with a 2-month history of low back pain, dull headaches several times a week, insomnia, fatigue, and irritability. She has always been healthy. Findings from her physical examination are all within normal limits, and a review of systems is noncontributory. Routine laboratory tests such as a chemistry panel, CBC, and thyroid function tests are all normal. The most likely diagnosis is:

(A) major depressive disorder.
(B) generalized anxiety disorder.
(C) pain disorder.
(D) hypochondriasis.
(E) somatization disorder.

340

A 29-year-old patient with borderline personality disorder is being seen in psychotherapy twice weekly. The psychiatrist realizes that the patient is unconsciously trying to coerce her into acting in a judgmental way. This phenomenon is best described as:

(A) identification with the aggressor.
(B) projection.
(C) projective identification.
(D) regression.
(E) splitting.

341

Which of the following is NOT FDA-approved for the treatment of acute mania?

(A) Carbamazepine
(B) Gabapentin
(C) Divalproex
(D) Olanzapine
(E) Risperidone

342

The term "four D's of negligence"—duty, dereliction, direct, and damages—refers to:

(A) the questions a defendant physician will be asked at deposition.
(B) what a patient/plaintiff must prove to win a malpractice suit.
(C) the calculation of punitive versus compensatory damages.
(D) the level of care that would be expected of a reasonable physician under similar circumstances.

343

In a psychotherapy session, a patient reveals that he has been having trouble obtaining an orgasm with his partner. He states that he has always felt aroused when traveling to work on a crowded bus, and he used to think that this enhanced his sexual life. He never thought it was a problem, but now he thinks it is interfering with his relationship. What is the most likely diagnosis?

(A) Exhibitionism
(B) Fetishism
(C) Frotteurism
(D) Pedophilia
(E) Voyeurism

344

Which of the following comparisons regarding the incidence and prevalence of posttraumatic stress disorder (PTSD) is the most accurate?

(A) The condition is more prevalent in men.
(B) The presence of a psychiatric disorder does not predispose a person to PTSD.
(C) Older individuals have a higher prevalence than younger individuals.
(D) Certain types of trauma are more likely to cause PTSD.

345

Which of the following statements is correct about the concordance of schizophrenia in the twin of an individual with schizophrenia?

(A) 50% if twin is monozygotic
(B) 75% if twin is monozygotic
(C) Almost 100% if twin is monozygotic
(D) 50% if twin is dizygotic
(E) 75% if twin is dizygotic

346

A 33-year-old woman with a diagnosis of borderline personality disorder was recently discharged from medical service after an aspirin overdose. She describes having had thoughts of suicide off and on since early adolescence and has made two previous suicide attempts. In addressing her suicidality in treatment, which of the following approaches would be most appropriate?

(A) Partial hospitalization or brief inpatient hospitalization
(B) Outpatient psychoanalysis
(C) Gabapentin pharmacotherapy
(D) Valproic acid pharmacotherapy

347

In addition to a stimulant trial for attention deficit hyperactivity disorder symptoms, the parents of an 8-year-old boy ask what other treatment would be most helpful for managing his refusal to cooperate at home. Which of the following is the best recommendation?

(A) Biofeedback
(B) Behavior therapy
(C) Cognitive behavior therapy
(D) Family therapy
(E) Psychodynamic psychotherapy

348

A 15-year-old girl is brought in for an emergency evaluation because she has been out all night and refuses to tell her parents where she has been. The parents report that for several months the girl has been irritable and oppositional with severe mood swings. She has been leaving home and school without permission. The girl admits that she has been somewhat moody but insists that her parents are making a big deal about nothing. A preliminary diagnosis of bipolar disorder is made. Which of the following is the most common comorbid condition with bipolar disorder?

(A) Conduct disorder
(B) Generalized anxiety disorder
(C) Oppositional defiant disorder
(D) Posttraumatic stress disorder
(E) Substance use disorder

349

A 29-year-old woman is admitted to the hospital with acute herpes simplex encephalitis. Which of the following is the most common residual deficit upon recovery?

(A) Apraxia
(B) Aphasia
(C) Amnesia
(D) Ataxia
(E) Dysarthria

350

Which of the following is most effective for the psychotherapeutic treatment of obsessive-compulsive disorder?

(A) Biofeedback
(B) Exposure and response prevention
(C) Psychodynamic psychotherapy
(D) Relaxation and visualization
(E) Interpersonal therapy

351

Rebound insomnia is most severe after abrupt withdrawal of which of the following medications?

(A) Alprazolam
(B) Clonazepam
(C) Diazepam
(D) Chlordiazepoxide
(E) Quazepam

352

All of the following are symptom clusters of posttraumatic stress disorder (PTSD) EXCEPT:

(A) reexperiencing.
(B) avoidance/numbing.
(C) hyperarousal.
(D) derealization/depersonalization.

353

In clinical or forensic evaluations when financial compensation or special benefits may be available, a psychiatrist must consider the diagnosis of:

(A) factitious disorder.
(B) malingering.
(C) somatization.
(D) hypochondriasis.

354

Avoidance symptoms in posttraumatic stress disorder (PTSD) include which of the following?

(A) Hypervigilance
(B) Intrusive images of the event
(C) Sense of reliving the event or experience
(D) Difficulty recalling important aspects of the event

355

Weight gain is LEAST likely to be a side effect of which of the following?

(A) Lithium
(B) Lamotrigine
(C) Divalproex
(D) Olanzapine

356

In Erikson's epigenetic model, each life stage has an identity crisis that must be navigated. Intimacy vs. isolation is the developmental crisis associated with:

(A) school age.
(B) adolescence.
(C) young adulthood.
(D) adulthood.
(E) old age.

357

Trichotillomania is a difficult symptom to treat with either psychotherapy or medication. Emerging evidence indicates that medication plus which of the following types of psychotherapy is effective?

(A) Exposure
(B) Flooding
(C) Habit reversal
(D) Interpersonal psychotherapy
(E) Psychodynamic psychotherapy

The following vignette applies to questions 358 and 359.

A 19-year-old woman presents to a clinic for treatment of chapped hands. She reports that for several months she has had "this notion in my head" that there are germs everywhere. At first she washed her hands more frequently, but as the thoughts have become more prominent, she now usually wears gloves and washes her hands with diluted bleach several times a day. She says that if she does not complete her cleansing rituals, she cannot stand the anxiety.

358

The most common comorbid condition with this disorder is:

(A) alcohol abuse.
(B) generalized anxiety disorder.
(C) major depressive disorder.
(D) social phobia.
(E) schizophrenia.

359

The structural brain abnormality that has been demonstrated most consistently in this disorder is:

(A) asymmetrical septal nuclei.
(B) decreased size of the caudate.
(C) enlarged lateral ventricles.
(D) hypertrophy of the amygdala.
(E) shrinkage of the hippocampus.

360

In which of the following disorders has reduced volume been observed in the prefrontal cortex?

(A) ADHD
(B) Delusional disorder
(C) Obsessive-compulsive disorder
(D) Panic disorder
(E) Schizophrenia

361

The first step in the evaluation of a patient with male erectile disorder is to:

(A) take a genetic history.
(B) rule out medical problems and substance use.
(C) refer the patient to a sex therapist.
(D) challenge with a test dose of a PDE-5 inhibitor.
(E) order a sleep study.

362

A 75-year-old woman with Parkinson's disease develops vivid dreams and night terrors. The most likely explanation for these symptoms is:

(A) the onset of dementia.
(B) a rapid progression of Parkinson's disease.
(C) a normal effect of aging.
(D) an anxiety disorder.
(E) side effects from carbidopa-levodopa.

363

In which of the following therapies, which has been studied for the treatment of patients with borderline personality disorder, is mindfulness training a central component?

(A) Cognitive behavior therapy
(B) Dynamic psychotherapy
(C) Dialectical behavior therapy
(D) Short-term group psychotherapy
(E) Interpersonal psychotherapy

364

Heightened arousal in posttraumatic stress disorder (PTSD) is associated with an increase in which of the following?

(A) Heart rate
(B) Constriction of pupils
(C) Weight
(D) Tidal volume

365

According to DSM-IV-TR, a mixed episode must meet diagnostic criteria for a manic episode and which of the following?

(A) Panic attacks
(B) Rapid cycling
(C) Brief psychotic episode
(D) Major depressive episode

366

A psychiatrist is called to see a 78-year-old female patient postoperatively on the surgical service who is said to be "manic." She is hardly sleeping, she is agitated and talking rapidly, and she believes she needs to talk with the President of the United States. Which of the following interventions is most likely to be effective?

(A) Transfer to a psychiatric unit
(B) Divalproex sodium
(C) Haloperidol
(D) ECT
(E) A benzodiazepine

367

Which of the following variables is most important to take into account when evaluating the score on a Mini-Mental State Exam (MMSE)?

(A) Educational level
(B) Gender
(C) History of alcohol use
(D) Medical history
(E) Past psychiatric history

368

The parents of a 5-year-old boy bring their child to a clinic with the complaint that he frequently awakens during the early part of the night screaming; he looks terrified, his pupils are dilated, and he hyperventilates. He is also sweating, agitated, and confused, and he cannot be comforted. When fully awakened, the child has no recall of the event. This presentation is most consistent with:

(A) narcolepsy.
(B) nightmare disorder.
(C) primary insomnia.
(D) sleep disordered breathing.
(E) sleep terror disorder.

369

A 6-year-old girl is brought to a clinic because of unusual stereotyped hand washing. Pregnancy, labor, and delivery were unremarkable, as were developmental milestones until the age of 8 months, when the child seemed to lose interest in her social environment. Thereafter, significant delays in development were noted. She did not walk until 2 years of age and has had no spoken language. Head growth has stagnated. Recently she has developed breath-holding spells. Examination reveals a small, noncommunicative child who demonstrates truncal ataxia and non-purposeful hand movements. EEG is abnormal. This presentation is most consistent with:

(A) Asperger's syndrome.
(B) autism.
(C) childhood schizophrenia.
(D) mild mental retardation.
(E) Rett's disorder.

370

Which of the following actions on the part of a psychiatrist constitutes abandonment?

(A) Failing to show up for a scheduled appointment with a patient
(B) Referring, with appropriate notification to the patient, an extremely difficult patient to a colleague with more experience in the treatment of the patient's disorder
(C) Terminating the treating relationship when a patient threatens to sue the psychiatrist
(D) Prematurely discharging a patient from the hospital

371

Common side effects of selective serotonin reuptake inhibitors include:

(A) orthostatic hypotension and dry mouth.
(B) confusion and disorientation.
(C) priapism and arrhythmia.
(D) seizures and hallucinations.
(E) nausea and sexual dysfunction.

372

Which of the following classes of medications is supported by well-designed studies as the first-line pharmacologic treatment of posttraumatic stress disorder (PTSD)?

(A) Mood stabilizers
(B) Benzodiazepines
(C) Tricyclic antidepressants
(D) Selective serotonin reuptake inhibitors (SSRIs)

373

A patient in early recovery from opiate dependence has been maintained on 40 mg/day of oral methadone for the last month. While the patient has not been experiencing any withdrawal symptoms at that dose, the weekly random urine drug tests begin showing a resumption of heroin use. Pharmacologically, the best change to make in medication would be to:

(A) increase the maintenance dose of methadone.
(B) decrease the maintenance dose of methadone.
(C) change the opiate agonist to levo-alpha-acetylmethadol (LAAM).
(D) augment with buprenorphine.

374

A 45-year-old man who travels frequently finds that on returning from his most recent trip to a distant city, he has had difficulty maintaining daytime alertness and falls asleep easily and at inappropriate times. Which of the following is the most likely diagnosis?

(A) Circadian rhythm sleep disorder
(B) Dissociative fugue
(C) Dyssomnia
(D) Parasomnia
(E) Narcolepsy

375

Compared with other dementias, the early presentation in Creutzfeldt-Jakob disease more often includes:

(A) choreoathetosis.
(B) dysarthria.
(C) extrapyramidal symptoms.
(D) frontal release signs.
(E) myoclonus.

376

A 27-year-old man has a 4-month history of persecutory delusions about being spied on at work by coworkers. Apart from the delusions, he functions reasonably well, and there is no evidence of medical illness or substance abuse. The most likely diagnosis is:

(A) brief psychotic disorder.
(B) delusional disorder.
(C) major depression with psychotic features.
(D) schizophrenia, paranoid type.
(E) schizophreniform disorder.

377

Nausea and other gastrointestinal side effects with SSRIs appear to be related to which receptor subtype?

(A) 5-HT$_2$ receptor
(B) DA-2 receptor
(C) DA-4 receptor
(D) H$_2$ receptor

378

Which of the following abilities is NOT directly relevant to a person's capacity to make medical decisions?

(A) Communicate or evidence a choice
(B) Understand the facts of the situation
(C) Appreciate how the facts of a situation apply to oneself
(D) Choose an option that reflects what most reasonable persons in that situation would do

379

An 18-year-old woman is starting her freshman year in college. She is living at home with her parents. On campus, she hopes to make friends but usually stays to herself, fearing that she will be rejected by her peers. When called on in class, she avoids eye contact with the professor. Although she almost always knows the answer to questions asked by the professor, she experiences inordinate anxiety that she will make a mistake. In private moments, she refers to herself as "the big nobody." This presentation is most consistent with:

(A) avoidant personality disorder.
(B) dependent personality disorder.
(C) paranoid personality disorder.
(D) schizoid personality disorder.
(E) schizotypal personality disorder.

380

The oncology team is concerned because a patient from another culture acts resigned when faced with a diagnosis of terminal cancer. The consulting psychiatrist points out that in the patient's culture illness and death are part of the normal cycle of life. Which of the following best describes the use of culture in this psychiatric formulation?

(A) Interpretive and explanatory tool
(B) Pathogenic and pathoplastic agent
(C) Diagnostic and nosologic factor
(D) Therapeutic and protective element
(E) Management and service instrument

381

According to DSM-IV-TR, which of the following characterizes acute stress disorder (ASD)?

(A) Lasts a maximum of 8 weeks
(B) Does not involve symptoms of hyperarousal
(C) Often occurs as a result of a minor threat
(D) Requires dissociative symptoms for a diagnosis

382

Olfactory hallucinations are most commonly associated with:

(A) grand mal seizures.
(B) hypoparathyroidism.
(C) parietal tumor.
(D) partial complex seizures.
(E) psychotic depression.

383

A new psychologist in town approaches an established psychiatrist and proposes that the psychiatrist refer therapy patients to the psychologist in return for a small percentage of fees collected by the psychologist from treating those patients. This practice is:

(A) not acceptable because it does not put the patients' interests first.
(B) not acceptable because psychiatrists should refer patients to psychiatrist therapists.
(C) acceptable because it provides incentives for all parties to benefit.
(D) acceptable because the psychologist is fairly compensating the psychiatrist.

384

In order for an individual to recover from PTSD after interpersonal violence, which of the following processes is likely to be most helpful?

(A) Go to court and see the perpetrator brought to justice.
(B) Wait for symptoms to subside with time.
(C) Emotionally engage with the memory of the trauma.
(D) Restore sleep with a benzodiazepine.
(E) Obtain treatment with eye movement desensitization techniques.

385

A hospital risk manager speaks with you about developing an educational seminar on suicide prevention contracts for emergency department staff. As part of the seminar, which of the following would be a most appropriate point to emphasize?

(A) A patient's willingness to enter into a suicide prevention contract indicates readiness for discharge from an emergency setting.
(B) In emergency settings, suicide prevention contracts are a helpful method for reducing suicide risk but should not be used to determine readiness for discharge.
(C) Using suicide prevention contracts in emergency settings is not recommended.
(D) Suicide prevention contracts can be useful for assessing the physician-patient relationship with individuals who are intoxicated, agitated, or psychotic.

386

A middle-aged man consults a psychiatrist at the recommendation of his primary care physician because he has been unable to recover from his deep grief and feelings of abandonment since his divorce 18 months ago. He endorses many symptoms of major depression and has withdrawn from the social activities that he used to enjoy, but he is not suicidal. Of the following things that this patient reports, which would be the most positive indicator that he would be able to benefit from psychodynamic psychotherapy?

(A) He is very angry at his ex-wife.
(B) He has no family history of psychiatric illness.
(C) He has been a successful writer.
(D) He gets significant support from his two best friends.
(E) He is very religious.

387

Lorazepam may be a better choice of a benzodiazepine than diazepam for an elderly patient because the:

(A) volume of distribution decreases with age.
(B) hepatic oxidation is unaffected by age.
(C) hepatic conjugation is unaffected by age.
(D) glomerular filtration rate is unaffected by age.
(E) hepatic blood flow is unaffected by age.

388

A patient who is an artist is severely depressed and has occasional passive suicidal thoughts. The patient tells the psychiatrist that health insurance benefits have been discontinued and that the patient is no longer able to pay the psychiatric bills. The psychiatrist has decided not to provide free care to this patient. The psychiatrist can avoid abandoning this patient by:

(A) giving the patient a written, 30-day notice of termination and terminating the patient at the end of the 30-day period.
(B) reducing the frequency of the patient's appointments to help make the patient's bill more affordable.
(C) arranging to commission an artwork by the patient in lieu of the professional fees.
(D) continuing to see the patient until acute depression-related crises are resolved and then discharging the patient to the local state-funded community agency clinic.

389

A primary substance abuse prevention program is being developed for adolescent girls in a large, metropolitan school district in the United States. The school district is diverse, with youths from African, Asian, Caucasian, Middle Eastern, and Native American families. Based on epidemiologic studies, which ethnic group of adolescent girls is at greatest risk of substance use?

(A) African American
(B) Asian American
(C) Caucasian
(D) Middle Eastern
(E) Native American

390

Posttraumatic stress disorder (PTSD) is considered to be chronic PTSD after:

(A) 1 month.
(B) 3 months.
(C) 6 months.
(D) 1 year.
(E) 3 years.

391

A 9-year-old boy is seen in the emergency department after attempting to jump out of a moving vehicle. His parents report that he has had a difficult time in the past year. Previously he had done well in school, but now he is struggling academically. He often says he does not want to go to school, "because I am so stupid and ugly." His teacher has contacted his parents and informed them that he is falling asleep in class, seems fatigued, has little to do with his peers, and often does not eat his lunch. The child used to play with friends in the neighborhood, but for the past 2 months has kept to himself, playing alone in his room or just sitting and looking out the window. A few days earlier, he informed his mother of what to do with his most important belongings should he die, but she did not make anything out of it. He has generally seemed very grouchy and "on edge." On questioning, he acknowledges that he was hoping to be killed when he tried to jump out of the car. The most likely diagnosis is:

(A) borderline personality disorder.
(B) major depressive disorder.
(C) oppositional defiant disorder.
(D) separation anxiety disorder.
(E) somatization disorder.

392

The family of a 40-year-old retired police officer reports that in the past year he has been increasingly isolative, withdrawn, and bizarre. He has accused his family of trying to poison him. He put tarps over the windows in his house. He is disheveled and carries a set of torn papers at all times. He has been observed mumbling and talking to himself. He has no history of substance abuse or prior depressive episodes. Which of the following is the most likely diagnosis?

(A) Bipolar disorder
(B) Delusional disorder
(C) Dementia of the Alzheimer's type
(D) Major depression with psychotic features or schizoaffective disorder
(E) Schizophrenia

393

Clinical signs of major depression may emerge for a patient during bereavement after a parent's death. According to DSM-IV-TR criteria, what is the earliest time interval after the parent's death that this diagnosis is generally made?

(A) 1 month
(B) 2 months
(C) 3 months
(D) 6 months

394

Involuntary hospitalization of a patient with schizophrenia who is hearing voices is justified in which of the following situations?

(A) The patient hears a voice that he cannot resist telling him to kill himself.
(B) Third-party payer deems hospitalization appropriate and will pay.
(C) The patient appears dirty and disheveled.
(D) The patient lacks insight into the nature of his illness.

395

Kidney stones are most likely to be a side effect of which of the following?

(A) Gabapentin
(B) Lithium
(C) Lamotrigine
(D) Topiramate

396

The CEO of a large company is fearful of speaking at a large stockholders' meeting. His fear of public speaking has been a lifelong disability, but he does not have anxiety in other social settings. Which of the following is the most reasonable agent to prescribe?

(A) A benzodiazepine
(B) A beta-blocker
(C) Buspirone
(D) A serotonin norepinephrine reuptake inhibitor (SNRI)
(E) An SSRI

397

A 49-year-old man with schizophrenia taking an antipsychotic asks to change medication because of intolerable side effects. He has had extrapyramidal side effects and has experienced a 24-pound weight gain. His body mass index is now 32.4. His family history is significant for obesity, diabetes, hypercholesterolemia, hypertension, and sudden cardiac death. Of the following medications, which would be the next best one in the management of this patient?

(A) Aripiprazole
(B) Olanzapine
(C) Quetiapine
(D) Risperidone
(E) Ziprasidone

398

A 34-year-old man who is comatose, has myoclonic twitching, and has a serum lithium level of 4.2 mEq/L should respond best to which of the following treatments?

(A) Activated charcoal
(B) Hemodialysis
(C) Intravenous sodium chloride
(D) Osmotic diuresis
(E) Plasmapheresis

399

Which of the following is the most common extrapyramidal side effect of antipsychotic medication?

(A) Akathisia
(B) Torticollis
(C) Oculogyric crisis
(D) Neuroleptic malignant syndrome
(E) Tardive myoclonus

400

The best legal protection for a psychiatrist who is accused of malpractice after a patient's suicide is:

(A) the documentation of the patient's risk factors for suicide recorded in the chart.
(B) the patient's documented history of an axis II disorder.
(C) a doctor-patient suicide prevention ("no-harm") contract.
(D) the patient's family having promised to supervise the patient closely.

Section 2: Answers and Explanations

1

A clinician is considering combination therapy for treatment-resistant depression. Which of the following combinations has the most potential for serious adverse reactions?

(A) Bupropion and fluoxetine
(B) Buspirone and nortriptyline
(C) Paroxetine and desipramine
(D) Phenelzine and lithium carbonate
(E) Venlafaxine and tranylcypromine

The correct response is option **E**: Venlafaxine and tranylcypromine

Serious adverse reactions, sometimes fatal, with features resembling serotonin syndrome and neuroleptic malignant syndrome have been reported when venlafaxine has been used with a monoamine oxidase inhibitor. While some adverse interactions could occur with the other combinations listed, none constitute contraindications.

Hodgman MJ, Martin TG, Krenzelok EP: Serotonin syndrome due to venlafaxine and maintenance tranylcypromine therapy. Hum Exp Toxicol 1997; 16:14–17
Diamond S, Pepper BJ, Diamond ML, Freitag FG, Urban GJ, Erdemoglu AK: Serotonin syndrome induced by transitioning from phenelzine to venlafaxine: four patient reports. Neurology 1998; 51:274–276

2

Which of the following conditions is most commonly comorbid with prepubertal bipolar disorder?

(A) Attention deficit hyperactivity disorder (ADHD)
(B) Autistic disorder
(C) Separation anxiety disorder
(D) Tourette's disorder

The correct response is option **A**: Attention deficit hyperactivity disorder (ADHD)

Studies of prepubertal bipolar disorder consistently find that attention deficit hyperactivity disorder (ADHD) is a common comorbid condition. For example, Geller et al. (1995) reported that about 90% of prepubertal (and 30% of adolescent) bipolar patients also had ADHD. Other studies had similar findings, namely, ADHD in 90% of children with mania and in 57% of adolescents with mania. These high proportions have not been accepted universally, and further study has been recommended (Reddy and Srinath, 2000). A study in adults found a much earlier onset of bipolar disorder in those with a history of childhood ADHD (12.1 years vs. 20 years) than in those without ADHD.

Sachs GS, Baldassano CF, Truman CJ, Guille C: Comorbidity of attention deficit hyperactivity disorder with early- and late-onset bipolar disorder. Am J Psychiatry 2000; 157:466–468
Geller B, Sun K, Zimerman B, Luby J, Frazier J, Williams M: Complex and rapid-cycling in bipolar children and adolescents: a preliminary study. J Affect Disorder 1995; 34:259–268
Reddy YCJ, Srinath S: Juvenile bipolar disorder. Acta Psychiatr Scand 2000; 102:162–170
Spencer TJ, Biederman J, Wozniak J, Faraone SV, Wilens TE, Mick E: Parsing pediatric bipolar disorder from its associated comorbidity with the disruptive behavior disorders. Biol Psychiatry 2001; 49:1062–1070
Geller B, Luby J: Child and adolescent bipolar disorder: a review of the past 10 years. J Am Acad Child Adolesc Psychiatry 1997; 36:1168–1176

3

A 39-year-old actuary for an insurance company is offered a substantial promotion that will require her to move to another city. Her new office will be on the 23rd floor of a high-rise building. She informs her psychiatrist that she is "terrified" of riding in an elevator and terrified of heights, but desperately wants the new job. Which of the interventions listed below is most likely to be successful for her?

(A) Cognitive therapy
(B) Hypnotherapy
(C) Insight-oriented psychotherapy
(D) Selective serotonin reuptake inhibitors
(E) Systematic desensitization

The correct response is option **E**: Systematic desensitization

This woman is suffering from a specific phobia. Although all of the therapies listed have been found to be at least of some use in the treatment of phobias, the method that has been most studied and found most effective is behavior therapy. The behavior therapy techniques that have been employed with phobias include systematic desensitization (serial exposure to a predetermined list of anxiety-provoking stimuli graded in a hierarchy from the least to the most frightening), imaginal flooding (intensive exposure to the phobic stimulus through imagery), and flooding (in vivo exposure to the actual phobic stimulus).

Stein DJ, Hollander E (eds): American Psychiatric Publishing Textbook of Anxiety Disorders. Washington, DC, American Psychiatric Publishing, 2002, p 350

4

During resettlement, a refugee takes on the values and attitudes of the new culture and does not retain his original cultural values. Which of the following best describes this process?

(A) Integration
(B) Assimilation
(C) Separation
(D) Marginalization

The correct response is option **B**: Assimilation

Assimilation entails making contacts with the new culture without retaining one's original cultural values. During resettlement, there are a number of ways to adapt to the new culture. Integration is retaining one's own cultural identity while maintaining contact with members of the newer culture. Separation is maintaining the original cultural identity and not seeking contact with the newer culture. Marginalization is shedding one's original identity and cultural values but not seeking contact with other cultural groups.

Fullilove MT: Psychiatric implications of displacement: contributions from the psychology of place. Am J Psychiatry 1996; 153:1516–1523

Lustig SL, Kia-Keating M, Knight WG, Geltman P, Ellis H, Kinzie JD, Keane T, Saxe GN: Review of child and adolescent refugee mental health. J Am Acad Child Adolesc Psychiatry 2004; 43:24–36

5

Parasomnias can be differentiated from dyssomnias because parasomnias involve abnormalities in which of the following aspects of sleep?

(A) Amount of sleep
(B) Initiation of sleep
(C) Physiological systems that occur during sleep
(D) Quality of sleep
(E) Timing of sleep

The correct response is option **C**: Physiological systems that occur during sleep

The factors listed in the other options are affected in dyssomnias.

American Psychiatric Association: Diagnostic and Statistical Manual of Mental Disorders, Fourth Edition, Text Revision (DSM-IV-TR). Washington, DC, American Psychiatric Association, 2000, pp 598, 630–631

6

A 27-year-old male patient with an initial episode of schizophrenia is treated with risperidone at an initial dose of 2 mg daily, and after 1 week of treatment he no longer experiences agitation. By the third week of treatment, with gradual titration of risperidone to 6 mg daily, his delusions and hallucinations are significantly improved. At week 4, he describes some trouble sleeping at night because of restlessness but reports that he is much less fearful and no longer hears voices. When seen for a scheduled appointment at week 6, however, he is noticeably drooling and is in constant motion, rocking back and forth and fidgeting in his chair. The side effect of treatment that he is most likely experiencing is:

(A) akathisia.
(B) neuroleptic malignant syndrome.
(C) restless leg syndrome.
(D) serotonin syndrome.
(E) tardive dyskinesia.

The correct response is option **A**: Akathisia

Akathisia consists of a subjective feeling of restlessness along with restless movements, usually in the legs or feet, which may be mistaken for ongoing psychosis with associated agitation. Akathisia is generally seen soon after the initiation of treatment, but it may become more prominent as the dose of antipsychotic medication is increased. In this vignette, the onset of restlessness soon after the start of antipsychotic treatment makes akathisia more likely than restless leg syndrome. Neuroleptic malignant syndrome and serotonin syndrome would be unlikely causes of this presentation, as they are associated with rigidity and motor twitching, respectively.

Hales RE, Yudofsky SC (eds): American Psychiatric Publishing Textbook of Clinical Psychiatry, Fourth Edition. Washington, DC, American Psychiatric Publishing, 2003, p 1087

American Psychiatric Association: Practice Guideline for the Treatment of Patients With Schizophrenia, 2nd ed. Am J Psychiatry 2004; 161(Feb suppl):1–56

7

A patient takes a medication for bipolar I disorder throughout pregnancy and delivery. The newborn is noted to be cyanotic and in respiratory distress. An echocardiogram reveals significant displacement of two leaflets of the tricuspid valve into the ventricle and a large atrial septal defect consistent with Ebstein's anomaly. Of the following medications, which was the woman most likely taking during her pregnancy?

(A) Carbamazepine
(B) Gabapentin
(C) Lithium
(D) Topiramate
(E) Valproate

The correct response is option **C**: Lithium

Lithium is the only psychoactive, non-anticonvulsant drug that is thought to be associated with the specific birth defect Ebstein's anomaly. This defect is 20 times more common in children born to mothers taking lithium than in the general population. Echocardiography and fetal ultrasonography can be used after the 16th week of pregnancy to check for the presence of cardiac abnormalities.

The general risk of major birth defect appears to be two to three times greater with lithium than in the general population. While initial information about the teratogenic risk of lithium treatment was derived from biased retrospective reports, more recent epidemiologic data indicate that the teratogenic risk of first-trimester lithium exposure is lower than previously suggested. The clinical management of women with bipolar disorder who have childbearing potential should be modified with this revised risk estimate. Valproate is more commonly associated with neural tube defects in the fetus, and carbamazepine with craniofacial defects, fingernail hypoplasia, neural tube defects, and developmental delays. Gabapentin and topiramate have not been systematically studied in pregnant women.

Schatzberg AF, Cole JO, DeBattista C: Manual of Clinical Psychopharmacology. Washington, DC, American Psychiatric Publishing, 2005, pp 260–261, 272, 281, 292
Cohen LS, Friedman JM, Jefferson JW, Johnson EM, Weiner ML: A reevaluation of risk of in utero exposure to lithium. JAMA 1994; 271:146

8

A forensic psychiatric evaluation differs from a general psychiatric evaluation in that a forensic evaluation:

(A) typically includes a mental status examination.
(B) does not have a doctor-patient relationship.
(C) requires a completed written report.
(D) requires the presence of a lawyer during the evaluation.

The correct response is option **B**: Does not have a doctor-patient relationship

A forensic evaluation essentially includes a general psychiatric evaluation within its context. Forensic evaluations are done for third parties and not for a "patient," and hence there is no doctor-patient relationship (therapeutic alliance). There is no requirement in forensic evaluations for the presence of an attorney or for a report. Forensic evaluations are not confidential in the same sense as a general evaluation in that the information is typically transmitted to the third party.

Simon RI: The law and psychiatry, in The American Psychiatric Publishing Textbook of Clinical Psychiatry, 4th ed. Edited by Hales RE, Yudofsky SC. Washington, DC, American Psychiatric Press, 2004, p 1618
Gutheil TG: Types of witnesses, in The Psychiatrist in Court: A Survival Guide. Washington, DC, American Psychiatric Press, 1998. Reprinted in FOCUS 2003; 1:385–388 (p 386)

9

A 30-year-old man reports that he is unable to sleep and hears noises and voices at night even though he lives alone. The symptoms started abruptly on the day preceding the visit. During the interview, he repeatedly brushes off his arms, muttering about bugs. The information that would be most helpful in determining initial interventions would be the history of:

(A) family disorders.
(B) medical problems.
(C) psychiatric hospitalization.
(D) recent stresses.

The correct response is option **B**: Medical problems

Psychotic symptoms may be due to a general medical condition, may be medication induced, or may be induced by substances of abuse. Medical reasons for psychotic symptoms should be ruled out, especially in the context of tactile and auditory hallucinations.

Sadock BJ, Sadock VA (eds): Kaplan and Sadock's Comprehensive Textbook of Psychiatry, 8th ed. Philadelphia, Lippincott Williams & Wilkins, 2005, p 989

10

The practice of obtaining informed consent from an individual prior to initiating any treatment fulfills which of the following ethical principles?

(A) Nonmaleficence
(B) Autonomy
(C) Justice
(D) Competence

The correct response is option **B**: Autonomy

Autonomy refers to the notion in medical ethics of individual self-rule or self-governance to make decisions. Nonmaleficence embodies the ethical principle of avoiding harm. Justice refers to fairness in the distribution or application of psychiatric treatment. Competence is generally considered a legal determination of a person's ability to make certain decisions, including but not limited to treatment-related decisions (e.g., competence to execute a will is termed "testamentary capacity"). Competence or decision-making capacity is a necessary requirement for informed consent but is not sufficient for informed consent, which has additional requirements (i.e., disclosure of relevant information and voluntariness).

Simon RI: A Concise Guide to Psychiatry and Law for Clinicians, 3rd ed. Washington, DC, American Psychiatric Publishing, 2001, pp 63–65
Beauchamp TL, Childress JF: Principles of Biomedical Ethics, 5th ed. New York, Oxford University Press, 2001, pp 77, 114, 189, 226
Kaplan HI, Sadock BJ: Synopsis of Psychiatry: Behavioral Sciences/Clinical Psychiatry, 9th ed. Baltimore, Lippincott Williams & Wilkins, 2003, pp 1365–1368

11

Which of the following psychotherapies has the best documented effectiveness in the treatment of major depressive disorder?

(A) Supportive
(B) Psychodynamic
(C) Interpersonal
(D) Psychoeducational
(E) Family

The correct response is option **C**: Interpersonal

Interpersonal and cognitive behavior therapy are the best documented psychotherapeutic treatments for major depressive disorder. Psychodynamic psychotherapy is usually used with patients who also have to work on some other life goals. Supportive and psychoeducational techniques can also be useful, depending on the severity of the depression.

Practice Guideline for the Treatment of Patients With Major Depressive Disorder, 2nd ed (2000), in American Psychiatric Association Practice Guidelines for the Treatment of Psychiatric Disorders, Compendium 2004. Washington, DC, APA, 2004, pp 464, 498–505

12

Which of the following antidepressants would be the best choice for a patient concerned about erectile dysfunction?

(A) Bupropion
(B) Fluoxetine
(C) Nortriptyline
(D) Imipramine
(E) Venlafaxine

The correct response is option **A**: Bupropion

Most antidepressants other than bupropion have significant rates of erectile dysfunction as well as other aspects of sexual dysfunction. Mirtazapine has lower rates of sexual dysfunction than the SSRIs.

Labbate LA, Croft HA, Oleshansky MA: Antidepressant-related erectile dysfunction: management via avoidance, switching antidepressants, antidotes, and adaptation. J Clin Psychiatry 2003; 64(suppl 10):11–19
Hales RE, Yudofsky SC (eds): The American Psychiatric Publishing Textbook of Clinical Psychiatry, 4th ed. Washington, DC, American Psychiatric Publishing, 2003, p 1058

13

The National Comorbidity Survey identified a number of gender differences in exposure and in the development of posttraumatic stress disorder (PTSD). Compared with females, males have:

(A) higher trauma exposure, and higher prevalence of PTSD.
(B) lower trauma exposure, and lower prevalence of PTSD.
(C) higher trauma exposure, and lower prevalence of PTSD.
(D) lower trauma exposure, and higher prevalence of PTSD.
(E) the same trauma exposure, and the same prevalence of PTSD.

The correct response is option **C**: Higher trauma exposure, and lower prevalence of PTSD

The National Comorbidity Survey found that males are more likely than females to be exposed to traumatic events (60% vs. 50%), while females are more likely than males to develop PTSD (12% vs. 6%). This finding may represent a gender difference in susceptibility to PTSD linked to biological, psychological, or social factors, or it may be a direct function of the differential in types of traumatic events to which men and women are exposed.

Yehuda R (ed): Treating Trauma Survivors With PTSD. Washington, DC: American Psychiatric Publishing, 2002, p 26

American Psychiatric Association: Practice Guideline for the Treatment of Patients With Acute Stress Disorder and Posttraumatic Stress Disorder. Am J Psychiatry 2004; 161(Nov suppl):20

Kessler RC, Sonnega A, Bromet E, Hughes M, Nelson CB: Posttraumatic stress disorder in the National Comorbidity Survey. Arch Gen Psychiatry 1995; 52:1048–1060

14

A cancer patient with significant nausea requires an antidepressant. Which of the following medications would be the best choice?

(A) Bupropion
(B) Duloxetine
(C) Mirtazapine
(D) Paroxetine
(E) Venlafaxine

The correct response is option **C**: Mirtazapine

With the exception of mirtazapine, all of the drugs listed have been shown in clinical trials to cause considerably more nausea than placebo. The reason that nausea is not a prominent side effect of mirtazapine is thought to be its 5-HT$_3$ receptor antagonism, an effect shared with antinausea drugs such as ondansetron and granisetron.

Nutt D: Mirtazapine: pharmacology in relation to adverse events. Acta Psychiatr Scand 1997; 96(suppl 391):31–37

McManis PG, Talley NJ: Nausea and vomiting associated with selective serotonin reuptake inhibitors: incidence, mechanisms, and management. CNS Drugs 1997; 8:394–401

Montgomery SA: Safety of mirtazapine: a review. Int Clin Psychopharmacol 1995; 10(suppl 4):37–45

15

When non-substance abusing men and women drink the same amount of alcohol, the women are likely to have higher alcohol blood levels than the men. The best explanation for this is that compared with men, women:

(A) have a larger volume of distribution.
(B) have lower excretion rates.
(C) only metabolize by first-order kinetics.
(D) metabolize less alcohol in the gut.
(E) are deficient in acetaldehyde dehydrogenase.

The correct response is option **D**: Metabolize less alcohol in the gut

Alcohol metabolism, regardless of gender, is based on zero-order kinetics. However, a number of factors contribute to higher blood alcohol concentrations in women than in men after consumption of the same amount of alcohol per unit of body weight. This includes a woman's lower body water content relative to men (alcohol is distributed in the total body water, and women have less water in their body to dilute the alcohol); an increased ratio of fat-to-water content as women age; lower quantities of alcohol dehydrogenase in the gastric mucosa of women compared with men; a tendency for women's bodies to absorb more of the alcohol they drink than do men's bodies; and variation in blood alcohol concentration related to menstrual cycle.

Romans SE, Seeman MV: Women's Mental Health: A Life-Cycle Approach. Philadelphia, Lippincott Williams & Wilkins, 2006, pp 182–183

Cyr MG, McGarry KA: Alcohol use disorders in women: screening methods and approaches to treatment. Postgrad Med 2002; 112(6):31–32, 39–40, 43–47

16

Which of the following situations best describes when weight considerations should determine hospitalization for anorexia nervosa in children and young adolescents?

(A) Weight is less than 20% of recommended healthy body weight.
(B) Weight is less than 25% of ideal body weight.
(C) Weight is being rapidly lost and outpatient efforts are ineffective, regardless of actual weight.
(D) The family asks for hospitalization.
(E) Weight is fluctuating unpredictably over 2–3 months.

The correct response is option **C**: Weight is being rapidly lost and outpatient efforts are ineffective, regardless of actual weight

For patients whose initial weight falls 25% below expected weight, hospitalization is often necessary to ensure adequate intake and to limit physical activity. In younger children and adolescents hospitalization should be considered even earlier whenever the patient is losing weight rapidly and before too much weight is lost, since early intervention may avert rapid physiological decline and loss of cortical white and gray matter. Generally, specialized eating disorder units yield better outcomes than general psychiatric units because of nursing expertise and effectively conducted protocols.

Yager J, Devlin MJ, Halmi KA, Herzog DB, Mitchell JE, Powers PS, Zerbe KJ: Eating disorders. Focus 2005; 3:502–510

Practice Guideline for the Treatment of Patients With Eating Disorders, 2nd ed (2000), in American Psychiatric Association Practice Guidelines for the Treatment of Psychiatric Disorders, Compendium 2004. Washington, DC, APA, 2004

17

Which of the following antipsychotic drugs is most likely to be associated with hyperprolactinemia?

(A) Aripiprazole
(B) Clozapine
(C) Olanzapine
(D) Quetiapine
(E) Risperidone

The correct response is option **E**: Risperidone

Risperidone causes prolactin elevations that are similar to those caused by high-potency dopamine antagonist antipsychotic medications. The other atypical antipsychotics cause minimal or no increase in prolactin levels.

Maguire GA: Prolactin elevation with antipsychotic medications: mechanisms of action and clinical consequences. J Clin Psychiatry 2002; 63(suppl 4):56–62
Compton MT, Miller AH: Antipsychotic-induced hyperprolactinemia and sexual dysfunction. Psychopharmacol Bull 2002; 36:143–164
American Psychiatric Association: Practice Guideline for the Treatment of Patients With Schizophrenia, 2nd ed. Am J Psychiatry 2004; 161(Feb suppl):1–56

18

Which of the following atypical antipsychotic drugs is a D_2 receptor partial agonist?

(A) Aripiprazole
(B) Olanzapine
(C) Quetiapine
(D) Risperidone
(E) Ziprasidone

The correct response is option **A**: Aripiprazole

Aripiprazole is a partial agonist. A partial agonist is an agonist that cannot maximally activate a receptor regardless of the concentration of drug present. While this feature of aripiprazole suggests a mechanism of action that differs from other atypical antipsychotics, there is no evidence to date that aripiprazole is any more or less effective than the other drugs.

Shapiro DA, Renock S, Arrington E, Chiodo LA, Liu LX, Sibley DR, Roth BL, Mailman R: Aripiprazole, a novel atypical antipsychotic drug with a unique and robust pharmacology. Neuropsychopharmacology 2003; 28:1400–1411

19

A 33-year-old man started twice-weekly psychodynamic psychotherapy 6 months ago with the goal of exploring issues stemming from his distant relationship with his father and his inability to form adequate mentoring relationships in his work as a research chemist. He reports an increasing preoccupation with his therapist's unwillingness to see him more frequently. The patient has been speaking in therapy of his wish that the therapist see him on Sunday. He believes that the therapist refuses to have extra sessions because he prefers other patients. Which of the following best explains the patient's behavior?

(A) Transference neurosis
(B) Delusional system
(C) Obsessional diathesis
(D) Erotomania
(E) Psychotic distortion

The correct response is option **A**: Transference neurosis

Over 6 months of intensive therapy, the patient has developed a pervasive transference that reenacts aspects of his childhood relationship with his father. This is an example of a classic transference neurosis at the core of traditional long-term psychodynamic psychotherapies.

Olds DD: Psychotherapy, in Psychiatry. Edited by Cutler JL, Marcus ER. Philadelphia, WB Saunders, 1999, pp 281–307

20

Which of the following disorders has the highest relative risk for first-degree relatives?

(A) Alcoholism
(B) Anorexia
(C) Bipolar disorder
(D) Panic disorder
(E) Somatization disorder

The correct response is option **C**: Bipolar disorder

The relative risk for bipolar disorder is around 25. For schizophrenia, it is 18; panic disorder, 10; anorexia, 5; alcoholism, around 7; and somatization, around 3. A relative risk for psychiatric disorders is defined as the probability that a first-degree relative of a patient with an illness will also develop that illness.

Knowles JA: Genetics, in The American Psychiatric Publishing Textbook of Clinical Psychiatry, 4th ed. Edited by Hales RE, Yudofsky SC. Washington, DC, American Psychiatric Publishing, 2003, pp 5–7

21

A 68-year-old man has a grand mal seizure that is attributed to an abrupt hyponatremia, with a serum sodium concentration of 110 mmol/L. Which of the following medications is the most likely cause?

(A) Gabapentin
(B) Lithium
(C) Oxcarbazepine
(D) Topiramate
(E) Valproate

The correct response is option **C**: Oxcarbazepine

According to the oxcarbazepine package insert, clinically significant hyponatremia (serum sodium <125 mmol/L) developed in 2.5% of patients in controlled studies of epilepsy. Several possible mechanisms have been proposed, but none are well substantiated. Risk factors include older age, high doses or blood levels, low pretreatment sodium levels, other drugs that cause hyponatremia, and possibly cigarette smoking.

Valproate can cause elevated liver function test results and increased ammonia levels. There have been some reports of hyponatremia with valproate, but this occurs rarely. Topiramate can cause a hyperchloremic, non-ion-gap metabolic acidosis (elevated chloride level and reduced bicarbonate level). Lithium may lead to diabetes insipidus, which in turn can cause hypernatremia. Gabapentin is not associated with any alterations in serum electrolytes.

Steinhoff BJ, Stoll KD, Stodieck SR, Paulus W: Hyponatremic coma under oxcarbazepine therapy. Epilepsy Res 1992; 11:67–70

Van Amelsvoort T, Bakshi R, Devaux CB, Schwabe S: Hyponatremia associated with carbamazepine and oxcarbazepine therapy: a review. Epilepsia 1994; 35:181–188

Sachdeo RC, Wasserstein A, Mesenbrink PJ, D'Souza J: Effects of oxcarbazepine on sodium concentration and water handling. Ann Neurol 2002; 51:613–620

Trileptal (oxcarbazepine) prescribing information (package insert), 2005

22

Social rhythm therapy, which is designed specifically for bipolar disorder, is based on which of the following models?

(A) Psychoeducation
(B) Object relations and self psychology theory
(C) Circadian regulation and interpersonal psychotherapy
(D) Cognitive therapy techniques to address social dysfunction
(E) Supportive psychotherapy

The correct response is option **C**: Circadian regulation and interpersonal psychotherapy

Social rhythm therapy grew from a chronobiological model of bipolar disorder. It modulates both biological and psychosocial factors to mitigate a patient's circadian and sleep-wake cycle vulnerabilities. Object relations theory is psychodynamic theory based on Melanie Klein's metapsychology. Psychoeducation entails offering the patient education about the patient's disorder. Cognitive therapy is a treatment designed to help people learn to identify and monitor negative ways of thinking and then alter this tendency and think in a more positive manner.

Frank E, Swartz HA, Kupfer DJ: Interpersonal and social rhythm therapy: managing the chaos of bipolar disorder. Biol Psychiatry 2000; 48:593–604

Rapaport M, Hales D: Relapse prevention and bipolar disorder: a focus on bipolar depression. FOCUS 2003; 1:15–31 (p 21)

23

Rapid cycling in bipolar I or II disorder is associated with:

(A) menopause.
(B) antidepressant use.
(C) cocaine abuse.
(D) early onset.
(E) alcohol abuse.

The correct response is option **B**: Antidepressant use

Rapid cycling is associated with antidepressant use. Rapid cycling in bipolar disorder is defined as four or more mood episodes in the previous 12 months. Rapid cycling is not related to any phase of the menstrual cycle. It occurs in both pre- and postmenopausal women. On the other hand, women constitute 70% to 90% of the patients affected by rapid cycling. The syndrome can appear or disappear at any time during the course of bipolar I or II disorder. By definition, substance abuse excludes the diagnosis of rapid cycling.

American Psychiatric Association: Diagnostic and Statistical Manual of Mental Disorders, 4th Edition, Text Revision (DSM-IV-TR). Washington, DC, American Psychiatric Association, 2000, pp 427–428

American Psychiatric Association: Practice Guideline for the Treatment of Patients With Bipolar Disorder (Revision). Am J Psychiatry 2002; 159(April suppl). Reprinted in FOCUS 2003; 1:64–110 (p 94)

24

A 65-year-old woman has a history of a left frontal lobe stroke. Which of the following psychiatric symptoms is most commonly associated with a stroke in this area of the brain?

  (A) Panic
  (B) Mania
  (C) Depression
  (D) Obsessions
  (E) Anxiety

The correct response is option **C**: Depression

Poststroke depression has been documented after cerebrovascular accidents occurring in many areas in the brain. However, anterior left hemisphere lesions, particularly large lesions and in the early recovery period, appear to carry a higher risk of poststroke depression. Other factors, such as history of depression and degree of disability after stroke, are also associated with poststroke depression.

Sadock BJ, Sadock VA (eds): Kaplan and Sadock's Comprehensive Textbook of Psychiatry, 8th ed. Philadelphia, Lippincott Williams & Wilkins, 2005, pp 349–357

Whyte EM, Mulsant BH: Post stroke depression: epidemiology, pathophysiology, and biological treatment. Biol Psychiatry 2002; 52:253–264

25

Genetic studies of obsessive-compulsive disorder have revealed linkages to which of the following disorders?

  (A) Alcohol dependence
  (B) Schizophrenia
  (C) Shared psychotic disorder
  (D) Somatoform disorder
  (E) Tourette's syndrome

The correct response is option **E**: Tourette's syndrome

Genetic studies of patients with obsessive-compulsive disorder have revealed high family rates of depression and anxiety disorders and Tourette's syndrome.

Hales RE, Yudofsky SC (eds): The American Psychiatric Publishing Textbook of Clinical Psychiatry, 4th ed. Washington, DC, American Psychiatric Publishing, 2003, p 32

26

A psychiatrist proposes to use an FDA-approved drug not previously used for the treatment of mania because it has biochemical properties similar to known antimanic agents. The psychiatrist has also read several articles describing open-label studies suggesting efficacy of the drug. The patient in question has not responded to any agent thus far. The psychiatrist must do which of the following?

  (A) Get an institutional review board approval, since what is proposed is clinical research.
  (B) Notify the FDA, since the drug is being used for a non-FDA-approved purpose.
  (C) Obtain informed consent from the patient or from an appropriate proxy agent.
  (D) Wait until there is higher-quality data to support this use of the drug.

The correct response is option **C**: Obtain informed consent from the patient or from an appropriate proxy agent

While obtaining explicit informed consent for any treatment is important, it is especially important when the treatment has not become standard. When all available treatments have failed, a nonstandard approach based on limited evidence may be all that is available, provided that proper precautions are taken. Unless the psychiatrist's intent is to demonstrate generalizable knowledge, a nonstandard treatment is usually not considered research. Physicians routinely and permissibly use drugs for non-FDA-approved indications using their best clinical judgment. While it is probably wise to wait until higher quality data support the use of a nonstandard treatment, it is not a "must."

Simon RI: A Concise Guide to Psychiatry and Law for Clinicians, 3rd ed. Washington, DC, American Psychiatric Publishing, 2001, pp 91–98

27

A 75-year-old retired physicist who is suffering from metastatic cancer is referred to a psychiatrist by the primary care physician because the patient wants to die and has requested assistance in suicide. On evaluation, the psychiatrist finds that the patient's cognition is intact. The most appropriate next step for the psychiatrist is to:

(A) be as persuasive as possible so that the patient accepts the cancer treatment.
(B) find out whether there are areas of suffering that can be addressed by available palliative care measures.
(C) tell the referring physician that the patient can be given assistance in suicide because the patient is a competent adult.
(D) tell the referring physician that even though the patient's cognition appears intact, the patient is probably incapacitated by virtue of the unreasonable choice that is being made.

The correct response is option **B**: Find out whether there are areas of suffering that can be addressed by available palliative care measures

While sometimes direct persuasion to accept a medically indicated treatment may be acceptable, the main issue is to identify the sources of the patient's suffering. Most patients who request assisted suicide eventually change their minds when the sources of their suffering are better addressed. To recommend assistance in suicide at this stage of the patient's cancer ignores the complexity of the situation. To use incapacity as a reason for paternalism (option D) is also unacceptable.

Block SD, Billings JA: Evaluating patient requests for euthanasia and assisted suicide in terminal illness: the role of the psychiatrist, in End of Life Decisions: A Psychosocial Perspective. Edited by Steinberg MD, Youngner SJ. Washington, DC, American Psychiatric Press, 1998, pp 205–233
Bascom P, Tolle SW: Responding to requests for physician-assisted suicide. JAMA 2002; 288:91–98

28

Of the following ethnic groups, which is at lowest risk of completed suicide?

(A) African Americans
(B) Asian Americans
(C) Caucasian Americans
(D) Hispanic Americans
(E) Native Americans

The correct response is option **B**: Asian Americans

With regard to ethnicity, most studies have demonstrated that Caucasians are at highest risk of suicide, followed in order by Native Americans, African Americans, Hispanic Americans, and Asian Americans.

Garlow SJ, Purselle D, Heninger M: Ethnic differences in patterns of suicide across the life cycle. Am J Psychiatry 2005; 162:319–323
Hales RE, Yudofsky SC (eds): The American Psychiatric Publishing Textbook of Clinical Psychiatry, 4th ed. Washington, DC, American Psychiatric Publishing, 2003, p 1458

29

A 15-year-old boy is referred for psychiatric evaluation after taking an overdose of an over-the-counter cold medication. The patient denies that this was a suicide attempt. The patient acknowledges that he has been having difficulties for about a year, since the separation of his parents. He often feels angry and irritable, has difficulty sleeping, has little appetite, has lost weight, has little interest in his usual activities, and often wishes he was dead. His grades have dropped to the point that he is failing his courses. Over the past year, he has been smoking 1–2 packs of cigarettes a day, drinking to the point of intoxication on the weekends, and taking over-the-counter cold medication to enhance the effects of the alcohol. His past psychiatric history is significant for attention deficit hyperactivity disorder (ADHD), for which he has a prescription for a stimulant medication. He has not taken his medication as prescribed. Instead, he hoards the medication and then takes large quantities to experience a euphoric effect. Which of the following medications would be the most efficacious in addressing this patient's symptom constellation?

(A) Bupropion
(B) Citalopram
(C) Desipramine
(D) Trazodone
(E) Venlafaxine

The correct response is option **A**: Bupropion

Bupropion is effective in the treatment of many types of depression. It is metabolized to a number of amphetamine-like products, which are effective in the treatment of ADHD. Bupropion has also been demonstrated to decrease nicotine use. In adolescents who have depression, nicotine dependence, substance abuse, and ADHD, bupropion might be the first-line treatment, as it has been shown to be effective in assisting with both smoking cessation and improving the core symptoms of ADHD. Citalopram and other SSRIs as well as trazodone have not demonstrated these added benefits. Venlafaxine and desipramine have been found to be effective in both childhood and adult ADHD, but they lack the potential of bupropion to assist with smoking cessation.

Schatzberg AF, Cole JO, DeBattista C: Manual of Clinical Psychopharmacology. Washington, DC, American Psychiatric Publishing, 2005, pp 85–89

30

A psychiatrist attends a dinner lecture sponsored by a major pharmaceutical company, the maker of a newly approved drug for major depression. The company's representative approaches the psychiatrist after the lecture and says, "I hope we can count on you to prescribe our medication. This is a great medication!" The psychiatrist does not know what to say and later feels troubled by this encounter. Which of the following statements reflects the psychiatrist's ethical obligation in this situation?

(A) The psychiatrist can accept dinners and "repay" the company with favorable prescribing practices if the psychiatrist chooses to do so.
(B) The psychiatrist should report the pharmaceutical representative's behavior to the local APA branch's ethics committee.
(C) The psychiatrist should be aware that "strings attached" industry-sponsored activities are unethical.
(D) The psychiatrist must repay the representative for the cost of the dinner, since there are apparent, though unstated, ethical conflicts.

The correct response is option **C**: The psychiatrist should be aware that "strings attached" industry-sponsored activities are unethical

The American Medical Association Code of Medical Ethics states that "Gifts should not be accepted if strings are attached." In this question, the psychiatrist's attendance at a dinner whose purpose was educational may be problematic if there are implicit or explicit strings attached. Most psychiatrists would not consider the psychiatrist's behavior in this situation unethical, although it would be unethical to promise to prescribe a certain medication in return for drug company favors, such as free dinners or concert tickets. Clearly, the blurring of the boundaries between educational activities and pharmaceutical company promotions continues to be a difficult issue facing the psychiatric community, and ethical psychiatrists may disagree about whether participation in any educational activities provided by pharmaceutical companies is ethical.

American Psychiatric Association: Ethics Primer of the American Psychiatric Association. Washington, DC, American Psychiatric Association, 2001, pp 48–49
Chren MM, Landefeld CS, Murray TH: Doctors, drug companies, and gifts. JAMA 1989; 262:3448–3451
American Medical Association Council on Ethical and Judicial Affairs: Code of Medical Ethics, Current Opinions With Annotations, 2000–2001. Chicago, American Medical Association, 2000

31

More severe and prolonged forms of conduct disorder are most often associated with which of the following comorbid disorders?

(A) Anxiety disorders
(B) Attention deficit hyperactivity disorder
(C) Depression
(D) Eating disorder
(E) Tic disorder

The correct response is option **B**: Attention deficit hyperactivity disorder

More severe and prolonged conduct disorder is associated with early onset, comorbid ADHD, and conduct symptoms that are more frequent, numerous, and varied.

Dulcan MK, Martini DR, Lake MB: Concise Guide to Child and Adolescent Psychiatry, 3rd ed. Washington, DC, American Psychiatric Publishing, 2003, p 49

32

A 62-year-old man is taking desipramine for depression. He presents with marked sedation, tachycardia, and postural hypotension about 10 days after the addition of a second antidepressant. Which of the following medications is most likely responsible?

(A) Venlafaxine
(B) Mirtazapine
(C) Citalopram
(D) Sertraline
(E) Fluoxetine

The correct response is option **E**: Fluoxetine

Desipramine is a substrate for cytochrome P450 2D6. Of the drugs listed, only fluoxetine is a potent inhibitor of this enzyme. In this patient, taking fluoxetine resulted in a marked increase in his blood levels of desipramine, which accounted for his new physical symptoms.

Greenblatt DJ, von Moltke LL, Harmatz JS, Shader RI: Drug interactions with newer antidepressants: role of human cytochromes P450. J Clin Psychiatry 1998; 59(suppl 15):19–27
Preskorn SH, Alderman J, Chung M, Harrison W, Messig M, Harris S: Pharmacokinetics of desipramine coadministered with sertraline or fluoxetine. J Clin Psychopharmacol 1994; 14:90–98
Schatzberg AF, Nemeroff CB (eds): The American Psychiatric Publishing Textbook of Psychopharmacology, 3rd ed, Washington, DC, American Psychiatric Publishing, 2004, pp 223–224

33

Which of the following diseases associated with dementia characteristically has early changes in personality and a late decline in memory?

   (A) HIV infection
   (B) Creutzfeldt-Jakob disease
   (C) Parkinson's disease
   (D) Lewy body dementia
   (E) Pick's disease

The correct response is option **E**: Pick's disease

Pick's disease specifically affects the frontal and temporal lobes, accounting for the early signs of personality changes, loss of social skills, and emotional blunting. Other features of dementia, such as memory loss and apraxia, come later. Specific diagnosis of Pick's disease is usually made only on autopsy. The medical illnesses Huntington's disease, Parkinson's disease, and HIV infection precede those dementias. Creutzfeldt-Jakob disease often has a clinical triad associated with dementia, involuntary movement, and periodic EEG activity. Lewy body dementia often presents first with hallucinations and psychosis.

American Psychiatric Association: Diagnostic and Statistical Manual of Mental Disorders, Fourth Edition, Text Revision (DSM-IV-TR). Washington, DC, American Psychiatric Association, 2000, pp 148–151

Practice Guideline for the Treatment of Patients With Alzheimer's Disease and Other Dementias of Late Life (1997), in American Psychiatric Association Practice Guidelines for the Treatment of Psychiatric Disorders, Compendium 2004. Washington, DC, APA, 2004, pp 82–83

34

Which of the following features best distinguishes anorexia nervosa from bulimia nervosa?

   (A) Amenorrhea
   (B) Decreased body weight
   (C) Calluses on the dorsum of the hand
   (D) Dental enamel erosion
   (E) Enlarged parotid glands

The correct response is option **B**: Decreased body weight

Decreased body weight is a defining feature of anorexia nervosa, whereas persons with bulimia nervosa typically have normal body weight. All of the other features listed may be present in both disorders.

American Psychiatric Association: Diagnostic and Statistical Manual of Mental Disorders, Fourth Edition, Text Revision (DSM-IV-TR). Washington, DC, American Psychiatric Association, 2000, pp 583–595

35

Which of the following aspects of cognitive performance is most likely to decline in the course of normal aging?

   (A) Short-term memory
   (B) Speed of performance
   (C) Store of knowledge
   (D) Syntax
   (E) Vocabulary

The correct response is option **B**: Speed of performance

Speed of learning, processing speed, and speed of performance of cognitive tasks tend to decline with normal aging. The other functions listed do not decline with normal aging, and a decline in any of them may be an indication for a thorough or formal assessment for cognitive impairment.

Spar JE, La Rue A: Concise Guide to Geriatric Psychiatry, 3rd ed. Washington, DC, American Psychiatric Publishing, 2002, pp 25–26

36

Disorders with significant psychiatric symptoms that can be linked to a single gene include:

   (A) attention deficit hyperactivity disorder.
   (B) bipolar disorder.
   (C) fragile X syndrome.
   (D) major depression.
   (E) schizophrenia.

The correct response is option **C**: Fragile X syndrome

All of these disorders have evidence of genetic transmission, although only fragile X syndrome is due to a single gene.

Sadock BJ, Sadock VA (eds): Kaplan and Sadock's Comprehensive Textbook of Psychiatry, 8th ed. Philadelphia, Lippincott Williams & Wilkins, 2005, pp 237–240

37

The rule of confidentiality is waived in a psychiatrist-patient interaction when the treatment or evaluation includes:

(A) a minor.
(B) a forensic consultation.
(C) an impaired physician.
(D) a patient who reveals a past felony.

The correct response is option **B**: A forensic consultation

Ethically, confidentiality is required in psychiatric treatment. However, there are some instances in which confidentiality is waived. When a psychiatrist is examining a patient for forensic purposes, the individual must be informed that information collected during the examination will be shared with the party that engaged the psychiatrist, such as the patient's lawyer or the court. In addition, common situations that require a waiver of the confidentiality rule include the reporting of child abuse and, in some states, elder abuse and spouse abuse.

Also, in most states, the psychiatrist evaluating a potentially violent patient is required to warn a potential victim of violence. However, in most states, a psychiatrist treating an impaired physician, unlike the physician's colleagues, is not required to report the physician if the physician is a private patient of the psychiatrist. On the other hand, if the psychiatrist is treating the patient under the auspices of a state diversion program, the relationship becomes more complicated and depends on the arrangement with the specific state's diversion program.

A patient who reveals past dangerousness but is not currently dangerous would not likely meet requirements for a breach of confidentiality. Finally, a minor's confidentiality would also be respected unless there was an emergent situation in which either the minor or another person was likely to be harmed. In summary, the rule of confidentiality is waived when there is a threat of harm to the patient or another person.

Rosner R: Principles and Practice of Forensic Psychiatry, 2nd ed. New York: Oxford University Press, 2003, pp 8–9, 177

38

The highest percentage of persons with mental retardation have an intelligence quotient of:

(A) <20.
(B) 20 to 35.
(C) 35 to 50.
(D) 50 to 70.
(E) 70 to 90.

The correct response is option **D**: 50 to 70

Up to 85% of persons with mental retardation have an IQ between 50 and 70, which is mild mental retardation. Patients with an IQ between 70 and 90 are not considered mentally retarded.

Dulcan MK, Martini DR, Lake MB: Concise Guide to Child and Adolescent Psychiatry, 3rd ed. Washington, DC, American Psychiatric Publishing, 2003, p 180

39

A 4-year-old girl who has been cared for in seven different foster homes since the age of 6 months, now exhibits excessive familiarity with strangers. Her current foster parents, with whom she has lived for the past 5 months, state that she does not seem to be particularly close to them. The girl's biological mother is reported to have used alcohol in a binge pattern during her pregnancy. Which of the following is the most likely diagnosis?

(A) Attention deficit hyperactivity disorder
(B) Fetal alcohol syndrome
(C) Oppositional defiant disorder
(D) Pervasive developmental disorder
(E) Reactive attachment disorder

The correct response is option **E**: Reactive attachment disorder

The girl's indiscriminate sociability is behavior typical of reactive attachment disorder, disinhibited type. DSM-IV-TR also specifies an inhibited type of this disorder. Often children with this disorder have experienced a series of caregivers or prolonged separation from a caregiver in early childhood. Symptoms of "markedly disturbed and developmentally inappropriate social relatedness" must be present before age 5 years.

Sadock BJ, Sadock VA (eds): Kaplan and Sadock's Comprehensive Textbook of Psychiatry, 8th ed. Philadelphia, Lippincott Williams & Wilkins, 2005, pp 3248–3252
American Psychiatric Association: Diagnostic and Statistical Manual of Mental Disorders, Fourth Edition, Text Revision (DSM-IV-TR). Washington, DC, American Psychiatric Association, 2000, pp 127–130

40

An 8-year-old girl insists on keeping a rigid routine when dressing, will wear only certain clothes, insists on recopying her homework if there are any mistakes, and has temper tantrums when the items on her desk are moved. During a discussion of the diagnosis and treatment options, her parents express reluctance to use medication and want to explore other options. The first recommendation would be:

(A) cognitive behavior therapy.
(B) family therapy.
(C) interpersonal psychotherapy.
(D) parent training.
(E) supportive psychotherapy.

The correct response is option **A**: Cognitive behavior therapy

Cognitive behavior therapy has been demonstrated to benefit children with obsessive-compulsive disorder. Uncontrolled trials of cognitive behavior therapy have shown excellent response in up to three-fourths of patients treated. Many experts recommend cognitive behavior therapy as the first-line approach for the majority of children and adolescents with obsessive-compulsive disorder.

Sadock BJ, Sadock VA (eds): Kaplan and Sadock's Comprehensive Textbook of Psychiatry, 8th ed. Philadelphia, Lippincott Williams & Wilkins, 2005, p 3285

41

Which of the following are common hyperarousal symptoms in posttraumatic stress disorder (PTSD)?

(A) Intense psychological distress at exposure to external cues resembling the trauma
(B) Difficulty falling or staying asleep
(C) Intrusive images of the event
(D) Feelings of estrangement from others

The correct response is option **B**: Difficulty falling or staying asleep

Difficulty falling or staying asleep is a symptom of hyperarousal. In the DSM-IV-TR, posttraumatic stress disorder symptoms are clustered into three categories: reexperiencing, avoidance and numbing, and hyperarousal. Options A and C are symptoms of reexperiencing the event. Option D falls into category C of the DSM-IV-TR criteria for PTSD, that is, "Persistent avoidance of stimuli associated with the trauma and numbing of general responsiveness."

American Psychiatric Association: Diagnostic and Statistical Manual of Mental Disorders, 4th Edition, Text Revision (DSM-IV-TR). Washington, DC, American Psychiatric Association, 2000, pp 467–468
Kaplan HI, Sadock BJ: Synopsis of Psychiatry: Behavioral Sciences/Clinical Psychiatry, 9th ed. Baltimore, Lippincott Williams & Wilkins, 2003, p 626
Shalev AY: What is posttraumatic stress disorder? J Clin Psychiatry 2001; 62(suppl 17):4–10

42

Which of the following medications is considered first-line monotherapy for posttraumatic stress disorder?

(A) Clonazepam
(B) Sertraline
(C) Olanzapine
(D) Valproate
(E) Propranolol

The correct response is option **B**: Sertraline

Sertraline is FDA approved for the treatment of PTSD. The other medications are less well established as beneficial. Clonazepam, widely used as an anxiolytic, has FDA approval only for use as an anticonvulsant and treatment for panic disorder, for which it is a second-line choice. Olanzapine has not been reported as a treatment for PTSD. Propranolol has been tried experimentally to diminish the autonomic arousal associated with the trauma. The rationale for its use is that it will curtail the body's emotional/autonomic response to the trauma by diminishing the body's "memory" of the heightened emotional state. The beta-blockers, theoretically, will prevent or at least minimize the PTSD syndrome.

Albucher RC, Liberzon I: Psychopharmacological treatment in PTSD: a critical review. J Psychiatr Res 2002; 36:355–367
Friedman MJ, Donnelly CL, Mellman TA: Pharmacotherapy for PTSD. Psychiatr Ann 2003; 31:57–62
Stein DJ, Hollander E (eds): American Psychiatric Publishing Textbook of Anxiety Disorders. Washington, DC, American Psychiatric Publishing, 2002, p 397

43

A 50-year-old woman has a long history of difficulty with driving because she worries that she might hit a car or a person accidentally. She also worries excessively about her son getting hurt or attacked when he goes out. Her husband can often reassure her. Which of the following diagnoses is most appropriate?

(A) Agoraphobia
(B) Delusional disorder
(C) Generalized anxiety disorder
(D) Obsessive-compulsive disorder
(E) Panic disorder

The correct response is option **C**: Generalized anxiety disorder

The worries that occur in generalized anxiety disorder are about everyday events and are responsive to reassurance. Obsessive-compulsive disorder involves obsessions, which are intrusive unrealistic ideas that may be recognized as being absurd but cannot be resisted. Panic disorder involves anxiety episodes without specific content. Agoraphobia involves being in situations from which escape might be difficult or embarrassing or for which help may not be available in the event of panic.

American Psychiatric Association: Diagnostic and Statistical Manual of Mental Disorders, Fourth Edition, Text Revision (DSM-IV-TR). Washington, DC, American Psychiatric Association, 2000, pp 472–476

44

A 40-year-old woman with chronic headaches has undergone trials with several narcotic and nonnarcotic agents with variable success. Her physician elects to try her on a newer antidepressant medication. Which of the following medications is most likely to be effective?

(A) Bupropion
(B) Mirtazapine
(C) Nefazodone
(D) Sertraline
(E) Venlafaxine

The correct response is option **E**: Venlafaxine

Venlafaxine is seen to be more promising as an analgesic than nefazodone, mirtazapine, or bupropion. Although the precise mechanism of action for analgesia is unknown, it is believed that agents that increase serotonin and norepinephrine are more effective than those that only increase serotonin.

King SA: Pain disorders, in The American Psychiatric Publishing Textbook of Clinical Psychiatry, 4th ed. Edited by Hales RE, Yudofsky SC. Washington, DC, American Psychiatric Publishing, 2003, p 1038

45

Echolalia and echopraxia are most likely manifestations of which of the following disorders?

(A) Hypochondriasis
(B) Bipolar disorder, mixed episode
(C) Depression with catatonic features
(D) Lewy body dementia
(E) Frontotemporal dementia

The correct response is option **C**: Depression with catatonic features

Echolalia and echopraxia can characterize catatonic depression. A mood disorder with catatonic features must have two or more of the following features: "Motoric immobility,…extreme agitation; extreme negativism; peculiarities of voluntary movement; and echolalia or echopraxia" (APA Practice Guideline).

Practice Guideline for the Treatment of Patients With Major Depressive Disorder, 2nd ed (2000), in American Psychiatric Association Practice Guidelines for the Treatment of Psychiatric Disorders, Compendium 2004. Washington, DC, APA, 2004, p 469

46

An adolescent female took an unknown drug at an all-night dance party. She was brought to the emergency department for evaluation of altered mental status and marked hyperthermia. Which of the following was most likely the drug that was ingested?

(A) Ketamine
(B) Methylenedioxymethamphetamine (MDMA)
(C) Flunitrazepam
(D) Gamma-hydroxybutyrate (GHB)
(E) Phencyclidine (PCP)

The correct response is option **B**: Methylenedioxymethamphetamine (MDMA)

All of these drugs are commonly known as "club drugs" and are frequently used at all-night dance parties. MDMA has been reported in some instances to cause severe adverse effects, including altered mental status, convulsions, hypo- or hyperthermia, cardiovascular instability, hepatotoxicity, and death.

GHB is a dopamine enhancer that causes euphoria. Higher doses of GHB can make the user feel sleepy and may cause vomiting, muscle spasms, and loss of consciousness. If mixed with alcohol, GHB can slow breathing to a dangerously low rate, which has caused a number of deaths.

Phencyclidine and ketamine are related substances. They belong to a class of drugs called "dissociative anesthetics," which have the effect of separating perception from sensation. At lower doses ketamine causes a dreamy feeling similar to nitrous oxide and may produce numbness in the extremities. Higher doses of ketamine may produce a hallucinogenic effect.

Flunitrazepam, a short-acting benzodiazepine, also known as Rohypnol (a trade name) or "roofies," has been characterized as the "date rape drug." Flunitrazepam is prescribed in Latin America and Europe as a short-term treatment for insomnia and as a pre-anesthetic medication. Flunitrazepam can cause a chemically induced amnesia and may cause decreased blood pressure, drowsiness, visual disturbances, dizziness, confusion, gastrointestinal disturbances, and urinary retention.

McDowell DM: MDMA, ketamine, GHB, and the "club drug" scene, in The American Psychiatric Publishing Textbook of Substance Abuse Treatment, 3rd ed. Edited by Galanter M, Kleber HD. Washington, DC, American Psychiatric Publishing, 2004, pp 321–331

47

A 23-year-old man who is hospitalized for psychosis displays prominent, excessive, and purposeless motor activity together with peculiar voluntary movements. On one occasion, he stands in the middle of the ward immobile and mute. He demonstrates waxy flexibility. The appropriate medical intervention is:

(A) benztropine.
(B) clonidine.
(C) lorazepam.
(D) propranolol.
(E) ziprasidone.

The correct response is option **C**: Lorazepam

Lorazepam, by a variety of routes of administration, improves catatonia dramatically, although temporarily. Major depression and schizophrenia (catatonic type) are the most frequently observed psychiatric disorders that are associated with catatonia. Possible medical causes include hypercalcemia and hepatic encephalopathy. Catatonia may also appear as an adverse drug effect of a neuroleptic medication or phencyclidine (PCP). Neurological causes of catato-

nia, such as parkinsonism and encephalitis, should also be considered.

Schatzberg AF, Cole JO, DeBattista C: Manual of Clinical Psychopharmacology, 4th ed. Washington, DC, American Psychiatric Publishing, 2003, p 350
Lee JW, Schwartz DL, Hallmayer J: Catatonia in a psychiatric intensive care facility: incidence and response to benzodiazepines. Ann Clin Psychiatry 2000; 12:89–96

48

A 49-year-old woman is referred for treatment of chronic, severe major depression. Which of the following treatment approaches is most likely to be associated with sustained improvement in her symptoms?

(A) Antidepressant medication plus psychotherapy
(B) Psychotherapy alone
(C) Antidepressant medication alone
(D) ECT alone
(E) ECT plus psychotherapy

The correct response is option **A**: Antidepressant medication plus psychotherapy

Since the publication in 2000 of the APA Practice Guideline for the Treatment of Patients With Major Depression, additional studies now support combined psychotherapy and antidepressant therapy for chronic depression. The evidence for this approach in treating mild or moderate depression is less compelling. While ECT is highly effective, ECT alone usually does not produce sustained improvement. There have been few controlled studies of ECT plus psychotherapy.

Pampallona S, Bollini P, Tibaldi G, Kupelnick B, Munizza C: Combined pharmacotherapy and psychological treatment for depression: a systematic review. Arch Gen Psychiatry 2004; 61:714–719
Hegerl U, Plattner A, Moller HJ: Should combined pharmaco- and psychotherapy be offered to depressed patients? A qualitative review of randomized clinical trials from the 1990s. Eur Arch Psychiatry Clin Neurosci 2004; 254:99–107
Thase ME, Greenhouse JB, Frank E, Reynolds CF III, Pilkonis PA, Hurley K, Grochocinski V, Kupfer DJ: Treatment of major depression with psychotherapy or psychotherapy-pharmacotherapy combinations. Arch Gen Psychiatry 1997; 54:1009–1015
De Jonghe F, Kool S, van Aalst G, Dekker J, Peen J: Combining psychotherapy and antidepressants in the treatment of depression. J Affect Disord 2001; 64(2-3):217–229
Arnow BA, Constantino MJ: Effectiveness of psychotherapy and combination treatment for chronic depression. J Clin Psychol 2003; 59:893–905
Casacalenda N, Perry JC, Looper K: Remission in major depressive disorder: a comparison of pharmacotherapy, psychotherapy, and control conditions. Am J Psychiatry 2002; 159:1354–1360
Segal Z, Vincent P, Levitt A: Efficacy of combined, sequential, and crossover psychotherapy and pharmacotherapy in improving outcomes in depression. J Psychiatry Neurosci 2002; 27:281–290
UK ECT Review Group: Efficacy and safety of electroconvulsive therapy in depressive disorders: a systematic review and meta-analysis. Lancet 2003; 361(9360):799–808

49

In people with typical left-brain dominance, the ability to interpret the emotional tone of speech is a function of the:

    (A) left premotor cortex (Broca's area).
    (B) right premotor cortex.
    (C) left parietotemporal cortex (Wernicke's area).
    (D) right parietotemporal cortex.
    (E) anterior cingulate gyrus.

The correct response is option **D**: Right parietotemporal cortex

Just as Wernicke's area in the dominant hemisphere is involved in understanding language, the corresponding area in the nondominant hemisphere interprets the emotional tone of speech, or prosody. Analogous to Broca's area in the left hemisphere, the right premotor cortex is involved in expressive language production, providing the "music" for the semantic content.

Kaufman DM: Clinical Neurology for Psychiatrists. Philadelphia, WB Saunders, 2001, p 175
Panksepp J: Affective Neuroscience: The Foundations of Human and Animal Emotions. New York, Oxford University Press, 1998, p 334

50

Which of the following psychotherapies has the greatest body of evidence demonstrating efficacy for social phobia?

    (A) Insight-oriented psychotherapy
    (B) Interpersonal psychotherapy
    (C) Brief psychodynamic psychotherapy
    (D) Cognitive behavior psychotherapy
    (E) Supportive psychotherapy

The correct response is option **D**: Cognitive behavior psychotherapy

The most effective commonly used treatment for social phobia is based on cognitive behavior therapy principles and techniques. Other theoretical approaches have been used, but little research has been done to establish their usefulness. The major problem in social phobia is negative evaluation. Mere exposure to the social interaction does not produce anxiety reduction. The individual with social phobia must alter dysfunctional beliefs and biased perceptions. Therefore, cognitive input must be included in the intervention for treatment success.

Stein DJ, Hollander E (eds): American Psychiatric Publishing Textbook of Anxiety Disorders. Washington, DC, American Psychiatric Publishing, 2002, pp 323–324, 330–332

51

A patient who is completely deaf arrives with an interpreter at the outpatient clinic for an evaluation of depressed mood. You wish to know about the patient's sleep quality. Of the following, which is the most appropriate way to work with the interpreter and the patient?

    (A) Ask the interpreter, "How is she sleeping?"
    (B) Ask the interpreter, "Please ask her how she is sleeping."
    (C) Look at the patient and ask, "How are you sleeping?"
    (D) Loudly enunciate "How are you sleeping?" to the patient.
    (E) Write out "How are you sleeping?" and give it to the patient.

The correct response is option **C**: Look at the patient and ask, "How are you sleeping?"

One should always address the patient directly while speaking in a regular manner. It is the job of the interpreter to translate the words into sign language and vice versa. The interpreter is not to be addressed directly.

Haskins BG: Serving deaf adult psychiatric inpatients. Psychiatr Serv 2004; 55:439–441
Phelan M, Parkman S: How to work with an interpreter. BMJ 1995; 311:555–557
Steinberg A: Issues in providing mental health services to hearing-impaired persons. Hosp Community Psychiatry 1991; 42:380–389

52

An internist consults a psychiatrist because of his frustration with an elderly patient who has a diagnosis of hypochondriasis. Medical tests are negative, but the patient is unable to accept that he is not ill. The psychiatrist confirms the diagnosis of hypochondriasis. Which of the following is the best management strategy for a patient with hypochondriasis?

    (A) Refer the patient to a more psychologically minded internist colleague.
    (B) Have regularly scheduled appointments with limited reassurance.
    (C) See the patient as needed, but for a limited time.
    (D) Instruct the patient to call only for urgent matters.
    (E) Refer the patient for psychotherapy.

The correct response is option **B**: Regularly scheduled appointments with limited reassurance

The management of hypochondriasis is a challenge for the internist. Regularly scheduled appointments with limited reassurance appears to be the management strategy of choice. A more psychologically minded internist might facilitate dependency, which might result in more visits and greater preoccupation with the symptoms. The other approaches do not provide enough structure to help the patient contain his anxiety.

American Psychiatric Association: Diagnostic and Statistical Manual of Mental Disorders, Fourth Edition, Text Revision (DSM-IV-TR). Washington, DC, American Psychiatric Association, 2000, pp 504–507

Wise MG, Rundell JR (eds): The American Psychiatric Publishing Textbook of Consultation-Liaison Psychiatry: Psychiatry in the Medically Ill, 2nd ed. Washington, DC, American Psychiatric Publishing, 2002, pp 377–378

53

A 29-year-old woman presents for an initial evaluation. She describes periods of mood lability and unstable interpersonal relationships, particularly with men. During periods of stress, she reports feeling angry and "empty" and sometimes scratches herself with sharp items. Sleep is often a problem, and alprazolam has been helpful. In developing a treatment plan, which of the following principles would be most appropriate?

(A) Restrict pharmacotherapy to antidepressants and mood stabilizers.
(B) Treat with multiple classes of medications for potential future symptoms.
(C) Target specific symptoms that are currently causing disruption.
(D) Refuse to prescribe a benzodiazepine.
(E) Withhold medications if the patient engages in acting out behavior.

The correct response is option **C**: Target specific symptoms that are currently causing disruption

Of the options listed, C is the most germane to the management of borderline personality disorder. Patients require a flexible, targeted approach. Many patients will need multiple classes of medications to target different domains of difficulty (affective, behavioral, and cognitive). Due to the heterogeneity of presentation, however, clinicians must be flexible in their pharmacotherapeutic approach.

Practice Guideline for the Treatment of Patients With Borderline Personality Disorder (2001), in American Psychiatric Association Practice Guidelines for the Treatment of Psychiatric Disorders, Compendium 2004. Washington, DC, APA, 2004, pp 755–757

54

A 45-year-old woman with bipolar disorder who has been successfully maintained on lithium presents at the clinic with the complaint of swelling in her ankles. Examination reveals 2+ pitting edema. Her serum lithium level is 0.8 mEq/L. The physician prescribes a thiazide diuretic. Four days later the patient presents at the emergency department with confusion, a coarse tremor in her extremities, and ataxia. Her serum lithium level is now 2.6 mEq/L. Urinalysis reveals a slightly elevated specific gravity and an absence of blood, ketones, and protein. Which of the following best explains the patient's lithium toxicity?

(A) Acute nephrogenic diabetes insipidus
(B) Increased reabsorption in the proximal tubules
(C) Decreased glomerular filtration rate
(D) Glomerulonephritis
(E) Tubulointerstitial nephropathy

The correct response is option **B**: Increased reabsorption in the proximal tubules

The patient has developed acute lithium toxicity after the administration of a thiazide diuretic. Lithium is excreted through the kidneys and is reabsorbed in the proximal tubules with sodium and water. When the body has a sodium deficiency, such as occurs with the administration of sodium-depleting diuretics, the kidneys compensate by reabsorbing more sodium, and along with it, lithium. This, and the loss of fluid volume, results in elevated serum lithium levels and toxicity. Lithium may induce nephrogenic diabetes insipidus. However, this would cause production of large volumes of dilute urine. Paradoxically, the administration of a thiazide diuretic reduces urine output. Cumulative exposure to lithium may result in a tubulointerstitial nephropathy and a decrease in the glomerular filtration rate; however, this is an insidious rather than an acute process and is unrelated to the introduction of a thiazide diuretic. Finally, lithium may cause a glomerulonephritis, resulting in a nephrotic syndrome. This is characterized by the presence of large quantities of protein in the urine.

Schatzberg AF, Cole JO, DeBattista C: Manual of Clinical Psychopharmacology. Washington, DC, American Psychiatric Publishing, 2005, pp 250, 259–265

Andreasen NC, Black DW: Introductory Textbook of Psychiatry, 3rd ed. Washington, DC, American Psychiatric Press, 2001

55

A random community sample contains 100 individuals who meet diagnostic criteria for borderline personality disorder. Which of the following is the best estimate of the gender ratio of the sample?

(A) 50% men and 50% women
(B) 40% men and 60% women
(C) 25% men and 75% women
(D) 10% men and 90% women

The correct response is option **C**: 25% men and 75% women

Borderline personality disorder is the most common personality disorder in clinical settings. It is present in 10% of individuals seen in outpatient mental health clinics, 15%–20% of psychiatric inpatients, and 30%–60% of clinical populations with a personality disorder. It occurs in an estimated 2% of the general population. Borderline personality disorder is diagnosed predominantly in women, with an estimated female-to-male ratio of 3:1. The disorder is present in cultures around the world. It is approximately five times more common among first-degree biological relatives of those with the disorder than in the general population. There is also a greater familial risk of substance-related disorders, antisocial personality disorder, and mood disorders.

Practice Guideline for the Treatment of Patients With Borderline Personality Disorder (2001), in American Psychiatric Association Practice Guidelines for the Treatment of Psychiatric Disorders, Compendium 2004. Washington, DC, APA, 2004

56

The Child Behavior Checklist is a commonly used instrument completed by parents about their children's behaviors. In a study comparing the results from subject groups obtained from multiple cultures, girls scored higher than boys across all cultures on which behavior scale?

(A) Aggression
(B) Anxious/depressed
(C) Attention problems
(D) Delinquency
(E) Thought problems

The correct response is option **B**: Anxious/depressed

Across all studied cultures, girls scored higher on the somatic complaints and anxious/depressed scales, while boys were higher on attention problems, delinquent behavior, and aggressive behavior scales. There was no significant difference between boys and girls on thought problems.

Crijnen AA, Achenbach TM, Verhulst FC: Problems reported by parents of children in multiple cultures: the Child Behavior Checklist syndrome constructs. Am J Psychiatry 1999; 156:569–574

57

Characteristic cognitive processes in persons with obsessive-compulsive disorder include:

(A) above average spatial recognition.
(B) better memory for pleasant events.
(C) decreased capacity for selective attention.
(D) impaired reality testing.
(E) normal confidence in one's own memory.

The correct response is option **C**: Decreased capacity for selective attention

In persons with obsessive-compulsive disorder, a decreased capacity for selective attention is hypothesized to be related to the difficulties in dismissing obsessions. Persons with the disorder have negative beliefs about responsibility, memory biases for disturbing themes, and decreased confidence in their memory, and they may show deficits in spatial recognition.

Hollander E, Simeon D: Anxiety disorders, in American Psychiatric Publishing Textbook of Clinical Psychiatry, Fourth Edition. Edited by Hales RE, Yudofsky SC. Washington, DC, American Psychiatric Publishing, 2003, p 586

58

In family studies of patients with schizophrenia, the personality disorder that has been found to occur most frequently in first-degree relatives is:

(A) borderline.
(B) histrionic.
(C) paranoid.
(D) schizoid.
(E) schizotypal.

The correct response is option **E**: Schizotypal

Although all cluster A personality disorders (paranoid, schizoid, and schizotypal) are more common in the biological relatives of patients with schizophrenia than in control groups, the greatest correlation has been found between schizotypal personality disorder and schizophrenia. There is increasing evidence, primarily from twin studies, that genetic factors contribute to personality disorders. Other evidence to support a genetic link is the relationship between certain axis I disorders and personality disorders.

Sadock BJ, Sadock VA: Kaplan and Sadock's Synopsis of Psychiatry, 9th ed. Philadelphia, Lippincott Williams & Wilkins, 2003, p 800

The following vignette applies to questions 59 and 60.

A 25-year-old woman presents to the emergency department with the chief complaint, "I think I'm having a heart attack." She reports that while grocery shopping she suddenly felt "scared to death." Her heart was racing, she felt short of breath and dizzy, and she was nauseated and broke out in a sweat. Her fingers and hands and the area around her mouth felt numb. The episode lasted about 10 minutes and dissipated on its own. She managed to drive herself to the emergency department. Physical examination and laboratory studies, including a chest X-ray, blood chemistries, cardiac enzymes, and electrocardiogram, are normal.

59

In the lab, which of the following substances would be most likely to induce an episode with these symptoms?

(A) Carbon monoxide
(B) Sodium lactate
(C) Physostigmine
(D) Propranolol
(E) Sodium pyruvate

The correct response is option **B**: Sodium lactate

The patient is exhibiting the classic signs and symptoms of panic disorder. Women are two to three times more likely to be affected than men; the mean age at presentation is about 25 years, and onset is typically acute. A number of panic-inducing substances (panicogens) have been identified. Respiratory panicogens shift the acid-base balance. They include carbon dioxide, sodium lactate, and bicarbonate. Neurochemical panicogens act through specific neurotransmitter systems.

Kaplan HI, Sadock BJ: Synopsis of Psychiatry. Philadelphia, Lippincott Williams & Wilkins, 2003, p 262

60

The medication that is most likely to be effective in the long-term treatment of her condition with the best tolerance of side effects is:

(A) alprazolam.
(B) buspirone.
(C) paroxetine.
(D) propranolol.
(E) imipramine.

The correct response is option **C**: Paroxetine

This patient is presenting with the classic symptoms of panic disorder. All of the medications listed have been used in the treatment of this condition. In general, experience is showing the superiority of the SSRIs and clomipramine over the benzodiazepines, monoamine oxidase inhibitors, and tricyclic and tetracyclic drugs in terms of effectiveness and tolerance of adverse effects. The beta-adrenergic receptor antagonists have not been found to be particularly useful for panic disorder.

Stein DJ, Hollander E (eds): American Psychiatric Publishing Textbook of Anxiety Disorders. Washington, DC, American Psychiatric Publishing, 2002, p 265
Stein DJ (ed): Clinical Manual of Anxiety Disorders. Washington, DC, American Psychiatric Publishing, 2004, pp 25–29

61

A 38-year-old man with migraine headaches had successfully obtained relief by taking codeine. Recently his physician started him on a trial of paroxetine for suspected depression. The patient notes improvement in his symptoms of depression and now has headaches less frequently, but when he does have one, he must take twice the amount of codeine for pain relief. Which of the following best describes this drug interaction?

(A) Cytochrome P450 enzymes: inhibition
(B) Cytochrome P450 enzymes: induction
(C) Increased protein binding
(D) Decreased absorption
(E) Increased excretion

The correct response is option **A**: Cytochrome P450 enzymes: inhibition

Codeine's analgesic effect is a result of its metabolism to morphine. This transformation is accomplished by a cytochrome P450 enzyme, CYP2D6. If that enzyme is inhibited—such as occurs with some drugs, including paroxetine—thereby interfering with available substrate (codeine) for transformation to the active metabolite (morphine), the dose of codeine must be increased above usual levels.

Hales RE, Yudofsky SC (eds): The American Psychiatric Publishing Textbook of Clinical Psychiatry, 4th ed. Washington, DC, American Psychiatric Publishing, 2003, pp 1117, 1034, 1057

62

Which of the following antidepressants is most likely to be associated with substantial weight gain?

(A) Bupropion
(B) Fluoxetine
(C) Sertraline
(D) Venlafaxine
(E) Mirtazapine

The correct response is option **E**: Mirtazapine

Appetite increase and weight gain have been more consistently associated with mirtazapine than with the other listed antidepressants, perhaps because of its potent H_1 antihistamine effect and its antagonism of the serotonin 5-HT$_2$ receptor.

Fava M: Weight gain and antidepressants. J Clin Psychiatry 2000; 61(suppl 11):37–41
Sussman N, Ginsberg DL: Weight effects of nefazodone, bupropion, mirtazapine, and venlafaxine: a review of available evidence. Primary Psychiatry 2000; 7:33–34, 47–48
Schatzberg AF, Nemeroff CB (eds): The American Psychiatric Publishing Textbook of Psychopharmacology, 3rd ed, Washington, DC, American Psychiatric Publishing, 2004, Tables 52–56, p 858

63

Expert consensus suggests that the length of time for a pharmacological trial in obsessive-compulsive disorder should be at least:

(A) 3 weeks.
(B) 6 weeks.
(C) 9 weeks.
(D) 12 weeks.

The correct response is option **D**: 12 weeks

The latency for responses to medications is longer in patients with obsessive-compulsive disorder than in those with depression; response may take 10 to 12 weeks. There is less agreement on what is acceptable as an adequate dose. Some fixed-dose trials suggest that higher doses are more effective. Trials of medications used for obsessive-compulsive disorder indicate that a daily dose for 10–12 weeks is optimal (e.g., clomipramine, 150 mg; fluvoxamine, 150 mg; fluoxetine, 40 mg; sertraline, 150 mg; paroxetine, 40 mg).

Stein DJ, Hollander E (eds): American Psychiatric Publishing Textbook of Anxiety Disorders. Washington, DC, American Psychiatric Publishing, 2002, pp 208–209

64

A 35-year-old man presents with a 4-week history of low mood, crying spells, poor sleep with early morning awakening, poor appetite with a 12-pound weight loss, and difficulty in concentrating at work. At age 27 he had been hospitalized with an episode of mania, but shortly thereafter he decided not to continue in outpatient follow-up treatment. He has no medical problems and takes no medications. As initial pharmacotherapeutic treatment, which of the following is most appropriate?

(A) Lamotrigine
(B) Nortriptyline
(C) Sertraline
(D) Valproate
(E) Venlafaxine

The correct response is option **A**: Lamotrigine

According to the APA Practice Guideline for the Treatment of Patients With Bipolar Disorder (Revised), the first-line pharmacological treatment for bipolar depression is the initiation of either lithium or lamotrigine. The treatment goals are the remission of the symptoms of major depression and to avoid precipitation of a manic or hypomanic episode. Antidepressant monotherapy is not recommended given the risk of precipitating a switch into mania. Small studies have suggested that interpersonal therapy and cognitive behavior therapy may also be useful when added to pharmacotherapy during depressive episodes in patients with bipolar disorder.

American Psychiatric Association: Practice Guideline for the Treatment of Patients With Bipolar Disorder (Revision). Am J Psychiatry 2002; 159(April suppl). Reprinted in FOCUS 2003; 1:64–110 (p 71)

65

A patient with borderline personality disorder is in dialectical behavior therapy. She has left messages on the therapist's voice-mail while he is on vacation despite an agreement that she would not call him at all during his vacation and would go to the emergency department if she became suicidal. The best approach in dialectical behavior therapy is for the therapist to:

(A) explain that a treatment boundary has been violated and therapy will have to end.
(B) wait for the patient to bring up the issue before discussing the implications for therapy.
(C) explain to the patient that the treatment plan will have to change if she cannot keep the agreement.
(D) make an exception since there is a history of serious attempts and safety is an issue.

The correct response is option **C**: Explain to the patient that the treatment plan will have to change if she cannot keep the agreement

Boundary issues are a significant aspect of treatment of patients with borderline personality disorder. Therapists should be alert to the occurrence of boundary violations and proactive in dealing with them—both in terms of ascertaining their meaning and in terms of restoring the boundaries to maintain the patient's safety and the effectiveness of therapy.

Practice Guideline for the Treatment of Patients With Borderline Personality Disorder (2001), in American Psychiatric Association Practice Guidelines for the Treatment of Psychiatric Disorders, Compendium 2004. Washington, DC, APA, 2004, p 763

66

A patient being treated with interferon for hepatitis C complains of depression, anxiety, and irritability. Which of the following pharmacological agents has the most evidence for efficacy in treating those symptoms?

(A) Trazodone
(B) Haloperidol
(C) Risperidone
(D) Nefazodone
(E) Sertraline

The correct response is option **E**: Sertraline

The treatment of choice for interferon's psychiatric side effects of depression, anxiety, and irritability is currently a selective serotonin reuptake inhibitor such as sertraline or one of the other commonly used agents. Nefazodone would be contraindicated because of its reported hepatic toxicity. The antipsychotics listed, risperidone and haloperidol, are not the first choice for symptoms of depression and anxiety. Finally, trazodone, a strong soporific, is used more commonly as a sleep medication than as an antidepressant drug.

Wise MG, Rundell JR (eds): The American Psychiatric Publishing Textbook of Consultation-Liaison Psychiatry: Psychiatry in the Medically Ill, 2nd ed. Washington, DC, American Psychiatric Publishing, 2002, p 1065

67

An 11-year-old girl is referred for an evaluation of school problems. Her teachers and parents describe her as argumentative, hostile, disrespectful, and difficult. The girl often refuses to listen, will not obey instructions, does not do her work, has temper tantrums, and insists on having her own way. She has been this way since preschool. The most likely diagnosis is:

(A) antisocial personality disorder.
(B) attention deficit hyperactivity disorder.
(C) conduct disorder.
(D) intermittent explosive disorder.
(E) oppositional defiant disorder.

The correct response is option **E**: Oppositional defiant disorder

The features of oppositional defiant disorder include a recurrent pattern of negativistic, defiant, disobedient, and hostile behavior toward authority figures. Children with conduct disorder demonstrate a repetitive and persistent pattern of behavior in which the basic rights of others and major age-appropriate societal norms or rules are violated. Oppositional behavior is not part of the criteria of ADHD. These behaviors do not meet the criteria for antisocial personality disorder, which, moreover, cannot be diagnosed in an 11-year-old. These behaviors also do not fit the criteria of intermittent explosive disorder.

Loeber R: Oppositional defiant and conduct disorder: a review of the last 10 years, part I. J Am Acad Child Adolesc Psychiatry 2000; 39:1468–1484
American Psychiatric Association: Diagnostic and Statistical Manual of Mental Disorders, Fourth Edition, Text Revision (DSM-IV-TR). Washington, DC, American Psychiatric Association, 2000, pp 85–102, 701–706, 663–667

68

Patients with end-stage renal disease who are on hemodialysis are most likely to present with which of the following psychiatric symptoms?

(A) Major depression
(B) Delirium
(C) Psychosis
(D) Panic attacks
(E) Generalized anxiety

The correct response is option **A**: Major depression

While various psychiatric symptoms can occur in hemodialysis patients, depression is the most prevalent.

Rouchell AM, Pounds R, Tierney JG: Depression, in The American Psychiatric Publishing Textbook of Consultation-Liaison Psychiatry: Psychiatry in the Medically Ill, 2nd ed. Edited by Wise MG, Rundell JR. Washington, DC, American Psychiatric Publishing, 2002, pp 313–314

69

A 27-year-old woman has had five hospitalizations over the 3-year period since she was initially diagnosed with schizophrenia. On each occasion, recurrent psychotic symptoms have been associated with treatment nonadherence. Which of the following strategies is supported by the greatest body of research evidence as the most likely to improve medication adherence for this patient?

(A) Cognitive-motivational interventions
(B) Insight-oriented psychotherapy
(C) Psychoeducational interventions
(D) Family therapy
(E) Supportive group psychotherapy

The correct response is option **A**: Cognitive-motivational interventions

A review of 39 studies of psychosocial interventions for improving medication adherence showed that programs that focus on the attitudinal and behavioral aspects of taking medications generally have better outcomes. Psychoeducation alone and family therapy alone were ineffective. There is no evidence-based data on insight-oriented psychotherapy.

Zygmunt A, Olfson M, Boyer CA, Mechanic D: Interventions to improve medication adherence in schizophrenia. Am J Psychiatry 2002; 159:1653–1664
Mueser KT, Corrigan PW, Hilton DW, Tanzman B, Schaub A, Gingerich S, Essock SM, Tarrier N, Morey B, Vogel-Scibilia S, Herz MI: Illness management and recovery: a review of the research. Psychiatr Serv 2002; 53:1272–1284. Reprinted in FOCUS 2004; 2:37–43

70

Which of the following is the most likely symptom in cocaine intoxication?

(A) Paranoid delusions
(B) Hypotension
(C) Bradycardia
(D) Depersonalization

The correct response is option **A**: Paranoid delusions

Cocaine intoxication can produce hypertension, tachycardia, seizures, paranoid delusions, and delirium. Depersonalization is more commonly associated with hallucinogen intoxication.

Mack AH, Frances RJ: Substance-related disorders. FOCUS 2003; 1:125–146 (p 129)
American Psychiatric Association: Practice Guideline for the Treatment of Patients With Substance Use Disorders: Alcohol, Cocaine, Opioids. Am J Psychiatry 1995; 152(Nov suppl)

71

A consultation-liaison psychiatrist, on arriving on the internal medicine hospital unit, learns that the patient's nurse requested the consultation and that the attending internist does not want the consultation. Of the following, the best action for the psychiatrist would be to:

(A) talk briefly with the nurse about why he or she considered the consultation important.
(B) apologize to the attending internist and leave the unit.
(C) talk with the nurse's supervisor about the correct way to request a consultation.
(D) proceed with the consultation and make treatment recommendations.
(E) ask to have a case conference about the patient with the physician and nursing staff.

The correct response is option **A**: Talk briefly with the nurse about why he or she considered the consultation important

The liaison process includes case-finding and fostering the development of greater psychiatric knowledge in nonpsychiatric medical care providers, as opposed to simply providing patient care recommendations when asked. The discrepancy between the internist's and the nurse's perceptions suggests an opportunity for teaching.

Strain JJ: Liaison psychiatry, in The American Psychiatric Publishing Textbook of Consultation-Liaison Psychiatry: Psychiatry in the Medically Ill, 2nd ed. Edited by Wise MG, Rundell JR. Washington, DC, American Psychiatric Publishing, 2002, pp 38–46

72

Which of the following accurately describes the major quality that fundamentally distinguishes brief dynamic psychotherapy from long-term dynamic psychotherapy? Brief therapy has:

(A) no more than five sessions.
(B) limited focus and goals.
(C) less demonstrated efficacy.
(D) no transference or countertransference phenomena.
(E) fewer demands on the therapist.

The correct response is option **B**: Limited focus and goals

While brief therapy is intended to be shorter-term, it can vary from one to 40 sessions, with the average close to six. Brief therapy is not just a shorter version of long-term therapy but is structured to address a specific, limited focus with the least-radical intervention and generally does not aim for character change. Outcome data have not demonstrated superior efficacy for time-unlimited therapy. Transference and countertransference occur in all therapies, although they may be less emphasized in brief therapy. The therapist requires at least equal psychotherapeutic skills as in classical long-term dynamic therapy and must be much more active.

Levenson H, Bujtler SF, Powers TA, Beitman BD: Concise Guide to Brief Dynamic and Interpersonal Therapy, 2nd ed. Washington, DC, American Psychiatric Publishing, 2002

73

A 68-year-old man with bipolar I disorder has been adequately maintained on lithium. His most recent serum lithium level was 0.8 mEq/L. He has a variety of medical problems for which he takes several medications. He now presents with pressured speech, racing thoughts, increased energy, and little sleep. His serum lithium level is 0.3 mEq/L. His wife reports that the patient has been adherent to his medication regimen, but she began to notice a change 2 weeks after his primary care physician started him on a new medication. What was the most likely class of medication added to his regimen?

(A) Angiotensin-converting enzyme inhibitors
(B) Beta-blockers
(C) Nonsteroidal anti-inflammatory drugs
(D) Thiazide diuretics
(E) Xanthine bronchodilators

The correct response is option **E**: Xanthine bronchodilators

Drugs that may decrease lithium levels include xanthine bronchodilators such as theophylline and aminophylline. Because the kidney excretes lithium, any medication that alters renal function can affect lithium levels. Thiazide diuretics reduce lithium clearance and hence may increase lithium levels. Certain nonsteroidal anti-inflammatory medications, such as ibuprofen, may increase lithium levels. Beta-blockers do not affect lithium levels. Angiotensin-converting enzyme inhibitors may increase lithium levels.

Marangell LB, Silver JM, Goff DC, Yudofsky SC: Psychopharmacology and electroconvulsive therapy, in The American Psychiatric Publishing Textbook of Clinical Psychiatry, 4th ed. Edited by Hales RE, Yudofsky SC. Washington, DC, American Psychiatric Publishing, 2003, p 1109

74

A patient with an alcohol problem is ambivalent about starting acamprosate. The psychiatrist explores the patient's thoughts about the advantages and disadvantages of taking and not taking the medication, attempting to tip the patient's decisional balance in favor of taking the medication. Which of the following techniques is the physician using?

(A) Cognitive reframing
(B) Contingency management
(C) Motivational enhancement
(D) Pessimistic anticipation
(E) Rational emotion

The correct response is option **C**: Motivational enhancement

Motivational enhancement therapy is a form of psychotherapy that has been shown to be effective in the treatment of substance use disorders. It uses directive, empathic, patient-centered techniques to address ambivalence and denial.

Mack AH, Franklin JE, Frances RJ: Substance use disorders, in The American Psychiatric Press Textbook of Clinical Psychiatry. Edited by Hales RE, Yudofsky SC. Washington, DC, American Psychiatric Publishing, 2003, p 353
Polcin DL, Galloway GP, Palmer J, Mains W: The case for high-dose motivational enhancement therapy. Subst Use Misuse 2004; 39:331–343

75

Which of the following differentiates Lewy body dementia from dementia of the Alzheimer's type?

(A) Apraxia
(B) Choreiform movements
(C) Executive dysfunction
(D) Gradual progression of deficits
(E) Recurrent visual hallucinations

The correct response is option **E**: Recurrent visual hallucinations

Of the core criteria that are part of the consensus criteria for the diagnosis of dementia with Lewy bodies, visual hallucinations (usually well-formed) are a particularly important finding in the differentiation. Other core criteria are fluctuation in cognitive function and spontaneous motor features of parkinsonism. In a prospective study that aimed to validate these core criteria using neuropathology at autopsy, the sensitivity and specificity of these clinical criteria were 0.83 and 0.95, respectively.

McKeith IG, Perry EK, Perry RH: Report of the second Dementia With Lewy Body International Workshop: diagnosis and treatment. Neurology 1999; 53:902–905
McKeith IG, Ballard CG, Perry RH, Ince PG, O'Brien JT, Neill D, Lowery K, Jaros E, Barber R, Thompson P, Swann A, Fairbairn AF, Perry EK: Prospective validation of consensus criteria for the diagnosis of dementia with Lewy bodies. Neurology 2000; 54:1050–1058

76

The symptom of "flashbacks" is a manifestation of which of the following psychological states?

(A) Psychosis
(B) Fugue
(C) Hyperarousal
(D) Dissociation

The correct response is option **D**: Dissociation

Flashback experiences are best understood as dissociative states. Uncommonly, the individual suffering from PTSD experiences flashbacks that can last from a few seconds to hours or days. During flashbacks, parts of the traumatic event are reexperienced and the patient behaves as though the event was occurring at that moment. There is no evidence of psychosis during flashbacks associated with PTSD. Flashbacks can also result from the toxic effects of LSD and other hallucinogenic agents. Flashbacks associated with hallucinogenic agents are usually characterized by repeated psychedelic experiences, usually visual, and occur after the drug use has stopped. Fugue states include sudden unexpected travel away from one's home or customary activities, with amnesia for some or all of one's past. Hyperarousal is described by persistent symptoms of anxiety or increased arousal, including difficulty falling or staying asleep, irritability, difficulty concentrating, hypervigilance, and exaggerated startle response.

American Psychiatric Association: Diagnostic and Statistical Manual of Mental Disorders, Fourth Edition, Text Revision (DSM-IV-TR). Washington, DC, American Psychiatric Association, 2000, pp 464–468
Wise MG, Rundell JR (eds): Textbook of Consultation/Liaison Psychiatry, 2nd ed. Washington, DC, American Psychiatric Publishing, 2002, pp 403–404

77

Response prevention is a useful psychotherapeutic technique for which of the following disorders?

(A) Generalized anxiety disorder
(B) Intermittent explosive disorder
(C) Obsessive-compulsive disorder
(D) Pedophilia
(E) Schizophrenia

The correct response is option **C**: Obsessive-compulsive disorder

Response prevention techniques that decrease the frequency of rituals have been shown in several controlled clinical trials to be useful in the treatment of patients with obsessive-compulsive disorder. The patient is prevented from engaging in compulsive acts, such as hand washing after exposure to situations that the patient considers contaminating. The patient is gradually exposed to the feared situation and is helped to abstain from engaging in compulsive behavior after the exposure. The patient begins with the easiest situation and gradually moves toward more difficult tasks.

Hales RE, Yudofsky SC (eds): The American Psychiatric Publishing Textbook of Clinical Psychiatry, 4th ed. Washington, DC, American Psychiatric Publishing, 2003, p 594

78

A patient with alcoholism wants a psychiatrist to bill the patient's insurance company under another diagnosis because the patient is afraid of the stigma attached to the diagnosis. The psychiatrist should:

(A) tell the patient that this would be lying and refuse to comply.
(B) comply with the request because stigmas are inherently unfair to patients.
(C) comply with the request provided the patient's fears are adequately addressed.
(D) explore the reasons behind the request and explain why this is something the psychiatrist is reluctant to do.

The correct response is option **D**: Explore the reasons behind the request and explain why this is something the psychiatrist is reluctant to do

The issue of therapeutic benefit to the patient must guide the manner in which the psychiatrist works within the limits of ethics and the law. Making a false insurance claim is both illegal and unethical; thus options B and C are not appropriate. Option A considers only the letter of the law without an overall consideration of how to incorporate one's response into the therapeutic relationship.

Lo B: Avoiding deception and nondisclosure, in Resolving Ethical Dilemmas: A Guide for Clinicians, 2nd ed. Philadelphia, Lippincott Williams & Wilkins, 2000 (chap 6)

79

In a patient experiencing bereavement, which of the following suggests the diagnosis of major depression?

(A) A poor appetite
(B) Initial insomnia
(C) A feeling of worthlessness
(D) Hallucinations of the deceased
(E) Sadness

The correct response is option **C**: A feeling of worthlessness

The symptoms that would prompt one to consider a diagnosis of major depressive episode include feelings of worthlessness and generalized guilt, not guilt about "missed opportunities" with the deceased. The usual signs of bereavement include feelings of sadness as well as insomnia, poor appetite, and weight loss. The bereaved patient often believes that the depressed mood is normal. Additional symptoms of major depression include general preoccupation with death (not wishes to die to join the deceased), psychomotor retardation, extended functional impairment, and hallucinatory experiences other than about the deceased.

American Psychiatric Association: Diagnostic and Statistical Manual of Mental Disorders, Fourth Edition, Text Revision (DSM-IV-TR). Washington, DC, American Psychiatric Association, 2000, pp 740–741

80

Which CNS structure is most responsible for arousal and sleep-wake cycles?

(A) Amygdala
(B) Hippocampus
(C) Hypothalamus
(D) Reticular activating system
(E) Ventral striatum

The correct response is option **D**: Reticular activating system

The reticular activating system is a collection of fibers and nuclei that include the main monoamine nuclei, extending from the medulla oblongata to the thalamus. Structures within the reticular activating system modulate arousal, sleep-wake cycles, and conscious activity. The amygdala is associated with fear, anxiety, and aggression. The hippocampus is associated with memory and anxiety. The hypothalamus is related to hormonal regulation, eating, and drinking. The ventral striatum is associated with motivation.

Cummings JL, Trimble MR: Concise Guide to Neuropsychiatry and Behavioral Neurology, 2nd ed. Washington, DC, American Psychiatric Association, 2002, pp 28–32
Neylan TC, Reynolds CF, Kupfer DJ: Sleep disorders, in The American Psychiatric Press Textbook of Clinical Psychiatry. Edited by Hales RE, Yudofsky SC. Washington, DC, American Psychiatric Publishing, 2003, p 976

81

A 38-year-old patient provides a 12-year history of obsessive concerns about dirt, germs, and contamination and spends more than 3 hours a day with washing and cleaning rituals. Which of the following would be preferred as an initial medication treatment?

(A) Desipramine
(B) Duloxetine
(C) Paroxetine
(D) Phenelzine
(E) Venlafaxine

The correct response is option **C**: Paroxetine

The patient's history is consistent with a diagnosis of obsessive-compulsive disorder. Selective serotonin reuptake inhibitors (SSRIs) are the preferred initial treatment for this condition, and fluoxetine, fluvoxamine, paroxetine, and sertraline have FDA approval for this indication. The FDA has also approved clomipramine for obsessive-compulsive disorder, but this agent has a more adverse side effect profile than the SSRIs.

Jenicke MA: Obsessive-compulsive disorder. N Engl J Med 2004; 350:259–265
Schruers K, Koning K, Luermans J, Haack MJ, Griez E: Obsessive-compulsive disorder: a critical review of therapeutic perspectives. Acta Psychiatr Scand 2005; 111:261–271

82

A 59-year-old woman is seen for an initial outpatient psychiatric assessment. Her husband says that increasingly over the past 2 years she has seemed less like her usual outgoing self. She has been increasingly apathetic and uninterested in her usual activities, and more recently she has behaved inappropriately in social interactions, making unusual comments and returning home with items that do not belong to her. Recently, her husband has had to begin helping her dress in the morning, and he notes that she is occasionally incontinent of urine. On mental status examination, her affect is blunted and her speech is sparse, although she does not report specific psychotic symptoms or changes in mood. She knows the year and the season but not the month or date, and she has particular difficulty in naming objects. MRI shows prominent frontal and some temporal atrophy with relative sparing of other cortical regions. Which of the following diagnoses is most likely in this patient?

(A) Dementia of the Alzheimer's type
(B) Creutzfeldt-Jakob disease
(C) Dementia associated with Huntington's disease
(D) Dementia associated with Parkinson's disease
(E) Pick's disease

The correct response is option **E**: Pick's disease

Of the diagnoses listed, only Pick's disease is among the frontotemporal dementias. It typically begins insidiously, with onset at an earlier age than dementia of the Alzheimer's type. Incontinence and abnormalities of speech and language occur relatively early in the illness course. Symptoms of frontal lobe dysfunction, including apathy and socially inappropriate behaviors, are common. Unlike dementia of the Alzheimer's type, which is generally associated with more diffuse atrophy, changes seen on MRI and single photon emission computed tomography in Pick's disease are more localized to the frontotemporal regions. With Huntington's disease and Parkinson's disease, characteristic neurological findings are prominent. Neurological findings are also observed in Creutzfeldt-Jakob disease, but the progression of dementia is more fulminant than with Pick's disease and MRI may show changes in basal ganglia in addition to cerebral atrophy.

Spar JE, La Rue A: Concise Guide to Geriatric Psychiatry, 3rd ed. Washington, DC, American Psychiatric Publishing, 2002, p 198

83

A psychiatrist decides that a patient with alcohol dependence would benefit from regular laboratory monitoring. Which of the following single tests would best provide information about heavy alcohol use over the preceding 7 to 10 days?

(A) Aspartate aminotransferase (AST)
(B) Carbohydrate-deficient transferrin (CDT)
(C) Exhaled ethanol concentration (e.g., Breathalyzer)
(D) Mean corpuscular volume (MCV)

The correct response is option **B**: Carbohydrate-deficient transferrin (CDT)

CDT is more sensitive and specific than the other tests listed. However, better results may be obtained with combined tests (e.g., CDT and gamma-glutamyltransferase—GGT). Because of interpatient variability in the CDT test result, the individual patient is best used as his or her own baseline for CDT levels.

Franklin JE, Leamon MH, Frances RJ: Substance-related disorders, in The American Psychiatric Publishing Textbook of Consultation-Liaison Psychiatry, 2nd ed. Edited by Wise MG, Rundell JR. Washington, DC, American Psychiatric Publishing, 2002, pp 417–454

84

A patient with major depression shows no improvement after an adequate trial (in dose and duration) of an antidepressant. The best next step is to:

(A) augment the antidepressant with thyroid hormone.
(B) augment with lithium.
(C) augment with both thyroid hormone and lithium.
(D) switch to a different class of antidepressant.
(E) conduct a "washout" by stopping all medication for 4 weeks, and then reassess.

The correct response is option **D**: Switch to a different class of antidepressant

If a patient shows not even a partial response despite full therapeutic doses of a particular antidepressant, augmentation is not recommended. Switching to a different drug, either within a class (if there has not been another trial within the same class) or in a different class is warranted. The addition of psychotherapy is also an option. Washing out by suddenly stopping all medications will probably precipitate discontinuation symptoms that will worsen the patient's status.

Practice Guideline for the Treatment of Patients With Major Depressive Disorder, 2nd ed (2000), in American Psychiatric Association Practice Guidelines for the Treatment of Psychiatric Disorders, Compendium 2004. Washington, DC, APA, 2004, p 455, Figure 3

85

Of the following, which is the most common reason psychiatrists are sued for malpractice?

(A) Sexual improprieties with patients
(B) Suicide
(C) Failure to obtain informed consent
(D) Tardive dyskinesia
(E) Unnecessary commitment

The correct response is option **B**: Suicide

Of the answer choices, suicide is the most common reason for malpractice litigation against a psychiatrist. Documentation of a proper assessment with consultation helps to provide a reasonable defense. Sexual improprieties are viewed most often as torts and are not usually covered by malpractice, because a law has not been broken. Failure to obtain informed consent, especially when prescribing a conventional antipsychotic that could produce tardive dyskinesia, can be a cause for litigation. The best protection against malpractice is a documented comparison of risks versus benefits in the decision about treatment and an indication that this comparison has been shared with the patient or, if the patient is incompetent, with a member of the patient's family.

Gutheil TG: Liability issues and liability prevention in suicide, in The Harvard Medical School Guide to Suicide Assessment and Intervention. Edited by Jacobs DG. San Francisco, Jossey-Bass, 1999, pp 561–578, p 561
Simon RI: A Concise Guide to Psychiatry and Law for Clinicians, 3rd ed. Washington, DC, American Psychiatric Publishing, 2001, p 143

86

Anorexia nervosa is most commonly comorbid with which of the following personality disorders?

(A) Dependent
(B) Paranoid
(C) Schizotypal
(D) Obsessive-compulsive
(E) Histrionic

The correct response is option **D**: Obsessive-compulsive

The association between personality disorders and other psychiatric disorders is important because of implications for treatment. Anorexia nervosa has been demonstrated to be associated with obsessive-compulsive personality disorder. Anorexia nervosa has not been associated with dependent, paranoid, schizotypal, or histrionic personality disorders.

Wonderlich S, Mitchell JE: The role of personality in the onset of eating disorders and treatment implications. Psychiatr Clin North Am 2001; 24:249–258

Practice Guideline for the Treatment of Patients With Eating Disorders, 2nd ed (2000), in American Psychiatric Association Practice Guidelines for the Treatment of Psychiatric Disorders, Compendium 2004. Washington, DC, APA, 2004, p 702

87

The use of which of the following has been associated with hyperparathyroidism?

(A) Lamotrigine
(B) Divalproex
(C) Lithium
(D) Topiramate

The correct response is option **C**: Lithium

Lithium-induced hypercalcemia and hyperparathyroidism are uncommon but well-established side effects associated with lithium therapy. Both hyperplasia and adenomas of the parathyroid glands have been described in association with lithium therapy.

McHenry CR, Lee K: Lithium therapy and disorders of the parathyroid glands. Endocrine Practice 1996; 2:103–109
Abdullah H, Bliss R, Guinea AI, Delbridge L: Pathology and outcome of surgical treatment for lithium-associated hyperparathyroidism. Br J Surg 1999; 86:91–93
Haden ST, Stoll AL, McCormick S, Scott J, Fuleihan G el-H: Alterations in parathyroid dynamics in lithium-treated subjects. J Clin Endocrinol Metab 1997; 82:2844–2848

88

Narcolepsy is characterized by which of the following signs and symptoms?

(A) Daytime nonrefreshing sleep episodes
(B) Bouts of urinary incontinence
(C) Early morning awakening
(D) Sleepwalking
(E) Sudden episodes of muscle tone loss

The correct response is option **E**: Sudden episodes of muscle tone loss

Cataplexy, or sudden loss of muscle tone, is often brought on by strong emotions in patients with narcolepsy. The other three components of the classic tetrad of narcolepsy are bouts of sleep attacks (that are refreshing), sleep paralysis, and hypnagogic or hypnopompic hallucinations that are abnormal intrusions of REM sleep.

American Psychiatric Association: Diagnostic and Statistical Manual of Mental Disorders, Fourth Edition, Text Revision (DSM-IV-TR). Washington, DC, American Psychiatric Association, 2000, pp 609–615

The four major components of a psychodynamic view of personality disorders are a biologically based temperament, a set of internalized object relations, an enduring sense of self, and:

(A) an assessment of reality testing.
(B) a punitive superego.
(C) an intact ego ideal.
(D) a specific constellation of defense mechanisms.

The correct response is option **D**: A specific constellation of defense mechanisms

The psychodynamic clinician views personality disorders as involving four major components: a biologically based temperament, a set of internalized object relations, an enduring sense of self, and a specific constellation of defense mechanisms.

Gabbard GO: Psychodynamic approaches to personality disorders. FOCUS 2005; 3:363–367

The antidepressant duloxetine may simultaneously improve mood and:

(A) panic attacks.
(B) chronic pain.
(C) flashbacks.
(D) psychotic symptoms.
(E) night terrors.

The correct response is option **B**: Chronic pain

The antidepressant duloxetine is a serotonin/norepinephrine reuptake blocker with dopamine reuptake effects as well. It has been shown in several studies to have efficacy in major depression. Major depression is frequently comorbid with chronic pain, often without organic cause. Duloxetine appears to improve both depression and painful physical symptoms, particularly backache and shoulder pain. It is thought that descending norepinephrine and serotonin fibers from the brain via the spinal cord serve to dampen peripheral pain signals. Increased norepinephrine and 5-HT "tone" may thus simultaneously improve mood and comorbid pain. At this time, there are no studies to support duloxetine's use in treating panic attacks, flashbacks, psychotic symptoms, or night terrors.

Schatzberg AF: Recent studies of the biology and treatment of depression. FOCUS 2005; 3:14–24

A 48-year-old man with a medical history of gastroesophageal reflux disease (GERD) is referred for a psychiatric evaluation of his anxiety. For the past month, since the patient's initial evaluation and treatment for GERD, he complains of an increasing sense of unease, nervousness, restlessness, and inability to sit and read the paper. His medications include 20 mg/day of esomeprazole, 10 mg of metoclopramide q.i.d., and 0.5 mg of lorazepam t.i.d. orally or as needed. He is very concerned about his condition because a sibling who had a similar problem died from esophageal carcinoma. Other than being noticeably fidgety, his mental status exam is unremarkable. What is the most likely explanation?

(A) Development of generalized anxiety disorder
(B) Adjustment disorder with anxious features
(C) Somatoform disorder not otherwise specified (i.e., "sympathy symptoms" with deceased sibling)
(D) Akathisia from metoclopramide
(E) Benzodiazepine withdrawal

The correct response is option **D**: Akathisia from metoclopramide

The description and observation of the inability to be still—that is, motor restlessness—suggests akathisia rather than a simple anxiety or adjustment disorder. Metoclopramide, an aliphatic phenothiazine and a cousin of chlorpromazine, is the most likely culprit. Benzodiazepine withdrawal would be a second possibility, especially if the patient took lorazepam three times a day for 1 month and then stopped several days before the evaluation.

Stern TA, Fricchione GL, Cassem NH, Jellinek MS, Rosenbaum JF (eds): Massachusetts General Hospital Handbook of General Hospital Psychiatry, 5th ed. St Louis, Mosby, 2004, chapter 13, p 260

A 30-year-old patient with no prior history of mental health treatment presents with a major depressive episode. Which of the following elements would be the most important in choosing a medication for treatment?

(A) Co-occurring diagnosis of alcohol dependence in full sustained remission
(B) Good antidepressant response to fluoxetine in a first-degree relative
(C) History of a hypomanic episode
(D) Inactive hepatitis C infection
(E) Suicide attempt by aspirin overdose at age 16

The correct response is option **C**: History of a hypomanic episode

In deciding on pharmacotherapy of a major depressive episode, it is most important to rule out a diagnosis of a bipolar disorder. In such patients, initiation of either lithium or lamotrigine would be a reasonable option. Particularly in more seriously depressed individuals, some clinicians initiate simultaneous treatment with lithium and an antidepressant. In contrast to treatment of major depressive disorder, antidepressant monotherapy is not recommended for treating depression in patients with bipolar disorder.

Practice Guideline for the Treatment of Patients With Major Depressive Disorder, 2nd ed (2000), in American Psychiatric Association Practice Guidelines for the Treatment of Psychiatric Disorders, Compendium 2004. Washington, DC, APA, 2004, pp 477–478
Practice Guideline for the Treatment of Patients With Bipolar Disorder, 2nd ed (2002), in American Psychiatric Association Practice Guidelines for the Treatment of Psychiatric Disorders, Compendium 2004. Washington, DC, APA, 2004, p 534

93

A 32-year-old woman with bipolar I disorder has been adequately maintained on lamotrigine. Recently she has experienced an exacerbation of her manic symptoms, and her physician elects to add a second mood stabilizer. Instead of improving, the patient's symptoms worsen. Her serum lamotrigine levels are nearly undetectable. What was the most likely mood stabilizer that was added?

  (A) Olanzapine
  (B) Carbamazepine
  (C) Valproate
  (D) Topiramate
  (E) Lithium

The correct response is option **B**: Carbamazepine

Lamotrigine, which has been approved for the treatment of bipolar depression, is metabolized through the liver. Carbamazepine and oral contraceptives containing ethynyl estradiol, which induce hepatic enzyme systems, can rapidly decrease lamotrigine levels. Valproate, which inhibits these enzymes, could markedly increase lamotrigine levels. Olanzapine, topiramate, and lithium do not affect the hepatic enzyme system involved in the metabolism of lamotrigine.

Marangell LB, Silver JM, Goff DC, Yudofsky SC: Psychopharmacology and electroconvulsive therapy, in The American Psychiatric Publishing Textbook of Clinical Psychiatry, 4th ed. Edited by Hales RE, Yudofsky SC. Washington, DC, American Psychiatric Publishing, 2003, p 1114
Schatzberg AF, Nemeroff CB (eds): The American Psychiatric Publishing Textbook of Psychopharmacology, 3rd ed. Washington, DC, American Psychiatric Publishing, 2004, p 624

94

Obsessive-compulsive disorder is hypothesized to involve a neural circuit connecting the cortex and striatum with the:

  (A) amygdala.
  (B) hippocampus.
  (C) hypothalamus.
  (D) mammillary body.
  (E) thalamus.

The correct response is option **E**: Thalamus

Brain imaging studies suggest that obsessive-compulsive disorder involves abnormalities in a cortico-striatalthalamic circuit. A complementary model of obsessive-compulsive disorder has emphasized that the orbitofrontal cortex plays a major role in the "worry circuit." Data have indicated that hyperactivity of the orbitofrontal cortex as well as the anterior cingulate cortex diminishes with treatment.

Stein DJ, Hollander E (eds): American Psychiatric Publishing Textbook of Anxiety Disorders. Washington, DC, American Psychiatric Publishing, 2002, pp 194–195

95

Which of the following psychiatric disorders occurs most commonly as a comorbid disorder with anorexia nervosa?

  (A) Somatization disorder
  (B) Generalized anxiety disorder
  (C) Major depressive disorder
  (D) Obsessive-compulsive disorder
  (E) Social phobia

The correct response is option **C**: Major depressive disorder

Anorexia nervosa is associated with depression in 65% of cases, social phobia in 34% of cases, and obsessive-compulsive disorder in 26% of cases.

Sadock BJ, Sadock VA: Kaplan and Sadock's Synopsis of Psychiatry, 9th ed. Philadelphia, Lippincott Williams & Wilkins, 2003, p 739

Which of the following is the LEAST problematic for the psychiatrist according to ethical principles?

(A) A psychiatrist in a metropolitan area agrees to treat her financial adviser's child.
(B) A psychiatrist in a remote area with no other psychiatrists is involved in a romantic relationship with a patient's adult grandchild.
(C) A psychiatrist hires a current patient to perform clerical work in the psychiatrist's office.
(D) A psychiatrist convinces a patient who was sexually abused by a former clinician to file a suit against that former clinician and serves as the forensic expert for the patient.

The correct response is option **B**: A psychiatrist in a remote area with no other psychiatrists is involved in a romantic relationship with a patient's adult grandchild

Psychiatrists have an obligation in general to avoid roles that can compromise the primary fiduciary duty they have to their patients as well as roles that may increase the potential for exploitation of vulnerable patients. In option B, although a romantic relationship with a patient's adult grandchild may create a problematic dual role, the psychiatrist does not have the option of referring the patient to another competent clinician and thus lacks one possible way of avoiding the dual role. In options A and C, the psychiatrist is entering into avoidable roles that involve interests of the psychiatrist that could potentially conflict with the interests of the patient. In option D, the psychiatrist needs to distinguish between treatment and advocacy; the latter may not serve the patient while certainly serving the personal or professional interests or convictions of the psychiatrist in this case.

American Psychiatric Association: Opinions of the Ethics Committee on the Principles of Medical Ethics With Annotations Especially Applicable to Psychiatry. Washington, DC, American Psychiatric Association, 2001, pp 17–41 (section 2)
Simon RI: A Concise Guide to Psychiatry and Law for Clinicians, 3rd ed. Washington, DC, American Psychiatric Publishing, 2001, pp 26–28

In the initial assessment, a psychiatrist is consulted by a lesbian couple seeking help for some problems in their long-standing committed relationship. Which of the following is the best approach for the psychiatrist to take in assessing the possibility of domestic violence within the couple?

(A) Ask about it only when material is presented that suggests the problem.
(B) Ask routine questions about battering while taking the history.
(C) Obtain information from collateral sources.
(D) The topic need not be raised because domestic violence is low in lesbian couples.
(E) Wait until the therapy is well established before asking about it.

The correct response is option **B**: Ask routine questions about battering while taking the history

Domestic violence in general is underestimated, and it is particularly likely to be overlooked in lesbian couples because of the stereotype that battering is only an offense of men against women. Couples often do not bring it up spontaneously.

Cabaj RP, Stein TS: Textbook of Homosexuality and Mental Health. Washington, DC, American Psychiatric Press, 1996, pp 809–813
McClennen JC: Domestic violence between same-gender partners. J Interpers Violence 2005; 20:149–154
Owen SS, Burke TW: An exploration of prevalence of domestic violence in same-sex relationships. Psychol Rep 2004; 95:129–132

98

A patient is being treated for a cat phobia. The therapist encourages the patient to pass by a pet store that has cats in the window. From which of the following psychotherapy approaches does this strategy derive?

(A) Cognitive behavior
(B) Insight oriented
(C) Interpersonal
(D) Short-term anxiety-regulating
(E) Supportive

The correct response is option **A**: Cognitive behavior

Specific phobias are fears of specific objects, situations, or activities. The treatment of choice for specific phobias is exposure, a type of cognitive behavior therapy. The patient is encouraged to discuss the irrationality of the phobia and encouraged to expose him- or herself to the feared object. Interpersonal psychotherapy focuses on current interpersonal problems in depressed nonbipolar, nonpsychotic individuals. Insight psychotherapy attempts to make what is out of awareness conscious so that one can identify and work through patterns of behavior derived from childhood. Supportive psychotherapy emphasizes external events and is directed toward helping patients return to their previous best level of functioning. Short-term anxiety-regulating psychotherapy uses psychodynamic principles and techniques to effect change.

Hales RE, Yudofsky SC (eds): The American Psychiatric Publishing Textbook of Clinical Psychiatry, 4th ed. Washington, DC, American Psychiatric Publishing, 2003, pp 581, 1177–1198

99

Which of the following cognitive functions is most likely to remain stable with normal aging?

(A) Language syntax
(B) Recent memory
(C) Speed of information processing
(D) Topographic orientation
(E) Working memory

The correct response is option **A**: Language syntax

Syntax, vocabulary, communication, and store of knowledge tend to remain stable with normal aging, but the other functions listed tend to decline with age.

Spar JE, La Rue A: Concise Guide to Geriatric Psychiatry, 3rd ed. Washington, DC, American Psychiatric Publishing, 2002, pp 25–26

100

A consultation is requested for a 22-year-old man because of a gradual onset of behavioral symptoms that include irritability, aggression, and personality change. Associated findings include mild jaundice, dysarthria, and choreiform movements. The consultation-liaison psychiatrist also notices a golden-brown discoloration of the cornea. The most likely diagnosis is:

(A) Huntington's disease.
(B) Wilson's disease.
(C) Parkinson's disease.
(D) progressive supranuclear palsy.
(E) adrenoleukodystrophy.

The correct response is option **B**: Wilson's disease

Wilson's disease, or hepatolenticular degeneration, is an autosomal recessive disorder of copper metabolism characterized by CNS and hepatic manifestations. Copper deposition in the cornea results in the telltale Kayser-Fleischer ring.

Hefter H: Wilson's disease: review of pathophysiology, clinical features, and drug treatment. CNS Drugs 1994; 2:26–39

101

According to DSM-IV-TR, a patient with recurrent hypomanic episodes without intercurrent depressive features would receive which of the following diagnoses?

(A) Bipolar I disorder
(B) Bipolar II disorder
(C) Cyclothymic disorder
(D) Bipolar disorder, not otherwise specified

The correct response is option **D**: Bipolar disorder, not otherwise specified

Recurrent hypomania in the absence of depressive periods would be classified as bipolar disorder not otherwise specified. According to DSM-IV-TR, a diagnosis of bipolar I disorder requires at least one manic or mixed episode; a diagnosis of bipolar II disorder requires recurrent major depressive episodes with hypomanic episodes; and a diagnosis of cyclothymic disorder requires periods of hypomanic symptoms and periods of depressive symptoms.

American Psychiatric Association: Diagnostic and Statistical Manual of Mental Disorders, Fourth Edition, Text Revision (DSM-IV-TR). Washington, DC, American Psychiatric Association, 2000, pp 382–400

102

The ventral tegmentum, the nucleus accumbens, and the prefrontal cortex are brain structures or regions most involved in the neurobiology of:

(A) alcohol dependence.
(B) anorexia nervosa.
(C) bipolar disorder.
(D) panic disorder.
(E) schizophrenia.

The correct response is option **A**: Alcohol dependence

Dopaminergic and glutaminergic circuits in the tegmentum, accumbens, and prefrontal cortex are necessary in producing pleasure from drug use, in the development of addiction, and in the maintenance of drug craving, salience, and impaired control over use. The amygdala plays a more central role in anxiety disorders. The anterior cingulate gyrus, the thalamus, the cerebellum, and the temporal lobe regions are involved in schizophrenia. The hypothalamus has been suggested as a site of dysfunction in anorexia. A wide range of structures and regions have been studied in the neurobiology of bipolar disorder.

Hyman SE: Addiction: a disease of learning and memory. Am J Psychiatry 2005; 162:1414–1422
Miller LA, Taber KH, Gabbard GO, Hurley RA: Neural underpinnings of fear and its modulation: implications for anxiety disorders. J Neuropsychiatry Clin Neurosci 2005; 17:1–6
Hales RE, Yudofsky SC (eds): The American Psychiatric Publishing Textbook of Clinical Psychiatry, 4th ed. Washington, DC, American Psychiatric Publishing, 2003, pp 474, 1005, 408

103

A 32-year-old man with panic disorder treated with lorazepam for several years begins combination therapy (which includes ritonavir) for HIV infection. Two weeks later, his panic attacks increase in frequency. What is the most likely explanation?

(A) An HIV-related brainstem lesion
(B) An HIV-related lung infection
(C) A direct side effect of one of his HIV medications
(D) Ritonavir is decreasing blood lorazepam levels
(E) Failure to take lorazepam as directed

The correct response is option **D**: Ritonavir is decreasing blood lorazepam levels

Ritonavir induces the enzyme that metabolizes lorazepam and some other benzodiazepines (oxazepam and temazepam) that rely on glucuronyl transferase activity for clearance. Some other benzodiazepines (e.g., midazolam) are dependent on CYP 3A4 for metabolism. Potent inhibitors of this CYP isoform, such as protease inhibitors, can decrease clearance of these drugs and result in increased sedation. Therefore, lorazepam remains a good clinical choice for short-term use in patients who need treatment for panic disorder who must also take ritonavir for treatment of HIV infection.

Although the other options listed cannot be absolutely excluded, they are not as likely as the effect of ritonavir. Also, modern combination therapy in compliant patients tends to be quite effective in preventing secondary infections or lesions of HIV.

Practice Guideline for the Treatment of Patients With HIV/AIDS (2000), in American Psychiatric Association Practice Guidelines for the Treatment of Psychiatric Disorders, Compendium 2004. Washington, DC, APA, 2004, p 200
Hsu A, Frenneman GR, Bertz RJ: Ritonavir: clinical pharmacokinetics and interactions with other anti-HIV agents. Clin Pharmacokinet 1998; 35:275–291
Fernandez F: Ten myths about HIV infection and AIDS. FOCUS 2005; 3:184–193

104

A 24-year-old man who lives with his parents is being treated for schizophrenia in a continuing day treatment program. Since the onset of his illness at age 20, he has had three hospitalizations for recurrent psychosis. He is currently on quetiapine 300 mg b.i.d., and his auditory hallucinations have resolved, but he still has some concerns that a government conspiracy may be operating and spying on him. Apart from his family and the day treatment program, he has few interactions with others and no outside interests. If family therapy were instituted with this patient's parents, which of the following outcomes would be most likely to be observed?

(A) Improved employability
(B) Improved social functioning
(C) Reduced likelihood of psychotic relapse and rehospitalization
(D) Reduced number and severity of negative symptoms
(E) Reduced number and severity of positive symptoms

The correct response is option **C**: Reduced likelihood of psychotic relapse and rehospitalization

Like most of the psychosocial treatments for schizophrenia, family therapy results in improved outcomes in important but discrete areas. Although studies of family interventions have used varying approaches to treatment, all effective family interventions include education about the illness and its course, training in coping and problem-solving skills within the family, improved communication, and stress reduction. By teaching practical educative and behavioral methods in highly structured programs that last 9 months to several years, these interventions are designed to elicit family participation and collaboration in treatment planning, goal setting, and service delivery. They are also intended to complement and encourage the use of other treatments, such as having the patient adhere to a medication regimen, and to embed the psychiatrist's care within a multidisciplinary team approach to the patient and family. Meta-analyses and systematic reviews of such family programs have consistently shown reduced family burden and reductions in relapse rates, which are typically halved by structured family interventions compared with control treatments.

Bustillo JR, Lauriello J, Horan WP, Keith SJ: The psychosocial treatment of schizophrenia: an update. Am J Psychiatry 2001; 158:163–175

American Psychiatric Association: Practice Guideline for the Treatment of Patients With Schizophrenia, 2nd ed. Am J Psychiatry 2004; 161(Feb suppl):1–56

105

Biological relatives of individuals with antisocial personality disorder have an increased risk of having antisocial personality disorder and substance-related disorders. These relatives, especially if they are female, are also at greater risk of:

(A) autism.
(B) narcissistic personality disorder.
(C) bipolar disorder.
(D) schizophrenia.
(E) somatization disorder.

The correct response is option **E**: Somatization disorder

Family members of individuals with antisocial personality disorder have an increased risk of having somatization disorder. This is especially true for females, although the rate of this disorder is also higher among male family members than in the general population. There is no association between antisocial personality disorder and autism, schizophrenia, narcissistic personality disorder, or bipolar disorder.

American Psychiatric Association: Diagnostic and Statistical Manual of Mental Disorders, Fourth Edition, Text Revision (DSM-IV-TR). Washington, DC, American Psychiatric Association, 2000, p 704

106

Compared with younger adults, the elderly require lower doses of lithium to achieve a given serum lithium concentration because of:

(A) impaired hepatic metabolism.
(B) more complete absorption.
(C) reduced fat storage.
(D) reduced renal excretion.
(E) reduced serum protein binding.

The correct response is option **D**: Reduced renal excretion

Lithium is a water-soluble element that is not metabolized and has no meaningful protein binding. There is no evidence that drug absorption is more efficient in the elderly, and the slight decreases in absorptive abilities with advanced age are not thought to be clinically meaningful. Lithium is excreted unchanged almost entirely by the kidneys. Because there is a tendency for the glomerular filtration rate to decrease with age, excretion of lithium becomes less efficient.

Sproule BA, Hardy BG, Shulman KI: Differential pharmacokinetics of lithium in elderly patients. Drugs Aging 2000; 16:165–177

Jefferson JW: Genitourinary system effects of psychotropic drugs, in Adverse Effects of Psychotropic Drugs. Edited by Kane JM, Lieberman JA. New York, Guilford, 1992, pp 431–444

Iber FL, Murphy PA, Connor ES: Age-related changes in the gastrointestinal system. Drugs Aging 1994; 5:34–48

Gitlin M: Lithium and the kidney: an updated review. Drug Saf 1999; 20:231–233

107

Which of the following is the best description of the therapist's empathy?

(A) Envisioning what it would be like for the therapist to be in the patient's situation
(B) Mirroring the patient's presentations of a vulnerable self
(C) Understanding the patient's inner experience from the patient's perspective
(D) Maintaining an attitude of compassion and sympathy
(E) Avoiding making the patient anxious or uncomfortable

The correct response is option **C**: Grasping the patient's inner experience from the patient's perspective

When a therapist empathizes, he or she understands the patient's feelings without getting involved in them. The empathic response would be to imagine thinking and feeling from the patient's level of insight. Empathy, a critical skill for psychotherapy, may be confused with sympathy, or just being nice, or avoiding anything that the patient dislikes. A common source of error is the "almost right" notion of imagining how one would feel if one were in the patient's shoes.

Mohl PC, Warrick GD: Listening to the patient, in Psychiatry. Edited by Tasman A, Kay J, Lieberman JA. Philadelphia, WB Saunders, 1997, p 9

108

A 39-year-old secretary must do everything meticulously. Her work area is extremely neat and organized. However, she is not very productive, because she will restart any project if she makes an error. She typically works through lunch and rarely socializes with her coworkers. At home, she is in constant conflict with her children about the tidiness of their rooms, the neatness of their schoolwork, and the need to be frugal. Her children and coworkers tell her that her behaviors "drive them nuts." She does not believe she has a problem and in fact thinks her habits represent "strong moral values." Which term best describes the woman's lack of distress about her problems?

(A) Ambivalence
(B) Denial
(C) Ego-syntonic
(D) La belle indifference
(E) Projection

The correct response is option **C**: Ego-syntonic

Although there may be elements of each of these options contributing to the patient's lack of distress, the one term that best describes this phenomenon is "ego-syntonic." Personality disorder symptoms are described as alloplastic (i.e., able to adapt to, and alter, the external environment) and ego-syntonic (i.e., acceptable to the ego). Because individuals with personality disorders do not find their behaviors distressing, these individuals often seem uninterested in treatment.

Sadock BJ, Sadock VA: Kaplan and Sadock's Synopsis of Psychiatry, 9th ed. Philadelphia, Lippincott Williams & Wilkins, 2003, p 800

109

An 18-year-old female patient who is being evaluated for depression reveals that she worries excessively about her weight. She states that she is unable to diet and consumes large quantities of food about once a month. She appears to have normal weight for her height. What is the most likely diagnosis?

(A) Anorexia nervosa
(B) Body dysmorphic disorder
(C) Bulimia nervosa
(D) Eating disorder not otherwise specified
(E) Factitious disorder

The correct response is option **D**: Eating disorder not otherwise specified

The eating disorder not otherwise specified category is for disorders of eating that do not fully meet the criteria for a specific eating disorder. This patient appears to have normal weight and thus does not meet the criteria for anorexia nervosa. She describes binges, but they do not occur frequently enough to meet the criteria for bulimia nervosa, which is on average at least twice a week.

American Psychiatric Association: Diagnostic and Statistical Manual of Mental Disorders, Fourth Edition, Text Revision (DSM-IV-TR). Washington, DC, American Psychiatric Association, 2000, pp 583–595

110

Patients with bulimia nervosa who engage in binge/purge behaviors are at risk for which of the following medical disorders?

    (A) Hyperkalemia
    (B) Decreased serum amylase
    (C) Cardiomyopathy
    (D) Hypothyroidism
    (E) Osteopenia

The correct response is option **C**: Cardiomyopathy

In patients with bulimia nervosa, cardiomyopathy as a result of ipecac intoxication may occur and usually results in death. Patients who binge and vomit may have parotid gland enlargement associated with elevated serum amylase levels. They are susceptible to hypokalemic alkalosis. Unlike patients with anorexia nervosa, those with bulimia do not have a high risk of osteopenia.

Hales RE, Yudofsky SC (eds): The American Psychiatric Publishing Textbook of Clinical Psychiatry, 4th ed. Washington, DC, American Psychiatric Publishing, 2003, pp 1011–1012

Rushing JM, Jones LE, Carney CP: Bulimia nervosa: a primary care review. Prim Care Companion J Clin Psychiatry 2003; 5:217–224

111

A 76-year-old woman presents with weakness, fatigue, somnolence, and depression. Her husband has also noticed that there has been some cognitive slowing and her voice is hoarse. Which of the following endocrine disorders is the most likely diagnosis?

    (A) Cushing's disease
    (B) Hyperparathyroidism
    (C) Hypoparathyroidism
    (D) Hypothyroidism
    (E) Pheochromocytoma

The correct response is option **D**: Hypothyroidism

Hypothyroidism presents with fatigue, somnolence, weakness, dry skin, brittle hair, cold intolerance, and hoarse speech. Depression is common, and cognitive slowing can occur. Hypoparathyroidism and hyperparathyroidism can both result in anxiety, irritability, or depression. Hyperparathyroidism is commonly accompanied by weakness and anorexia, whereas hypoparathyroidism has mainly neuromuscular signs such as spasms, tetany, and hyperreflexia. Pheochromocytoma results in palpitations, panic attacks, headaches, and hypertension.

Sadock BJ, Sadock VA (eds): Kaplan and Sadock's Comprehensive Textbook of Psychiatry, 8th ed. Philadelphia, Lippincott Williams & Wilkins, 2005, pp 2154–2155

112

Early-onset Alzheimer's dementia due to mutations in the amyloid precursor protein genes, presenilin-1 and presenilin-2, are transmitted by what mode of inheritance?

    (A) Autosomal dominant
    (B) Autosomal recessive
    (C) X-linked
    (D) Trinucleotide repeat
    (E) Polygenic

The correct response is option **A**: Autosomal dominant

Three genes have been associated with early-onset Alzheimer's dementia: the β-amyloid precursor protein gene (APP) on chromosome 21, the presenilin-1 (PS1) gene on chromosome 14, and the presenilin-2 (PS2) gene on chromosome 1. All three missense mutations are autosomal dominantly inherited and together account for only about 5% of all cases of Alzheimer's dementia.

Stern TA, Herman JB: Massachusetts General Hospital Psychiatry Update and Board Preparation, 2nd ed. New York, McGraw-Hill, 2004, p 494

Blazer DG, Steffens DC, Bausse EW (eds): The American Psychiatric Publishing Textbook of Geriatric Psychiatry, 3rd ed. Washington, DC, American Psychiatric Publishing, 2004, pp 110–111

113

A 27-year-old man has a long-standing history of marked discomfort in social situations and avoids group discussions, parties, dating, and speaking at meetings. He also has a history of binge alcohol use, particularly when he has to engage in social activities. The class of medication preferred for treatment of this patient would be:

(A) benzodiazepines.
(B) beta-blockers.
(C) tricyclics.
(D) second-generation antipsychotics.
(E) selective serotonin reuptake inhibitors.

The correct response is option **E**: Selective serotonin reuptake inhibitors

The patient's history is consistent with a diagnosis of social anxiety disorder, generalized type. While beta-blockers may be useful prior to occasional public speaking events, they are not effective for generalized social anxiety disorder. Selective serotonin reuptake inhibitors (SSRIs) are well-established, effective treatments. Sertraline and paroxetine (as well as the non-SSRI venlafaxine) are FDA-approved for the treatment of social anxiety disorder. There have been some studies showing benefit with benzodiazepines, but these agents are not preferred for long-term use and none are FDA-approved for this indication. Particularly in light of this patient's history of binge drinking, benzodiazepine use would be a relative contraindication. A very small double-blind placebo-controlled study of olanzapine had promising results, but additional studies are necessary. Tricyclics have not been shown to be of benefit for social anxiety disorder.

Blanco C, Raza MS, Schneier FR, Liebowitz MR: The evidence-based pharmacological treatment of social anxiety disorder. Int J Neuropsychopharmacol 2003; 6:427–442

Barnett SD, Kramer ML, Casat CD, Connor KM, Davidson JR: Efficacy of olanzapine in social anxiety disorder: a pilot study. J Psychopharmacol 2002; 16:365–368

114

The consultation-liaison psychiatrist is called to the emergency department to evaluate a 17-year-old patient who is highly agitated and floridly psychotic with findings of ataxia, nystagmus, dysarthria, miosis, and elevated blood pressure. Intoxication with which of the following substances best explains this presentation?

(A) Heroin
(B) Psilocybin
(C) Cannabis
(D) LSD
(E) Phencyclidine

The correct response is option **E**: Phencyclidine

The patient's presentation is consistent with phencyclidine (PCP) intoxication. Hallucinogens such as LSD and psilocybin do not cause ataxia, dysarthria, and nystagmus. While miosis is characteristic of heroin intoxication, hypertension and agitation are not. Cannabis-induced psychosis is not characterized by miosis or the above-mentioned neurological findings.

Moore DP, Jefferson JW: Substance use and related disorders, in Handbook of Medical Psychiatry, 2nd ed. Philadelphia, Elsevier Mosby, 2004, pp 61–44

McCarron MM, Schulze BW, Thompson GA, Conder MC, Goetz WA: Acute phencyclidine intoxication: incidence of clinical findings in 1,000 cases. Ann Emerg Med 1981; 10:237–242

115

A 35-year-old nurse is admitted to the medical service with numerous ecchymoses on her body and a complaint of tarry stools. Her prothrombin time was 4 INR (international normalized prothrombin ratio) units (normal, 0.78–1.22). Several days after admission her prothrombin time was normal. A medical workup failed to identify the cause of her abnormal clotting time. Her stool was weakly positive for blood. Four days after admission, more ecchymoses appeared and her prothrombin time was again elevated. The patient expressed concern that she might have leukemia and inquired if she would need a bone marrow biopsy. On the fifth day of admission, a warfarin pill was found beneath her bed. The patient signed out of the hospital that evening. Which of the following is the most likely diagnosis?

(A) Somatization disorder
(B) Malingering
(C) Hypochondriasis
(D) Factitious disorder
(E) Body dysmorphic disorder

The correct response is option **D**: Factitious disorder

Factitious disorder is the most likely diagnosis for this patient because the negative workup and the discovery of the warfarin pill beneath the bed strongly suggest that her bleeding problems were self-induced. Such patients have a great need to be taken care of by physicians and even undergo serious procedures, such as a bone marrow biopsy. The diagnosis is often elusive unless evidence is found that the illness was self-inflicted. No clear motive for the behavior is present; the motive most often identified is a desire to assume the sick role. In malingering, by contrast, an individual presents with a disability claim or an illness motivated by a goal of getting out of prison, collecting insurance money, or some other secondary gain.

Somatization disorder is a polysystem disorder that is characterized by a combination of pain, gastrointestinal, sexual, and psychoneurological symptoms. Hypochondriasis is the chronic fear that one has a serious illness. The anxiety may be generated by an exaggeration of an actual mild illness or concerns in the absence of medical causes. Body dysmorphic disorder is characterized by a significant preoccupation with imagined or exaggerated physical defects.

American Psychiatric Association: Diagnostic and Statistical Manual of Mental Disorders, Fourth Edition, Text Revision (DSM-IV-TR). Washington, DC, American Psychiatric Association, 2000, pp 471–475

116

Patients who suffer from depression after a myocardial infarction should be treated with which of the following antidepressants?

(A) A monoamine oxidase inhibitor
(B) Bupropion
(C) Trazodone
(D) A tricyclic antidepressant
(E) An SSRI

The correct response is option **E**: An SSRI

Depression occurs in approximately 20% of patients who have had a myocardial infarction. Moreover, the mortality rate is much higher among post-myocardial infarction patients who have depression. Several studies have established that the SSRIs constitute the safest antidepressants to use in such circumstances. They have little effect on conduction time and do not cause orthostatic hypotension. Various tricyclic antidepressants are not ideal because they may cause orthostatic hypotension, anticholinergic side effects, and effects on conduction. Bupropion has been implicated in hypertension in some patients. Trazodone presents problems of alpha-adrenergic blockade and postural hypotension. Finally, the monoamine oxidase inhibitors may cause a hypertensive response when certain foods are eaten, and they have orthostatic hypotension as a side effect as well.

Wise MG, Rundell JR (eds): The American Psychiatric Publishing Textbook of Consultation-Liaison Psychiatry: Psychiatry in the Medically Ill, 2nd ed. Washington, DC, American Psychiatric Publishing, 2002, pp 542–545
Shulman J, Muskin P, Shapiro PA: Psychiatry and cardiovascular disease. FOCUS 2005; 2:208–224

117

Cocaine-induced euphoria is most highly associated with which of the following neurotransmitters?

(A) Serotonin
(B) Dopamine
(C) Norepinephrine
(D) Gamma-aminobutyric acid
(E) Acetylcholine

The correct response is option **B**: Dopamine

Cocaine is known to inhibit dopamine reuptake and increase extracellular dopamine concentration. These effects, which occur in the nucleus accumbens, are considered to be related to cocaine-induced euphoria. Cocaine also blocks the reuptake of norepinephrine and serotonin, although the behavioral effects are mediated primarily by the dopaminergic system. The inhibitory neurotransmitter gamma-aminobutyric acid also interacts with dopamine neurons in the nucleus accumbens and the ventral tegmental area. The binding of cocaine to the dopamine transporter correlates best with its behavioral potency.

Withers NW, Pulvirenti L, Koob GF, Gillin JC: Cocaine abuse and dependence. J Clin Psychopharmacology 1995; 15:63–78
Dackis CA, O'Brien CP: Cocaine dependence: a disease of the brain's reward centers. J Subst Abuse Treat 2001; 21:111–117

118

Which of the following is an example of an instrumental activity of daily living that becomes impaired in the mild to moderate stages of dementia?

(A) Ambulating
(B) Dressing
(C) Feeding oneself
(D) Remembering appointments
(E) Toileting

The correct response is option **D**: Remembering appointments

Instrumental activities of daily living (IADLs) include more complex daily tasks such as managing finances (e.g., writing checks), grocery shopping, preparing meals, keeping track of current events, remembering appointments, managing medications, using the phone, and traveling (e.g., taking the bus). A person's ability to manage these activities independently generally becomes impaired in the mild to moderate stages of dementia. As dementia progresses, the more basic activities of daily living (ADLs) become impaired, and most people need assistance with them. ADLs include feeding, dressing, toileting, grooming, physical ambulation and transferring, and bathing.

Coffey CE, Cummings JL: American Psychiatric Press Textbook of Geriatric Neuropsychiatry, 2nd ed. Washington, DC, American Psychiatric Press, 2000, p 26

119

A 66-year-old patient who is being treated for bipolar disorder presents comatose with a serum sodium concentration of 112 mmol/L. Which of the following is most likely to be the cause of the sodium imbalance?

(A) Divalproex
(B) Carbamazepine
(C) Lithium
(D) Olanzapine

The correct response is option **B**: Carbamazepine

Hyponatremia can be an adverse reaction of carbamazepine. Hyponatremic coma has been attributed to the drug. If lithium use is associated with dehydration, hypernatremia may be a complication.

Schatzberg AF, Nemeroff CB (eds): American Psychiatric Publishing Textbook of Psychopharmacology, 3rd ed. Washington, DC, American Psychiatric Publishing, 2004, pp 591–592

120

Which of the following features differentiates delirium from dementia of the Alzheimer's type?

(A) Acuity of onset and level of consciousness
(B) Level of consciousness and orientation
(C) Acuity of onset and orientation
(D) Visual hallucinations and memory
(E) Memory and level of consciousness

The correct response is option **A**: Acuity of onset and level of consciousness

Delirium is often confused with dementia or functional psychiatric disorders in elderly patients. Clinical features help in differentiating between delirium and dementia. Patients with delirium have an acute onset and exhibit fluctuation in the level of consciousness, cognition, and clinical symptoms, whereas patients with Alzheimer's dementia tend to have an insidious onset and an alert and stable level of consciousness, and cognitive and symptom fluctuation are infrequent. Orientation and memory are impaired in both disorders. Visual hallucinations are frequent in delirium and occur only occasionally in Alzheimer's dementia. EEG shows marked slowing in patients with delirium and either normal or mild slowing in patients with Alzheimer's dementia.

Cole MG: Delirium in elderly patients. Am J Geriatr Psychiatry 2004; 2:1, 7–21
Ajilore OA, Kumar A: Delirium and dementia. FOCUS 2004; 2:210–220

121

Which of the following sleep disorders is more common in males than females during childhood?

(A) Breathing-related sleep disorder
(B) Nightmare disorder
(C) Primary insomnia
(D) Sleep terror disorder
(E) Sleepwalking disorder

The correct response is option **D**: Sleep terror disorder

Only option D is correct. The other disorders either have no gender differentiation or are more common in females.

American Psychiatric Association: Diagnostic and Statistical Manual of Mental Disorders, Fourth Edition, Text Revision (DSM-IV-TR). Washington, DC, American Psychiatric Association, 2000, pp 599–604, 615–622, 631–644

122

A physician elects to treat a depressed patient with imipramine. Four days after the start of treatment, the physician receives a call from the emergency department reporting that the patient has fallen. The staff report that the patient stood up quickly after being in bed overnight, felt dizzy, and then lost consciousness, falling to the floor. Examination reveals a pulse of 76 bpm; blood pressure is 136/82 mm Hg lying and 84/46 mm Hg standing. An electrocardiogram is unremarkable. Which of the following best explains the patient's symptoms?

(A) α-Adrenergic receptor blockade
(B) Cholinergic receptor blockade
(C) Histamine receptor blockade
(D) First-degree atrioventricular block
(E) Prolongation of the QTc interval

The correct response is option **A**: α-Adrenergic receptor blockade

The tricyclic antidepressants block peripheral alpha-adrenergic receptors, delaying the reflexive constriction of peripheral blood vessels when a patient goes from lying to standing, and through this mechanism induce orthostatic hypotension. In this particular vignette, the patient has a period of loss of consciousness on rising and objective evidence of orthostatic hypotension in light of a normal ECG. The signs, symptoms, and ECG suggest that the patient's fall is secondary to orthostatic hypotension. The tricyclic antidepressants may cause a variety of side effects, including anticholinergic, cardiovascular, and central nervous system effects. Anticholinergic effects include dry mouth, constipation, urinary hesitancy, and blurred vision. Antihistaminic effects include sedation and weight gain. Cardiovascular effects tend to be the most worrisome. All tricyclics prolong cardiac conduction, much like quinidine or procainamide, and carry the risk of exacerbating existing conduction abnormalities, such as first-degree atrioventricular block.

Schatzberg AF, Cole JO, DeBattista C: Manual of Clinical Psychopharmacology. Washington, DC, American Psychiatric Publishing, 2005, pp 102, 114–115
Andreasen NC, Black DW: Introductory Textbook of Psychiatry, 3rd ed. Washington, DC, American Psychiatric Press, 2001, p 725

123

Soon after ECT, a patient is most likely to have problems with which of the following items on the Mini-Mental State Examination?

(A) Reporting the date
(B) Spelling "WORLD" backwards
(C) Repeating "no ifs ands or buts"
(D) Following a three-step command
(E) Writing a sentence

The correct response is option **A**: Reporting the date

ECT can cause a retrograde amnesia. While some anterograde memory impairment may be present, it can be difficult to separate from the impairments brought on by depression itself. Following a treatment, postictal/postanesthesia confusion is often present but generally resolves within several hours. Of the Mini-Mental State Examination components listed, reporting the date is the only one that potentially relies on material learned in the hours prior to a treatment.

Practice Guideline for the Treatment of Patients With Major Depressive Disorder, 2nd ed (2000), in American Psychiatric Association Practice Guidelines for the Treatment of Psychiatric Disorders, Compendium 2004. Washington, DC, APA, 2004, pp 495–496
UK ECT Review Group: Efficacy and safety of electroconvulsive therapy in depressive disorders: a systematic review and meta-analysis. Lancet 2003; 361(9360):799–808
American Psychiatric Association: The Practice of Electroconvulsive Therapy: Recommendations for Treatment, Training, and Privileging: A Task Force Report of the American Psychiatric Association, 2nd ed. Washington, DC, APA, 2001

124

Imaging genetics is a form of:

(A) association study.
(B) double-blind study.
(C) linkage study.
(D) randomized study.

The correct response is option **A**: Association study

An association study looks for a statistically significant link between two variables in comparison with a control. Imaging genetics uses neuroimaging methods—structural MRI, positron emission tomography (PET), functional MRI (fMRI), and magnetic resonance spectroscopy (MRS)—to assess the impact of genetic variation on the human brain in order to find aspects of brain function or structure that can be examined in association with genetic variations across individuals.

Kempf K, Meyer-Lindenberg A: Imaging genetics and psychiatry. FOCUS 2006; 4

125

Which of the following is the most appropriate indication for ECT in a patient with borderline personality disorder?

(A) Comorbid major depression
(B) Severe mood instability
(C) Poor response to valproate
(D) Noncompliance with medications
(E) Recurrent transient psychotic episodes

The correct response is option **A**: Comorbid major depression

The goal of ECT in patients with borderline personality disorder is to decrease depressive symptoms in individuals with a comorbid axis I mood disorder. Although ECT is not a recommended treatment for borderline personality disorder per se, it can be useful in treating comorbid major depression. The decision to use ECT in this patient group should be guided by the neurovegetative symptoms more than the psychological symptoms of depression, which are chronically present in many persons with borderline personality disorder. There is, unfortunately, little research specifically testing ECT for treatment of depression in borderline personality disorder.

Practice Guideline for the Treatment of Patients With Borderline Personality Disorder (2001), in American Psychiatric Association Practice Guidelines for the Treatment of Psychiatric Disorders, Compendium 2004. Washington, DC, APA, 2004, pp 817–818

126

A 70-year-old woman presents with a depression that has not responded to treatment with sertraline, paroxetine, or escitalopram. She has said that she would like to die, and she has a history of an overdose in the past 3 months. Although abdominal computerized tomography shows no abnormalities, she is convinced that a hole in her liver is causing her to lose weight. Mental status examination is also significant for severe psychomotor retardation, and physical examination shows evidence of dehydration. She is currently being treated with 150 mg/day of venlafaxine. Which of the following recommendations is most appropriate at the present time?

(A) Increase the dose of venlafaxine
(B) Recommend ECT
(C) Change to mirtazapine
(D) Add lamotrigine
(E) Obtain a liver scan to assess for evidence of carcinoma

The correct response is option **B**: Recommend ECT

The patient is experiencing a treatment-resistant episode of depression that has accompanying suicidal ideation, somatic delusions, severe psychomotor retardation, and probable dehydration. These clinical features make this patient a candidate for ECT, which has been shown to be an effective treatment for patients with severe major depression. ECT is typically recommended for depressed patients with severe symptoms, including psychosis, marked suicidal intent, and refusal to eat. Given this patient's history of nonresponse to, or inability to tolerate, multiple antidepressants during the current episode, the likelihood that her depression will respond to ECT is significantly greater than the likelihood that it will respond to an increased dose of venlafaxine or to a change to a different antidepressant (e.g., mirtazapine) or augmentation with an anticonvulsant (e.g., lamotrigine).

Although an occult carcinoma might also explain this patient's loss of weight, abdominal computerized tomography has not shown any hepatic abnormality, so obtaining a liver scan is not likely to be informative.

Sadock BJ, Sadock VA (eds): Kaplan and Sadock's Comprehensive Textbook of Psychiatry, 7th ed. Philadelphia, Lippincott Williams & Wilkins, 2000, p 507
Practice Guideline for the Treatment of Patients With Major Depressive Disorder, 2nd ed (2000), in American Psychiatric Association Practice Guidelines for the Treatment of Psychiatric Disorders, Compendium 2004. Washington, DC, APA, 2004, p 461

127

A 29-year-old unmarried woman is admitted to an acute inpatient unit after police spotted her wandering along a busy highway gesturing and muttering to herself. On admission, she was disheveled and bizarrely clothed. Her speech was tangential, and she reported auditory hallucinations commenting on her behavior and telling her that "criminal elements" were watching her. She had recently been residing with her parents and gave permission for staff to contact them. Her parents report that her first hospitalization was at age 25, just after she began working on her thesis for a Ph.D. in mathematics. She responded rapidly to treatment with risperidone 3 mg daily, and several months later, with the support of her adviser, she was able to resume work on her thesis. Over the past 6 months, after she decided to stop her medication, her symptoms have returned. In responding to the parents' questions about her prognosis, which of the following factors would be the best predictor of a good prognosis for this patient?

(A) Age at onset of illness
(B) Initial response to medication
(C) Marital status
(D) Number and duration of remissions between psychotic episodes
(E) Premorbid cognitive functioning

The correct response is option **B**: Initial response to medication

A better prognosis is indicated by late age at onset, good premorbid functioning, longer remission periods, and being married. The best predictor, however, is a good initial response to medication.

Stern TA, Herman JB: Massachusetts General Hospital Psychiatry Update and Board Preparation, 2nd ed. Boston, Massachusetts General Hospital, p 101
Quick reference for schizophrenia. FOCUS 2004; 2:13

128

A patient with a history of "manic and major depressive episodes" who has persistent delusions or hallucinations even when prominent mood symptoms are absent, would have which of the following diagnoses?

(A) Bipolar I disorder
(B) Delusional disorder, grandiose type
(C) Schizoaffective disorder
(D) Schizophrenia, disorganized type

The correct response is option **C**: Schizoaffective disorder

The DSM-IV diagnostic criteria for schizoaffective disorder, bipolar type, include at least one manic or mixed episode concurrent with symptoms of schizophrenia and with the persistence of delusions and hallucinations for at least 2 weeks when prominent mood symptoms are no longer present. Just having schizophrenic symptoms during a manic or mixed episode is insufficient for a diagnosis of schizoaffective disorder, because manic or mixed episodes in bipolar I disorder can be severe with psychotic features.

American Psychiatric Association: Diagnostic and Statistical Manual of Mental Disorders, Fourth Edition, Text Revision (DSM-IV-TR). Washington, DC, American Psychiatric Association, 2000, pp 319–323, 413–415

129

A patient with borderline personality disorder reports prominent lability, sensitivity to rejection, anger, outbursts, and "mood crashes." As an initial approach to pharmacotherapy, which of the following would be most appropriate?

(A) Gabapentin
(B) Sertraline
(C) Quetiapine
(D) Phenelzine
(E) Valproic acid

The correct response is option **B**: Sertraline

Of the options listed, initial treatment with SSRIs for symptoms of affective dysregulation in patients with borderline personality disorder has the most empirical support. Although the use of mood stabilizers is common with patients with borderline personality disorder, there are not enough data at this time to support their use as a first-line therapy for affective dysregulation.

Practice Guideline for the Treatment of Patients With Borderline Personality Disorder (2001), in American Psychiatric Association Practice Guidelines for the Treatment of Psychiatric Disorders, Compendium 2004. Washington, DC, APA, 2004, pp 770–773

130

Which of the following schools of therapy has its base in the idea that family problems are due to structural imbalances in family relationships and symptoms are communications?

(A) Cognitive behavior
(B) Insight oriented
(C) Psychoeducational
(D) Solution focused
(E) Strategic

The correct response is option **E**: Strategic

Structural/strategic/systematic therapies are based on the idea that the family has a problem because there is a structural imbalance and that symptoms are communications to control relationships when other strategies cannot be used. The therapist's role becomes one of highlighting problematic interaction patterns, encouraging substituting new behaviors to interrupt feedback cycles, and applying indirect strategies such as reframing and paradoxical interventions to alter the frame of reference and allow new choices.

Hales RE, Yudofsky SC (eds): The American Psychiatric Publishing Textbook of Clinical Psychiatry, 4th ed. Washington, DC, American Psychiatric Publishing, 2003, pp 1381–1385
Sadock BJ, Sadock VA (eds): Kaplan and Sadock's Synopsis of Psychiatry: Behavioral Sciences/Clinical Psychiatry, 9th ed. Philadelphia, Lippincott Williams & Wilkins, 2003, p 945
Szapocznik J, Williams RA: Brief strategic family therapy: twenty-five years of interplay among theory, research, and practice in adolescent behavior problems and drug abuse. Clin Child Fam Psychol Rev 2000; 3:117–134

131

Compared with depressed elderly individuals who had a first episode of depression in young adulthood, individuals with a first episode of depression in late life are more likely to have:

(A) brain imaging findings suggesting dementia.
(B) comorbid personality disorder.
(C) first-degree relatives with depression.
(D) good response to treatment.
(E) suicidal ideation.

The correct response is option **A**: Brain imaging findings suggesting dementia

Research suggests that compared with older patients with early-onset depression, elderly patients with late-life onset of depression are more likely to have chronic medical illness, brain imaging findings suggestive of dementia, and poorer response to treatment. Patients with early onset of depression are more likely to have first-degree relatives with depression.

Coffey CE, Cummings JL: American Psychiatric Press Textbook of Geriatric Neuropsychiatry, 2nd ed. Washington, DC, American Psychiatric Press, 2000, p 313

132

A 10-year-old boy has a well-documented episode of moderately severe non-bipolar major depression. Which of the following medications is FDA-approved for use in this patient?

(A) Bupropion
(B) Duloxetine
(C) Fluoxetine
(D) Sertraline
(E) Venlafaxine

The correct response is option **C**: Fluoxetine

While other antidepressants may be of benefit for treating children and adolescents with major depressive disorder, only fluoxetine has met FDA requirements for use in pediatric patients. FDA approval was based on two 8–9-week, placebo-controlled clinical trials. More recently, the Treatment of Adolescents with Depression Study (TADS) found fluoxetine alone to be more effective than cognitive behavior therapy alone, although the combination appeared to be most beneficial.

Whittington CJ, Kendall T, Fonagy P, Cottrell D, Cotgrove A, Boddington E: Selective serotonin reuptake inhibitors in childhood depression: systematic review of published versus unpublished data. Lancet 2004; 363:1341–1345

Treatment for Adolescents with Depression Study team: Fluoxetine, cognitive-behavioral therapy, and their combination for adolescents with depression. JAMA 2004; 292:807–820

Prozac (fluoxetine) prescribing information (package insert)

133

A 35-year-old man has a 10-year history of schizophrenia and poor adherence with outpatient treatment. He has been stabilized on 20 mg of olanzapine in the hospital, and he has previously done well on 10 mg of oral haloperidol. He has agreed to switch to haloperidol decanoate injections once a month. He is given an initial injection of 50 mg. Which of the following is the most likely amount of time he will need to continue taking the oral olanzapine?

(A) Two days
(B) Two weeks
(C) One month
(D) Three months
(E) One year

The correct response is option **D**: Three months

The haloperidol decanoate may require 3 to 6 months to reach a steady state. Hence, long-acting injectable first-generation antipsychotic medications are seldom used alone during acute treatment, when the psychiatrist is adjusting the dose in accordance with therapeutic effects and side effects.

Ereshefsky L, Mascarenas CA: Comparison of the effects of different routes of antipsychotic administration on pharmacokinetics and pharmacodynamics. J Clin Psychiatry 2003; 64(suppl 16):18–23

American Psychiatric Association: Practice Guideline for the Treatment of Patients With Schizophrenia, 2nd ed. Am J Psychiatry 2004; 161(Feb suppl):1–56

134

A 51-year-old woman presents to her physician with the chief complaint of feeling depressed over the past month. She has no energy, is disinterested in her children, and has lost 25 pounds. She is unable to fall asleep until the early morning hours. She has begun to feel that she is unworthy of her family. With the onset of these symptoms, she is quite certain that she has developed a degenerative nerve condition, although all investigations have been negative. The most appropriate first step in treating this patient is to start her on:

(A) a serotonin reuptake inhibitor alone.
(B) a serotonin-norepinephrine reuptake inhibitor alone.
(C) a serotonin reuptake inhibitor and an antipsychotic.
(D) a serotonin-norepinephrine reuptake inhibitor and a benzodiazepine.

The correct response is option **C**: A serotonin reuptake inhibitor and an antipsychotic

About 15% of individuals with a major depressive disorder will develop delusions. Since this woman's belief about having a degenerative nerve condition is quite fixed and unsupported by medical evaluation, it is probably delusional. In addition, her belief that she is unworthy of her family may reach delusional proportions. In the presence of psychotic features, major depression generally requires combined treatment with an antidepressant and an antipsychotic.

Sadock BJ, Sadock VA (eds): Kaplan and Sadock's Comprehensive Textbook of Psychiatry, 7th ed. Philadelphia, Lippincott Williams & Wilkins, 2000, pp 1354, 1379–1380

Practice Guideline for the Treatment of Patients With Major Depressive Disorder, 2nd ed (2000), in American Psychiatric Association Practice Guidelines for the Treatment of Psychiatric Disorders, Compendium 2004. Washington, DC, APA, 2004, p 469

135

Which of the following is NOT a predisposing risk factor for the development of posttraumatic stress disorder (PTSD) after a traumatic event?

(A) Recent life stressors
(B) Female gender
(C) Internal locus of control
(D) Past history of depression

The correct response is option **C**: Internal locus of control

Of the choices listed, all but option C are established personal vulnerability–related risk factors for the development of PTSD following trauma. When the type of trauma is controlled for, women appear to be at higher risk of developing PTSD compared with men. In one nationwide survey, the highest current (17.8%) and lifetime (38.5%) rates of PTSD were in women who had been exposed to physical assault or rape. PTSD is more common in younger than in older individuals, probably because of the higher incidence of physical violence and accidents in the younger population. Individuals who respond to the initial trauma with high levels of anxiety (e.g., a panic attack), also have a higher risk of developing PTSD after trauma, as are those who perceive an external (vs. internal) locus of control.

Kaplan HI, Sadock BJ: Synopsis of Psychiatry: Behavioral Sciences/Clinical Psychiatry, 9th ed. Baltimore, Lippincott Williams & Wilkins, 2003, p 624

Resnick HS, Kilpatrick DG, Dansky BS, Saunders BE, Best CL: Prevalence of civilian trauma and posttraumatic stress disorder in a representative national sample of women. J Consult Clin Psychol 1993; 61:984–991

Breslau N: The epidemiology of posttraumatic stress disorder: what is the extent of the problem? J Clin Psychiatry 2001; 62(suppl 17):16–22

Connor KM, Butterfield MI: Posttraumatic stress disorder. FOCUS 2003; 1:247–262

136

A patient with schizophrenia, paranoid type, and methamphetamine dependence receives mental health care through a community mental health clinic (CMHC). The patient has appeared to clinically deteriorate over a period of 6 weeks and is hospitalized with a psychotic decompensation. A drug screen on admission shows methamphetamine and amphetamine in the patient's urine. After a 3-day hospital stay, the patient is ready for discharge. The outpatient psychiatrist should do which of the following?

(A) Resume psychiatric care through the CMHC, deferring substance dependence treatment unless the patient resumes methamphetamine use.
(B) Resume psychiatric care at the CMHC, with increased emphasis on the provision of substance dependence treatment by the mental health team.
(C) Enroll the patient in a separate program specifically for substance dependence and continue to provide psychiatric care through the CMHC.
(D) Enroll the patient in a separate program specifically for substance dependence and resume psychiatric care at the CMHC once a period of sobriety is achieved.

The correct response is option **B**: Resume psychiatric care at the CMHC, with increased emphasis on the provision of substance dependence treatment by the mental health team

Integrated treatment, in which the same clinicians provide both mental health and substance abuse treatment, has better outcomes than treatment that is split either in a parallel or sequential fashion.

McHugo GJ, Drake RE, Teague GB, Xie H: Fidelity to assertive community treatment and client outcomes in the New Hampshire dual disorders study. Psychiatr Serv 1999; 50:818–824

Drake RE, Osher FC: Treating substance abuse in patients with severe mental illness, in Innovative Approaches for Difficult-to-Treat Populations. Edited by Henggeler SW, Santos AB. Washington, DC, American Psychiatric Press, 1997, pp 191–210

137

Which of the following is the most accurate way to diagnose early-stage dementia of the Alzheimer's type?

(A) Apolipoprotein E genotyping
(B) Brain MRI
(C) History of stepwise memory decline
(D) Neuropsychological testing
(E) Patient self-report of memory difficulties

The correct response is option **D**: Neuropsychological testing

Of the methods listed, neuropsychological testing is the most sensitive, even for very mild deficits in early dementia of the Alzheimer's type. History of stepwise memory decline is associated with vascular dementia. Patient self-report of memory difficulties is notoriously unreliable.

Salmon DP, Thomas RG, Pay MM, Booth A, Hofstetter CR, Thal LJ, Katzman R: Alzheimer's disease can be accurately diagnosed in very mildly impaired individuals. Neurology 2002; 59:1022–1028

138

A man reports that he avoids public urinals even when he has great urgency to urinate. This type of chief complaint is most consistent with a diagnosis of:

(A) body dysmorphic disorder.
(B) obsessive-compulsive disorder.
(C) panic disorder with agoraphobia.
(D) social phobia.
(E) posttraumatic stress disorder.

The correct response is option **D**: Social phobia

The inability to urinate in a public toilet is one of many performance-related anxieties of people with social phobia. Eating, writing, telephoning, and especially speaking in public are all behaviors during which persons with social phobia fear being scrutinized or humiliated. The other options listed could be reasons for avoiding a public toilet—for example, contamination fears (obsessive-compulsive disorder), concern that the penis is abnormal (body dysmorphic disorder), and prior sexual trauma in a public toilet (posttraumatic stress disorder)—but are clinically unlikely.

Stein DJ, Hollander E (eds): American Psychiatric Publishing Textbook of Anxiety Disorders. Washington, DC, American Psychiatric Publishing, 2002, pp 289–290

139

A patient with mild dementia of the Alzheimer's type is brought in by his wife, who is also his primary caregiver, for follow-up evaluation. She brings along a list of his medications. The patient is taking donepezil, hydrochlorothiazide, and warfarin. The use of which of the following herbal or over-the-counter products by this patient would be of the most concern?

(A) Ginkgo biloba
(B) Ginseng
(C) Hawthorn
(D) Vitamin C
(E) Vitamin E

The correct response is option **A**: Ginkgo biloba

Psychiatrists should routinely ask about the use of herbal and over-the-counter preparations, as these are often presumed by patients and caregivers to be safe. Although ginkgo biloba has been widely advertised as having cognitive-enhancing properties, the evidence for its slowing the progression of dementia of the Alzheimer's type is modest. Ginkgo biloba should be avoided by patients taking warfarin, because there have been case reports of intracranial bleeding and hematoma.

De Smet PA: Herbal remedies. N Engl J Med 2002; 347:2046–2056
Jacobson SA, Pies RW, Greenblatt DJ: Handbook of Geriatric Psychopharmacology. Washington, DC, American Psychiatric Publishing, 2002, pp 379–380

140

What diagnostic specifier would be most appropriate for a depressed patient who complains of a sense of leaden paralysis and difficulty being around other people but is able to enjoy himself when good things happen?

(A) With atypical features
(B) With catatonic features
(C) With melancholic features
(D) With psychotic features

The correct response is option **A**: With atypical features

Depression with atypical features includes symptoms of mood reactivity combined with some symptoms of increased sleep, appetite, weight, rejection sensitivity, phobic symptoms, and severe fatigue. Depression with melancholic features includes a loss of pleasure in almost all activities or a loss of enjoyment of usually pleasurable activities combined with some symptoms of depression that are worse in the morning, early morning awakening, weight loss, inappropriate guilt, and either psychomotor retardation or agitation. Depression with catatonic features includes at least two of the following: motor immobility, excessive motor activity, extreme negativism, peculiar voluntary movements, echolalia, or apraxia. Depression with psychotic features refers to the presence of delusions or hallucinations.

American Psychiatric Association: Diagnostic and Statistical Manual of Mental Disorders, Fourth Edition, Text Revision (DSM-IV-TR). Washington, DC, American Psychiatric Association, 2000, pp 420–422
Practice Guideline for the Treatment of Patients With Major Depressive Disorder, 2nd ed (2000), in American Psychiatric Association Practice Guidelines for the Treatment of Psychiatric Disorders, Compendium 2004. Washington, DC, APA, 2004, p 469

141

A 34-year-old woman with two previous episodes of major depressive disorder is treated with 100 mg/day of sertraline. Her most recent episode occurred 9 months ago. At that time sertraline was initiated, with the dose titrated up to 150 mg/day over a 2-week period. Her symptoms remitted after 6 weeks, but she experienced significant sexual side effects that resolved with a decrease in the sertraline dose to 100 mg/day. Over the past 7 months she has remained free of depressive symptoms and now inquires about decreasing her dose of medication. Which of the following recommendations is most appropriate?

(A) Continue sertraline at 100 mg/day.
(B) Decrease sertraline to 50 mg/day and continue at that dose.
(C) Discontinue sertraline after tapering the dose.
(D) Initiate psychotherapy and then decrease sertraline to 50 mg/day.
(E) Initiate psychotherapy and then gradually discontinue sertraline.

The correct response is option **A**: Continue sertraline at 100 mg/day

The same dose that was effective during the acute and continuation phases of treatment should be used during the maintenance phase. In this instance, the initial dose of sertraline was associated with side effects, but a therapeutic response was maintained with a lower dose of medication. While psychotherapy is often indicated, its use does not justify reducing or stopping medication.

Practice Guideline for the Treatment of Patients With Major Depressive Disorder, 2nd ed (2000), in American Psychiatric Association Practice Guidelines for the Treatment of Psychiatric Disorders, Compendium 2004. Washington, DC, APA, 2004, p 456

142

Which of the following antipsychotic drugs has the greatest effect on prolonging the QT interval on the electrocardiogram?

(A) Aripiprazole
(B) Haloperidol
(C) Olanzapine
(D) Thioridazine
(E) Ziprasidone

The correct response is option **D**: Thioridazine

Thioridazine prolongs the QT interval in a dose and blood level dependent fashion, and has a greater effect on the QT interval than most other antipsychotic drugs. In a comparative study, ziprasidone caused a modest QT prolongation, but it was considerably less than that caused by thioridazine.

Taylor DM: Antipsychotics and QT prolongation. Acta Psychiatr Scand 2003; 107:85–95
Harrigan EP, Miceli JJ, Anziano R, Watsky E, Reeves KR, Cutler NR, Sramek J, Shiovitz T, Middle M: A randomized evaluation of the effects of six antipsychotic agents on QTc, in the absence and presence of metabolic inhibition. J Clin Psychopharmacol 2004; 24:62–69
Yap YG, Camm AJ: Drug induced QT prolongation and torsades de pointes. Heart 2003; 89:1363–1372
Witchel HJ, Hancox JC, Nutt DJ: Psychotropic drugs, cardiac arrhythmia, and sudden death. J Clin Psychopharmacol 2003; 23:58–77
Glassman AH, Bigger JT Jr: Antipsychotic drugs: prolonged QTc interval, torsade de pointes, and sudden death. Am J Psychiatry 2001; 158:1774–1782

143

The therapeutic benefit of acamprosate is best established for which of the following conditions?

(A) Alcohol dependence
(B) Barbiturate dependence
(C) Cocaine withdrawal
(D) Heroin addiction
(E) Methamphetamine abuse

The correct response is option **A**: Alcohol dependence

Acamprosate is FDA-approved "for the maintenance of abstinence from alcohol in patients with alcohol dependence who are abstinent at treatment initiation" (Campral package insert). Its efficacy was established in three double-blind placebo-controlled studies ranging in duration from 90 to 360 days. "Acamprosate may not be effective in patients who are actively drinking at the start of treatment, or in patients who abuse other substances in addition to alcohol" (FDA talk paper). Currently no clinical trials of acamprosate for other psychiatric conditions are under way.

Saitz R: Unhealthy alcohol use. N Engl J Med 2005; 352:596–607
Bouza C, Angeles M, Munoz A, Amate JM: Efficacy and safety of naltrexone and acamprosate in the treatment of alcohol dependence: a systematic review. Addiction 2004; 99:811–828
Campral (acamprosate) prescribing information (package insert)
FDA talk paper: FDA approves new drug for treatment of alcoholism, July 29, 2004. Available at http://www.fda.gov/bbs/topics/ANSWERS/2004/ANS01302.html
Mack AH, Frances RJ: Substance-related disorders. FOCUS 2003; 1:125–146 (p 139)

144

A 25-year-old woman with bipolar disorder is about to be started on lamotrigine for maintenance therapy. She should receive one-half of the usual starting dose if she is taking which of the following medications?

(A) Carbamazepine
(B) Lithium
(C) Oral contraceptive
(D) Phenytoin
(E) Valproate

The correct response is option **E**: Valproate

Lamotrigine is metabolized outside the cytochrome P450 system. It undergoes phase II conjugation mainly to an inactive 2-N-glucuronide. Nonetheless, its pharmacokinetics can be altered by other drugs. Enzyme inducers such as carbamazepine, phenytoin, and oral contraceptives lower blood levels of lamotrigine. Lithium has no effect, but valproate inhibits lamotrigine metabolism and doubles its blood level. Dosage adjustment is especially important to minimize the risk of rash.

Jefferson JW: Lamotrigine in psychiatry: pharmacology and therapeutics. CNS Spectr 2005; 10:224–232
Sabers A, Buchholt JM, Uldall P, Hansen EL: Lamotrigine plasma levels reduced by oral contraceptives. Epilepsy Res 2001; 47:151–154
Practice Guideline for the Treatment of Patients With Bipolar Disorder, 2nd ed (2002), in American Psychiatric Association Practice Guidelines for the Treatment of Psychiatric Disorders, Compendium 2004. Washington, DC, APA, 2004, pp 572–573. Reprinted in FOCUS 2003; 1:64–110 (pp 91–92)

145

Of the following, which is the most important factor in determining whether a patient is suited to brief psychodynamic psychotherapy?

(A) Ability to recognize and discuss feelings
(B) Existence of multiple conflicts
(C) Compliance with medication
(D) Lack of meaningful relationships
(E) Failure of long-term psychodynamic psychotherapy

The correct response is option **A**: Ability to recognize and discuss feelings

Patient selection for brief psychodynamic psychotherapy requires that the patient has a focal conflict, is able to think in feeling terms, is highly motivated, has had at least one meaningful relationship, and has had a good response to a trial interpretation. Complex or deep-seated issues require more time. The patient who reports having had at least one meaningful relationship with another person during his or her life will have better object relations and be better able to tolerate the difficult feelings that can be stirred up by psychotherapy.

Ursano RJ, Sonnenberg SM, Lazar SG: Concise Guide to Psychodynamic Psychotherapy, 3rd ed. Washington, DC, American Psychiatric Publishing, 2004, p 179

146

Compared with men, women with schizophrenia taking equivalent doses per weight of antipsychotics are less likely to have which of the following?

(A) Acute dystonia
(B) Drug-drug interactions
(C) Lower serum drug levels
(D) Sedation

The correct response is option **C**: Lower serum drug levels

Studies indicate that women have higher serum levels of antipsychotic medications compared with men. Women are more likely to be taking other drugs, such as contraceptives, and hence are at greater risk of drug-drug interactions. On equivalent doses, women appear to have more acute dystonia. Sedation appears to occur equally in men and women.

Seeman MV: Gender differences in the prescribing of antipsychotic drugs. Am J Psychiatry 2004; 161:1324–1333. Reprinted in FOCUS 2006; 4:115–124

147

A 22-year-old man presents at the emergency department with agitated, guarded behavior, paranoid delusional thoughts, and a 7-month history consistent with a diagnosis of schizophrenia, paranoid type. Understanding the man's cultural background would be most helpful for:

(A) choosing his acute and maintenance medications.
(B) determining the cause of his disorder.
(C) determining safety issues and the need for hospitalization.
(D) understanding the content of the delusions and hallucinations.

The correct response is option **D**: Understanding the content of the delusions and hallucinations

Culture can influence the content of hallucinations and delusions. Schizophrenia is thought to occur at similar prevalence rates worldwide. The other options listed are generally decided on the basis of the patient's psychiatric status.

Sadock BJ, Sadock VA (eds): Kaplan and Sadock's Comprehensive Textbook of Psychiatry, 8th ed. Philadelphia, Lippincott Williams & Wilkins, 2005, pp 616–617

148

Hypertension is most associated with which of the following medications?

(A) Bupropion
(B) Fluvoxamine
(C) Mirtazapine
(D) Paroxetine
(E) Venlafaxine

The correct response is option **E**: Venlafaxine

Venlafaxine is the antidepressant most associated with a sustained hypertension (systolic blood pressure greater than 90 mm Hg and greater than 10 mm Hg above baseline for three consecutive visits). It tends to occur most frequently with doses above 300 mg but can occur at any dose. There is also a venlafaxine withdrawal syndrome that consists mainly of gastrointestinal and neurological symptoms. The other antidepressants listed do not have sustained or significant hypertensive effects.

Sadock BJ, Sadock VA (eds): Kaplan and Sadock's Comprehensive Textbook of Psychiatry, 7th ed. Philadelphia, Lippincott Williams & Wilkins, 2000, p 2430

149

A patient reports regularly taking a drug bought on the street. Its effect is pleasurable, but it sometimes causes nausea, restlessness, and teeth grinding. The drug is most likely:

(A) methamphetamine.
(B) flunitrazepam (Rohypnol).
(C) methylenedioxymethamphetamine (MDMA).
(D) cocaine.

The correct response is option **C**: Methylenedioxymethamphetamine (MDMA)

Methylenedioxymethamphetamine (MDMA, or "Ecstasy") both releases and inhibits the reuptake of serotonin. Although MDMA is a synthetic amphetamine derivative, its effects are quite different from those of its parent drug. Flunitrazepam, best known as Rohypnol, is a rapid-acting benzodiazepine that is available only illegally in the United States.

Morgan MJ: Ecstasy (MDMA): a review of its possible persistent psychological effects. Psychopharmacology 2000; 152:230–248
McDowell DM: MDMA, ketamine, GHB, and the "club drug" scene, in The American Psychiatric Press Textbook of Substance Abuse Treatment, 3rd ed. Edited by Galanter M, Kleber HD. Washington, DC, American Psychiatric Publishing, 2004 pp 321–333

150

Indications of caffeine withdrawal:

(A) are evident following an average intake of 50 mg/day.
(B) include symptoms that typically last 3 weeks.
(C) include a flushed face and diuresis.
(D) include headache.

The correct response is option **D**: Include headache

Caffeine withdrawal effects can be seen at doses as low as 100 mg/day. Withdrawal effects may include headache, fatigue, drowsiness, nausea, and vomiting. Withdrawal headaches can cause functional impairment. Flushing of the face and diuresis are characteristics of caffeine intoxication. Caffeine withdrawal effects usually begin within 12 hours, peak around 24 to 48 hours, and last up to 1 week.

Strain EC, Griffiths RR: Caffeine use disorders, in Psychiatry, 2nd ed. Edited by Tasman A, Kay J, Lieberman JA. Philadelphia, WB Saunders, 1997, pp 779–794

151

A 23-year-old college student from Ethiopia is admitted to the hospital for a psychotic disorder. His symptoms include paranoid ideation, hallucinations, and disorganized thinking. He is initially started on 0.5 mg of risperidone twice daily, which is rapidly titrated to 4 mg/day. Despite this treatment, there is no improvement in his symptoms. No detectable plasma levels of the parent compound are noted. What is the most likely explanation for these results?

(A) Binding of the drug to fatty tissue
(B) First-pass effect
(C) Impaired absorption of the drug
(D) Increased excretion
(E) Ultrarapid metabolism of the drug

The correct response is option **E**: Ultrarapid metabolism of the drug

The metabolism of risperidone is contingent on the activity of the CYP2D6 enzyme, which in turn is genetically determined. Nearly one-third of North Africans and Middle Easterners have multiple alleles for this enzyme and consequently are ultrarapid metabolizers of medications using the CYP2D6 enzyme. Treatment approaches may include the addition of medications such as paroxetine, which inhibits CYP2D6, thus allowing for therapeutic dosages of risperidone. Approximately 7% of Caucasians and 25% of East Asians lack this enzyme and are poor metabolizers of risperidone.

Tseng WS, Streltzer J: Cultural Competence in Clinical Practice. Washington, DC, American Psychiatric Publishing, 2004, pp 169–170
De Leon J, Armstrong SC, Cozza KL: Clinical guidelines for psychiatrists for the use of pharmacogenetic testing for CYP450 2D6 and CYP450 2C19. Psychosomatics 2006; 47:75–85

152

The preferred initial pharmacological treatment for a 26-year-old woman who was violently assaulted 3 years ago and suffers from recurrent nightmares about the event, hypervigilance, difficulty concentrating, and constricted range of affect would be:

(A) alprazolam.
(B) clomipramine.
(C) clonidine.
(D) valproate.
(E) sertraline.

The correct response is option **E**: Sertraline

According to the APA Practice Guideline for the Treatment of Acute Stress Disorder and Posttraumatic Stress Disorder, "Evidence from several large randomized, double-blind controlled trials suggests that SSRIs are first-line medication treatment for both men and women with PTSD." Sertraline and paroxetine are the only drugs approved by the FDA for this indication. The successful use of clonidine and valproate has been restricted to small, open-label studies. Alprazolam was demonstrated in a controlled trial to be ineffective in the treatment of posttraumatic stress disorder.

American Psychiatric Association: Practice Guideline for the Treatment of Acute Stress Disorder and Posttraumatic Stress Disorder. Am J Psychiatry 2004; 161(Nov suppl)
Schemed FB, Marmar CR, Neylan TC: Current concepts in pharmacotherapy for posttraumatic stress disorder. Psychiatr Serv 2004; 55:519–531
Hidalgo RB, Davidson JRT: Diagnostic and pharmacologic aspects of posttraumatic stress disorder. Psychiatr Ann 2004; 34:837–841

153

In the initial assessment of a depressed patient, what is the most critical decision that the psychiatrist must make?

(A) Type of psychotherapy
(B) Choice of medication
(C) Level of care
(D) Medical workup
(E) Involvement of family

The correct response is option **C**: Level of care

Patients who present to the psychiatrist must be assessed for suicidality, which will often determine the need for hospitalization. The initial determination of the safety of the patient is paramount.

Sadock BJ, Sadock VA (eds): Kaplan and Sadock's Comprehensive Textbook of Psychiatry, 7th ed. Philadelphia, Lippincott Williams & Wilkins, 2000, pp 662–663, 2038–2040

154

A 27-year-old patient announces that she is pregnant despite having taken an oral contraceptive for 4 years. Which of the following medications might account for the failure of her oral contraceptive?

(A) Lithium
(B) Divalproex
(C) Carbamazepine
(D) Lamotrigine
(E) Gabapentin

The correct response is option **C**: Carbamazepine

Carbamazepine as well as oxcarbazepine are inducers of the cytochrome P450 system and therefore can lower serum concentrations of estrogen in birth control pills. Gabapentin has few drug interactions, and it has been shown to have no effect on ethinyl estradiol levels. Carbamazepine and oxcarbazepine, by contrast, reduce ethinyl estradiol levels by about 50% and topiramate by 18% to 25%. Breakthrough bleeding and an increased risk of pregnancy are possible complications associated with a reduced ethinyl estradiol level. Lamotrigine does not have pharmacokinetic interactions that could potentially lead to decreased oral contraceptive efficacy. However, in a series of seven cases, oral contraceptives were found to decrease lamotrigine levels by a mean of 49%.

Wilbur K, Ensom MHH: Pharmacokinetic drug interactions between oral contraceptives and second-generation anticonvulsants. Clin Pharmacokinet 2000; 38:355–365
Sabers A, Buchholt JM, Uldall P, Hansen EL: Lamotrigine plasma levels reduced by oral contraceptives. Epilepsy Res 2001; 47:151–154

Schatzberg AF, Nemeroff CB (eds): The American Psychiatric Publishing Textbook of Psychopharmacology, 3rd ed. Washington, DC, American Psychiatric Publishing, 2004, pp 598–599

155

Screening for hepatitis C (HCV) infection is LEAST important in patients with:

(A) methamphetamine dependence.
(B) marijuana dependence.
(C) heroin dependence.
(D) history of blood transfusion (before 1992).
(E) hemodialysis.

The correct response is option **B**: Marijuana dependence

Injection drug use is more common among patients who abuse stimulants and opioids than among marijuana abusers. The most well established risk factors for HCV are intravenous drug use, blood or blood product transfusions prior to 1992, and hemodialysis. Screening for patients with one or more of these risk factors has been recommended by CDC.

Rifai MA, Rosenstein DL: Hepatitis C and Psychiatry. FOCUS 3:194-195
Hagan H, Des Jarlais DC: HIV and HCV infection among injecting drug users. Mt Sinai J Med 2000; 67:423–428

156

Which of the following is best characterized as a degenerative dementia?

(A) Systemic lupus erythematosus
(B) Korsakoff's syndrome
(C) Parkinson's disease
(D) HIV disease
(E) Cerebrovascular accident

The correct response is option **C**: Parkinson's disease

Degenerative dementias, such as Parkinson's disease and Huntington's disease, are distinguished from non-degenerative dementias by intrinsic genetic processes that lead to neuron destruction rather than complications from systemic medical conditions or insults.

Plizka SR: Neuroscience for the Mental Health Clinician. New York, Guilford, 2003, p 257
Levenson JL: American Psychiatric Publishing Textbook of Psychosomatic Medicine, Table 7-3, Disorders that may produce dementia syndromes. Washington, DC, American Psychiatric Publishing, 2005, p 133

157

In a urine test for phencyclidine, a false positive test result can occur if a person has ingested:

(A) dextromethorphan.
(B) ibuprofen.
(C) tonic water.
(D) phenylephrine.
(E) diphenhydramine.

The correct response is option **A**: Dextromethorphan

Dextromethorphan can cause a false positive test result for phencyclidine. Ibuprofen can cause a false positive test result for marijuana metabolites. Tonic water can cause a false positive test result for opiates. Phenylephrine can cause a false positive test result for amphetamines. Diphenhydramine does not affect urine drug tests.

Tests for drugs of abuse. Medical Letter on Drugs and Therapeutics 2002, vol 44 (W1137A), August 19

158

A 48-year-old man is admitted to the hospital with cholecystitis, and after diagnosis he consents to and undergoes a cholecystectomy. On the third hospital day he becomes angry at the nursing staff and wishes to leave the hospital against medical advice. In assessing this patient's capacity to refuse further medical care, which of the following questions would be most useful for the psychiatrist to ask?

(A) Have you discussed with your family your decision to leave?
(B) What is the danger of your going home at this time?
(C) Have you been troubled by depression?
(D) Are you able to name all of your medications?
(E) When did you first become ill, and do you remember your symptoms?

The correct response is option **B**: What is the danger of your going home at this time?

Central to the patient's ability to make health care decisions is the understanding of the risks and benefits of one choice over another. Certainly the other questions are helpful in gaining this understanding, but they are not the key concern. In addition, by day three of hospitalization, concern about the presence of a delirium, withdrawal syndrome, or other metabolic syndrome is raised. The patient had been agreeable for all treatments before this time, having already agreed to the surgery and postoperative treatments.

Appelbaum PS, Grisso T: Assessing patients' capacities to consent to treatment. N Engl J Med 1988; 319:1635–1668

159

Which of the following disorders has been shown to have genetic or familial links?

(A) Autistic disorder
(B) Dissociative amnesia
(C) Factitious disorder
(D) Hypoactive sexual desire disorder
(E) Pyromania

The correct response is option **A**: Autistic disorder

Data from twin studies suggests that a substantial portion of the liability to autism is genetic in origin. The other disorders have not been shown to have genetic risk.

Popper CW, Gammon, GD, West SA, Bailey CE: Disorders usually first diagnosed in infancy, childhood, or adolescence, in The American Psychiatric Publishing Textbook of Clinical Psychiatry, 4th ed. Edited by Hales RE, Yudofsky SC. Washington, DC, American Psychiatric Publishing, 2003, pp 894–895

160

A 45-year-old man and his monozygotic twin have been diagnosed as having the same personality disorder. Which of the following diagnoses is most likely?

(A) Histrionic personality disorder
(B) Obsessive-compulsive personality disorder
(C) Narcissistic personality disorder
(D) Antisocial personality disorder
(E) Avoidant personality disorder

The correct response is option **D**: Antisocial personality disorder

Antisocial personality disorder has the highest estimated heritability of the personality disorders listed (approximately 60%–70%). Borderline personality disorder, in particular the emotional dysregulation characteristic of this disorder, also has a strong heritability.

Fu Q, Heath AC, Bucholz KK, Nelson E, Goldberg J, Lyons MJ, True WR, Jacob T, Tsuang MT, Eisen SA: Shared genetic risk of major depression, alcohol dependence, and marijuana dependence: contribution of antisocial personality disorder in men. Arch Gen Psychiatry 2002; 59:1125–1132

Lieb K, Zanarini MC, Schmahl C, Linehan MM, Bohus M: Borderline personality disorder. Lancet 2004; 364:453–461

161

Which of the following medication classes is the preferred treatment for obsessive-compulsive disorder?

(A) Atypical antipsychotics
(B) Anticonvulsants
(C) Mood stabilizers
(D) SSRIs
(E) Benzodiazepines

The correct response is option **D**: SSRIs

Numerous double-blind, placebo-controlled studies have found serotonin reuptake inhibiting antidepressants to be effective in the treatment of obsessive-compulsive disorder (clomipramine and SSRIs). Several antidepressants have been approved by the Food and Drug Administration for this indication.

Stein DJ: Obsessive-compulsive disorder. Lancet 2002; 360:397–405
Park LT, Jefferson JW, Greist JG: Obsessive-compulsive disorder: treatment options. CNS Drugs 1997; 7:187–202
Hollander E, Simeon D: Concise Guide to Anxiety Disorders. Washington, DC, American Psychiatric Publishing, 2003, p 170

162

Which of the following interventions is the best first step in the management of agitation in the elderly patient?

(A) Haloperidol, 5 mg twice a day, whatever the cause of the agitation
(B) Physical restraints
(C) Evaluation of the patient's surroundings and daily schedule
(D) Diazepam, 5 mg every 6 hours, or until the patient is asleep
(E) Seclusion until the behavior ceases

The correct response is option **C**: Evaluation of the patient's surroundings and daily schedule

The initial assessment of a geriatric patient with agitation should begin with a thorough psychiatric and medical assessment, including initial laboratory assessments and collateral information from the patient's caregiver; a diurnal and longitudinal record of the behavior; an accounting of any changes in environment or routine; an assessment of functional ability; and a schedule of daily activity. All prescription and nonprescription medications should be reviewed. The patient should also be evaluated for trauma or pain.

Cheong JA: An evidence-based approach to the management of agitation in the geriatric patient. FOCUS 2004; 2:197–205 (pp 198–203)

163

Which of the following will double the blood level of lamotrigine?

(A) Carbamazepine
(B) Divalproex
(C) Phenytoin
(D) Phenobarbital

The correct response is option **B**: Divalproex

Valproate (divalproex) reduces the clearance of lamotrigine by about 50%, whereas the other three drugs listed actually increase lamotrigine clearance and reduce lamotrigine blood levels by 40% to 50%. The valproate/lamotrigine interaction is important, because unless dosage adjustments are made, the risk of serious rash will be increased.

Benedetti MS: Enzyme induction and inhibition by new antiepileptic drugs: a review of human studies. Fundam Clin Pharmacol 2000; 14:305–319
Kannen AM, Frey M: Adding valproate to lamotrigine: a study of their pharmacokinetic interaction. Neurology 2000; 55:588–591
Riva R, Albani F, Contin M, Baruzzi A: Pharmacokinetic interactions between antiepileptic drugs: clinical considerations. Clin Pharmacokinet 1996; 31:470–493

164

Buspirone has been found to be most consistently effective in the treatment of which of the following anxiety disorders?

(A) Generalized anxiety disorder
(B) Obsessive-compulsive disorder
(C) Panic disorder with agoraphobia
(D) Panic disorder without agoraphobia
(E) Social phobia

The correct response is option **A**: Generalized anxiety disorder

Although trials have been conducted on the use of buspirone in the treatment of all the anxiety disorders, efficacy in multiple trials has been shown only for generalized anxiety disorder.

Davidson JR: Pharmacotherapy of social phobia. Acta Psychiatr Scand Suppl 2003; 417:65–71
Hollander E, Simeon D: Anxiety disorders, in American Psychiatric Publishing Textbook of Clinical Psychiatry, 4th ed. Edited by Hales RE, Yudofsky SC. Washington, DC, American Psychiatric Publishing, 2003, pp 543–630

165

Which of the following parental transmissions of the fragile X trinucleotide repeat is most likely to result in an affected child?

- (A) Mother-to-daughter
- (B) Mother-to-son
- (C) Father-to-daughter
- (D) Father-to-son
- (E) No parental gender difference

The correct response is option **B**: Mother-to-son

The basic inheritance pattern of an X-linked disease is mother to son. Although females can inherit the gene, they are less likely to be affected because they usually have a normal X chromosome as well. As fragile X syndrome is an X-linked disease, fathers cannot pass it on to their sons.

Sadock BJ, Sadock VA (eds): Kaplan and Sadock's Comprehensive Textbook of Psychiatry, 8th ed. Philadelphia, Lippincott Williams & Wilkins, 2005, p 2283

166

Which of the following is NOT a relative contraindication for the use of disulfiram as an adjunct in the treatment of alcohol dependence?

- (A) Impulsive behavior
- (B) Psychotic symptoms
- (C) Suicidal thoughts
- (D) A family history of alcoholism
- (E) Impaired judgment

The correct response is option **D**: A family history of alcoholism

Patients with impulsive, psychotic symptoms and suicidal thoughts are poor candidates for disulfiram treatment, given the adverse effects of drinking alcohol while taking disulfiram. Disulfiram inhibits the activity of the enzyme aldehyde dehydrogenase, which metabolizes acetaldehyde, a major metabolite of alcohol. If alcohol is consumed in the presence of disulfiram, toxicity secondary to acetaldehyde accumulation may occur.

Patients who are intelligent, motivated, and not impulsive and whose drinking is often triggered by unanticipated internal or external cues that increase alcohol craving are the best candidates for disulfiram treatment. Poor candidates include patients who are impulsive, have poor judgment, or are suffering from a comorbid psychiatric illness (e.g., schizophrenia, major depression) whose severity makes them unreliable or self-destructive. Disulfiram treatment should be avoided in patients with moderate to severe hepatic dysfunction, peripheral neuropathies, pregnancy, renal failure, or cardiac disease.

American Psychiatric Association: Practice Guideline for the Treatment of Patients With Substance Use Disorders: Alcohol, Cocaine, Opioids. Am J Psychiatry 1995; 152(Nov suppl)

167

Which of the following signs and symptoms is more likely to occur in females than in males at first presentation of psychosis?

- (A) Amotivation
- (B) Cognitive impairment
- (C) Dysphoric mood state
- (D) Paranoid ideation
- (E) Social isolation

The correct response is option **C**: Dysphoric mood state

At first presentation of psychosis, it has been shown that males are more likely than females to show cognitive deficits and females are more likely than males to show depression. These sex differences are most prominent in the preadolescent and adolescent periods. Affective symptoms, particularly depression, are associated with a better prognosis for schizophrenia and psychotic disorders in general and may explain the more favorable prognosis for women with schizophrenia.

Romans SE, Seeman MV: Women's Mental Health: A Life-Cycle Approach. Philadelphia, Lippincott Williams & Wilkins, 2006, p 196
Burt VK, Hendrick VC: Gender Issues in the treatment of mental illness, in Clinical Manual of Women's Mental Health. Washington, DC, American Psychiatric Publishing, 2005, p 148. Reprinted in FOCUS 2006; 4:66–80
Quick reference for schizophrenia. FOCUS 2004; 2:13–16

168

A 45-year-old woman complains of blurred vision, ocular pain, and headache and was noted to have increased intraocular pressure. Which of the recently started medications is the most likely cause?

(A) Lamotrigine
(B) Oxcarbazepine
(C) Tiagabine
(D) Topiramate
(E) Valproate

The correct response is option **D**: Topiramate

Topiramate is the only drug of those listed whose use has been associated with acute secondary angle-closure glaucoma. Symptoms typically begin early in the course of treatment and include blurred vision, ocular pain, and headache. If recognized early, full recovery is likely after drug discontinuation.

Fraunfelder FW, Fraunfelder FT, Keates EU: Topiramate-associated acute, bilateral secondary angle-closure glaucoma. Ophthalmology 2004; 111:109–111
Topamax (topiramate) prescribing information (package insert)
Thambi L, Kapcala LP, Chambers W, Nourjah P, Beitz J, Chen M, Lu S: Topiramate-associated secondary angle-closure glaucoma: a case series. Arch Ophthalmol 2002; 120:1108

169

A married 50-year-old woman is admitted to the hospital with an acute myocardial infarction. It is recommended that she have a cardiac catheterization with a possible procedure based on the findings. The patient refuses. Which of the following would be a reasonable approach to the patient at this time?

(A) Discharge the patient to home so that she can make up her mind.
(B) Call for a family meeting with her husband and adult children to discuss the options.
(C) Tell her that there is no guarantee that she wouldn't die if she leaves the hospital without treatment.
(D) Consider treatment for depression since she does not seem to want to live.
(E) Recommend treatment against her will because of the seriousness of the condition.

The correct response is option **B**: Call for a family meeting with her husband and adult children to discuss the options

The patient needs an assessment of her capacity to make this decision. A relatively young woman, she is likely fearful and struggling with this new diagnosis. Her family would be able to help explain some of her long-standing health beliefs as well as to support her through this difficult time. Even though this is a serious condition, without evaluating her capacity and engaging the family, there are no grounds for treating her against her will at this time.

Schouten R: Legal aspects of consultation, in Massachusetts General Hospital Handbook of General Hospital Psychiatry, 5th ed. Edited by Stern TA, Fricchione GL, Cassem NH, Jellinek MS, Rosenbaum JF. St Louis, Mosby, 2004, pp 349–362

170

Which of the following treatments is most effective for patients with bulimia nervosa and major depressive disorder?

(A) Cognitive behavior therapy
(B) Fluoxetine
(C) Imipramine
(D) Bupropion
(E) Combined cognitive behavior therapy and fluoxetine

The correct response is option **E**: Combined cognitive behavior therapy and fluoxetine

Cognitive behavior psychotherapy is the psychosocial intervention for which there is the most evidence of efficacy. A high percentage of treatment-seeking patients with eating disorders report a lifetime history of unipolar depression. Depression can impair a patient's ability to become meaningfully involved in psychotherapy and may dictate the need for medication treatment for the mood symptoms from the beginning of treatment.

The only medication approved by the Food and Drug Administration for bulimia nervosa is fluoxetine. Imipramine has also demonstrated efficacy. Bupropion has been associated with seizures in purging bulimic patients, so its use is not recommended.

Practice Guideline for the Treatment of Patients With Eating Disorders, 2nd ed (2000), in American Psychiatric Association Practice Guidelines for the Treatment of Psychiatric Disorders, Compendium 2004. Washington, DC, APA, 2004, p 717
Schatzberg AF, Nemeroff CB (eds): The American Psychiatric Publishing Textbook of Psychopharmacology, 3rd ed, Washington, DC, American Psychiatric Publishing, 2004, pp 1032–1035
Kotler LA, Devlin MJ, Davies M, Walsh BT: An open trial of fluoxetine for adolescents with bulimia nervosa. J Child Adolesc Psychopharmacol 2003; 13:329–335

Which of the following describes the American Academy of Pediatrics statement regarding maternal lithium use during breast-feeding?

(A) Associated with significant side effects in some nursing infants; use with caution
(B) Unknown effects on nursing infants; may be of concern
(C) Absolutely contraindicated
(D) Usually compatible

The correct response is option **A**: Associated with significant side effects in some nursing infants; use with caution

The American Academy of Pediatrics Committee on Drugs has stated that lithium has been associated with significant effects on some nursing infants and should be given to nursing mothers with caution. Lithium concentrations in breast milk are approximately 40% of maternal serum concentrations, and infant serum concentrations may be similar to or lower than milk levels. Nonetheless, there is only one convincing case of lithium intoxication in a breast-feeding infant, and it was associated with an intercurrent infection. Many experts do not view this contraindication as absolute but rather recognize the need to balance benefits and risks on an individual basis.

Burt VK, Suri R, Altshuler L, Stowe Z, Hendrick VC, Muntean E: The use of psychotropic medications during breast-feeding. Am J Psychiatry 2001; 158:1001–1009
American Academy of Pediatrics: The transfer of drugs and other chemicals into human milk. American Academy of Pediatrics committee on drug policy statement. Pediatrics 2001; 108:776–789. Available at http://aappolicy.aappublications.org/cgi/content/full/pediatrics;108/3/776.

Treatment with which of the following cytokines has been linked to suicidal behavior?

(A) Erythropoietin
(B) Granulocyte colony-stimulating factor
(C) Interferon-α
(D) Interleukin-1 receptor agonist
(E) Anti-tumor-necrosis-factor antibodies

The correct response is option **C**: Interferon-α

Interferon-α has been associated with fatigue, depression, cognitive impairment, psychosis, and suicidal ideation. The other medications listed have a negligible or undetermined effect on mental state.

Kronfol Z, Remick DG: Cytokines and the brain: implications for clinical psychiatry. Am J Psychiatry 2000; 157:683–694

The amygdala is most specifically involved in which of the following brain functions?

(A) Determining social behavior
(B) Emotional coding of sensory cues
(C) Generating normal sleep patterns
(D) Recalling previously learned material
(E) Signaling reward by exogenous substances

The correct response is option **B**: Emotional coding of sensory cues

The amygdala plays an important role in emotional functioning. The hippocampus is involved in recalling previously learned material. The frontal cortex is more involved in determining social behavior. The thalamus is more involved in generating normal sleep patterns. The nucleus accumbens and the ventral tegmentum are more involved in signaling reward by exogenous substances.

Fudge JL, Emiliano AB: The extended amygdala and the dopamine system: another piece of the dopamine puzzle. J Neuropsychiatry Clin Neurosci 2003; 15:306–316
Mah LW, Arnold MC, Grafman J: Deficits in social knowledge following damage to ventromedial prefrontal cortex. J Neuropsychiatry Clin Neurosci 2005; 17:66–74
Taber KH, Wen C, Khan A, Hurley RA: The limbic thalamus. J Neuropsychiatry Clin Neurosci 2004; 16:127–132
Tekin S, Cummings JL: Frontal-subcortical neuronal circuits and clinical neuropsychiatry: an update. J Psychosom Res 2002; 53:647

174

A 22-year-old woman wants to take an antidepressant for treatment of her major depression but is concerned about possible sexual side effects. Which of the following medications is the best choice for her?

(A) Bupropion
(B) Clomipramine
(C) Escitalopram
(D) Sertraline
(E) Venlafaxine

The correct response is option **A**: Bupropion

In placebo-controlled clinical trials bupropion has been shown to be associated with far less orgasm dysfunction (similar to placebo) than fluoxetine, escitalopram, and sertraline. In general, the agents that increase serotonergic tone tend to be more likely to cause sexual dysfunction in both men and women. A large primary care survey also found more sexual dysfunction with venlafaxine than with bupropion. Sexual dysfunction is a common side effect of clomipramine.

Croft H, Settle E Jr, Houser T, Batey SR, Donahue RM, Ascher JA: A placebo-controlled comparison of the antidepressant efficacy and effects on sexual functioning of sustained-release bupropion and sertraline. Clin Ther 1999; 21:643–658

Clayton AH, Pradko JF, Croft HA, Montano CB, Leadbetter RA, Bolden-Watson C, Bass KI, Donahue RM, Jamerson BD, Metz A: Prevalence of sexual dysfunction among newer antidepressants. J Clin Psychiatry 2002; 63:357–366

Clayton A, Wightman D, Modell JG, Horrigan J, Richard NE: Effects in MDD on sexual functioning of bupropion XL, escitalopram, and placebo in depressed patients, in 2005 Annual Meeting New Research Program and Abstracts. Arlington, Va, American Psychiatric Association, 2003, number 821

175

Which of the following factors is UNRELATED to a positive treatment outcome for cocaine dependence?

(A) Counseling rapport
(B) Treatment retention
(C) Patient choice of program type
(D) Comorbid depressive symptoms

The correct response is option **C**: Patient choice of program type

A patient's choice of one program compared with another does not seem to have a significant impact on treatment outcome. Considerable research has been done in recent years to try to uncover useful correlations between treatment outcomes and patient characteristics, program characteristics, and interaction variables.

Joe GW, Simpson DD, Danserau DF, Rowan-Szal GA: Relationships between counseling rapport and drug abuse treatment outcomes. Psychiatr Serv 2001; 52:1223–1229

Gottheil E, Weinstein SP, Sterling RC, Lundy A, Serota RD: A randomized controlled study of the effectiveness of intensive outpatient treatment for cocaine dependence. Psychiatr Serv 1998; 49:782–787

Brown RA, Monti PM, Myers MG, Martin RA, Rivinus T, Dubreuil ME, Rohsenow DJ: Depression among cocaine abusers in treatment: relation to cocaine and alcohol use and treatment outcomes. Am J Psychiatry 1998; 155:220–225

Ritsher JB, Moos RH, Finney JW: Relationship of treatment orientation and continuing care to remission among substance abuse patients. Psychiatr Serv 2002; 53:595–601

176

Weight gain is most likely to occur with which of the following antipsychotic drugs?

(A) Aripiprazole
(B) Clozapine
(C) Haloperidol
(D) Ziprasidone
(E) Risperidone

The correct response is option **B**: Clozapine

Studies of the various antipsychotic drugs have found weight gain to be most likely to occur with clozapine and next most commonly with olanzapine. It is important to realize that not everyone who takes those drugs gains weight and that weight gain can complicate the use of other antipsychotic drugs as well. Olanzapine and clozapine are listed as having a comparable risk of weight gain in the summary table of the schizophrenia practice guideline, and the difference between them, if any, is minor.

Allison DB, Mentore JL, Heo M, Chandler LP, Cappelleri JC, Infante MC, Weiden PJ: Antipsychotic-induced weight gain: a comprehensive research synthesis. Am J Psychiatry 1999; 156:1686–1696

American Psychiatric Association: Practice Guideline for the Treatment of Patients With Schizophrenia, 2nd ed. Am J Psychiatry 2004; 161(Feb suppl):1–56

Zimmermann U, Kraus T, Himmerich H, Schuld A, Pollmacher T: Epidemiology, implications, and mechanisms underlying drug-induced weight gain in psychiatric patients. J Psychiatr Res 2003; 37:193–220

177

A 16-year-old female patient is admitted to the hospital for gastric rupture. On interview, she reports that in the past 2 months, whenever she has felt anxious, angry, or sad, she has eaten unusually large quantities of cookies, candy, crackers, "or whatever I can get my hands on like I'm a maniac, totally out of control." She reports that after gorging, she feels better emotionally but is afraid that she will "get fat." She gags herself to induce vomiting, and recently she has begun drinking ipecac as an emetic after such episodes. This morning, after an episode of self-induced vomiting, she developed severe abdominal pain and was brought to the emergency department by her parents. On physical examination, her height is 5'6" and her weight is 120 pounds. The psychotherapy that has been found to be most effective in treating her eating disorder is:

(A) cognitive behavior therapy.
(B) family therapy.
(C) group therapy.
(D) psychodynamically oriented individual therapy.

The correct response is option **A**: Cognitive behavior therapy

The characteristics of this teenage girl's eating disorder include frenzied binges in response to a dysphoric mood state; compensatory purging out of fear of becoming fat; and normal weight. This presentation is most consistent with bulimia nervosa. More than 35 controlled studies have found cognitive behavior therapy (CBT) to be the most effective treatment for bulimia nervosa, and CBT is now considered the first-line treatment for this disorder. Some empirical studies have demonstrated the efficacy of family and group therapy and the use of selective serotonin reuptake inhibitors in the treatment of bulimia. There is no research evidence to support the use of psychodynamically oriented individual therapy.

Lewis M (ed): Child and Adolescent Psychiatry: A Comprehensive Textbook, 3rd ed. Philadelphia, Lippincott Williams & Wilkins, 2002, p 697
Mehler PS: Bulimia nervosa. N Engl J Med 2003; 349:875–881

178

Despite intensive psychosocial treatment for alcohol dependence, a patient continues to drink alcohol. The psychiatrist decides to recommend adjunctive medication. Which of the following medications would NOT be an acceptable treatment?

(A) Disulfiram
(B) Bromocriptine
(C) Naltrexone
(D) Ondansetron
(E) Acamprosate

The correct response is option **B**: Bromocriptine

Bromocriptine has been tested for the treatment of cocaine dependence with inconsistent results. The other listed medications are used in the treatment of alcohol dependence. Use of ondansetron in treating alcohol dependence is off-label, and this agent is used less commonly than the other three.

Johnson BA, Roache JD, Javors MA, DiClemente CC, Cloninger CR, Prihoda TJ, Bordnick PS, Ait-Daoud N, Hensler J: Ondansetron for reduction of drinking among biologically predisposed alcoholic patients: a randomized controlled trial. JAMA 2000; 284:963–971
Schuckit MA, Tapert S: Alcohol, in The American Psychiatric Publishing Textbook of Substance Abuse Treatment, 3rd ed. Edited by Galanter M, Kleber HD. Washington, DC, American Psychiatric Publishing, 2004, p 162

179

The anxiety disorder that includes a dissociation-like phenomenon in its criteria is:

(A) generalized anxiety disorder.
(B) obsessive-compulsive disorder.
(C) panic disorder.
(D) posttraumatic stress disorder.
(E) social phobia.

The correct response is option **D**: Posttraumatic stress disorder

Intrusive episodes of recall account for one of the three major symptom complexes in PTSD. The others are avoidance with numbing and increased arousal. An integral part of the intrusive symptoms are flashbacks that are thought to be dissociative experiences. Dissociation may occur in other anxiety disorders, such as panic disorder and generalized anxiety disorder, but it is not a regular component of those syndromes.

Stein DJ, Hollander E (eds): American Psychiatric Publishing Textbook of Anxiety Disorders. Washington, DC, American Psychiatric Publishing, 2002, pp 362–363, 404

180

Patients with which of the following personality disorders would be expected to benefit most from adjunctive pharmacotherapy?

(A) Borderline
(B) Schizoid
(C) Antisocial
(D) Obsessive-compulsive
(E) Dependent

The correct response is option **A**: Borderline

Targeting specific symptoms with medications rather than disorders per se currently appears to be the most effective approach. Pharmacotherapy appears to be most helpful for borderline personality disorder, given that medications can be effective for problems with affective dysfunction, impulsive-behavioral issues, and cognitive-perceptual problems. There is little evidence for the utility of medications for treating the major symptoms of antisocial personality disorder. Obsessive-compulsive personality disorder and dependent personality disorder are treated with psychotherapy.

Phillips KA, Yen S, Gunderson JG: Personality disorders, in The American Psychiatric Publishing Textbook of Psychiatry, 4th ed. Edited by Hales RE, Yudofsky SC. Washington, DC, American Psychiatric Publishing, 2003, pp 810–825

181

When assessing a patient's suitability for short-term psychodynamic psychotherapy, of the following factors, which is the most important?

(A) The DSM-IV-TR diagnosis
(B) Family psychiatric history
(C) Level of education
(D) An identifiable focus
(E) Need for psychoactive medication

The correct response is option **D**: An identifiable focus

While different models for short-term dynamic therapy stress different selection criteria, there is general agreement that traditional diagnostic categories or patient characteristics are less important than the ability of therapist and patient to agree on and maintain a defined focus for the treatment.

Hollender MH, Ford CV: Dynamic Psychotherapy: An Introductory Approach. Washington, DC, American Psychiatric Press, 1990, pp 135–136

182

A psychiatrist is treating an 8-year-old child of a divorced single parent who is the child's custodial parent. The noncustodial parent wishes to be informed of the child's source of problems and progress of treatment. The psychiatrist should share clinical information with the noncustodial parent:

(A) without consent of the custodial parent or the child.
(B) only with the informed consent of the custodial parent and the child.
(C) only with informed consent of the custodial parent.
(D) only with the informed consent of the child.

The correct response is option **C**: Only with informed consent of the custodial parent

In order to share any clinical information with a third party, including the noncustodial parent, the psychiatrist needs the informed consent of the custodial parent. Although it may be clinically advisable to involve the child in the process, it is not required, since an 8-year-old cannot give legally valid informed consent.

American Academy of Child and Adolescent Psychiatry Code of Ethics, Principles X and XVII. Available at http://www.aacap.org/galleries/AboutUs/CodeOfEthics.PDF

183

Cerebral ventricular enlargement, one of the most consistent structural brain findings in patients with schizophrenia, is most closely associated with:

(A) prominent negative symptoms.
(B) rapid onset of the disorder.
(C) improved response rates to atypical antipsychotics.
(D) retained memory- and language-processing capabilities.
(E) increased risk of developing tardive dyskinesia.

The correct response is option **A**: Prominent negative symptoms

Prominent negative symptoms are associated with cerebral ventricular enlargement. The phenomena listed in options B through D are more associated with nonenlarged ventricles in patients with schizophrenia. Other factors have been more directly associated with the risk of tardive dyskinesia than structural abnormalities.

Ho B, Black D, Andreasen N: Schizophrenia and other psychotic disorders, in The American Psychiatric Publishing Textbook of Clinical Psychiatry, 4th ed. Edited by Hales RE, Yudofsky SC. Washington, DC, American Psychiatric Publishing, 2003, pp 405–407
Malhotra AK, Murphy GM Jr, Kennedy JL: Pharmacogenetics of psychotropic drug response. Am J Psychiatry 2004; 161:780–796

184

A patient with heroin dependence purchases a drug on the street. The patient feels a mild opiate high but then, despite continued injection of a sizable volume of drug, feels opiate withdrawal coming on. The drug injected is most likely:

(A) buprenorphine.
(B) heroin.
(C) methadone.
(D) naloxone.

The correct response is option **A**: Buprenorphine

Buprenorphine is a partial opiate agonist or a mixed agonist-antagonist. Rapidly injecting high doses of a partial agonist in a highly dependent patient who has recently used a full agonist (e.g., heroin) can produce mild withdrawal symptoms. As the dose is increased, a drug effect ceiling is reached, both with respect to any drug-induced euphoria and with drug-induced respiratory depression. As the dose continues to rise, the opiate antagonist effects become more predominant. Naloxone is a full antagonist and would produce an immediate full withdrawal syndrome.

Stine SM: Opiate dependence and current treatments, in New treatments for chemical addictions. Edited by McCance-Katz EF, Kosten TR. Washington, DC, American Psychiatric Press, 1998, pp 75–111
O'Brien CP, Kampman KM: Opioids: Antagonists and partial agonists, in The American Psychiatric Publishing Textbook of Substance Abuse Treatment, 3rd ed. Edited by Galanter M, Kleber HD. Washington, DC, American Psychiatric Publishing, 2004, pp 275, 305–320

185

Which of the following would be the most important consideration when evaluating an individual for a personality disorder?

(A) Culture
(B) Intelligence
(C) Gender
(D) Socioeconomic status
(E) Education

The correct response is option **A**: Culture

Personality disorders are defined as an enduring pattern of inner experience and behavior that deviates markedly from the expectations of the individual's culture. In general, intelligence, socioeconomic status, gender, and education have not been determined to be helpful in making a diagnosis of a personality disorder.

Cloninger CR, Svrakic DM: Personality disorders, in Kaplan and Sadock's Comprehensive Textbook of Psychiatry, 7th ed. Edited by Sadock BJ, Sadock VA. Philadelphia, Lippincott Williams & Wilkins, 2000, pp 1738–1741

186

Treatments shown to be effective for smoking cessation include all of the following EXCEPT:

(A) bupropion.
(B) brief advice intervention.
(C) 12-step programs.
(D) nicotine replacement therapy.

The correct response is option **C**: 12-step programs

Twelve-step programs have not demonstrated effectiveness in smoking cessation. All nicotine replacement therapies including gum, patch, nasal spray, and inhaler, have been found to be effective for smoking cessation. Brief advice techniques in which a personal benefit of cessation is identified and discussed in less than 10 minutes increase smoking cessation rates from 5% to 10%. Pharmacotherapy with bupropion has been shown to be effective.

Fiore MC, Bailey WC, Cohen SJ, et al: Treating Tobacco Use and Dependence. Clinical practice guideline. Rockville, MD, US Dept of Health and Human Services, June 2000. Available at http://www.surgeongeneral.gov/tobacco/treating_tobacco_use.pdf.

187

Based on the mental status examination, the psychiatrist believes that a patient is delirious. The examination reveals disorientation, changing levels of consciousness, and visual illusions. Which of the following tests has the greatest evidence supporting its use in confirming a diagnosis of delirium?

(A) Positron emission tomography
(B) Magnetic resonance imaging
(C) Computerized tomography
(D) EEG

The correct response is option **D**: EEG

In most delirious patients, the EEG demonstrates slowing and may be helpful in confirming the diagnosis. During alcohol withdrawal, the EEG may show an increased frequency. None of the other options listed has value in the differential diagnosis.

Wise MG, Rundell JR (eds): The American Psychiatric Publishing Textbook of Consultation-Liaison Psychiatry: Psychiatry in the Medically Ill, 2nd ed. Washington, DC, American Psychiatric Publishing, 2002, p 263

188

The diagnosis of shared psychotic disorder is most commonly found in which of the following groups?

- (A) Couple relationships
- (B) Groups larger than two people
- (C) Groups of men, rather than women
- (D) Family blood relations
- (E) Children and adolescents

The correct response is option **A**: Couple relationships

Shared psychotic disorder is more common in couples but is occasionally seen in groups. It often involves nonbizarre delusions and occurs more often in women than men. It has a low recovery rate.

American Psychiatric Association: Diagnostic and Statistical Manual of Mental Disorders, Fourth Edition, Text Revision (DSM-IV-TR). Washington, DC, American Psychiatric Association, 2000, pp 332–334

Sadock BJ, Sadock VA (eds): Kaplan and Sadock's Comprehensive Textbook of Psychiatry, 8th ed. Philadelphia, Lippincott Williams & Wilkins, 2005, p 1530

189

A colleague who is a cardiac surgeon asks for a psychiatrist's help in raising funds for a new wing of the local hospital. The cardiac surgeon asks the psychiatrist to solicit patients for charitable contributions. The psychiatrist's ethical response should be to agree to solicit funds from:

- (A) only former patients, because there is no longer a doctor-patient relationship.
- (B) only wealthy patients who have the means to contribute.
- (C) no patients, because of the nature of the psychiatrist-patient relationship.
- (D) both current and former patients, since patients can make autonomous decisions.

The correct response is option **C**: No patients, because of the nature of the psychiatrist-patient relationship

While the psychiatrist could be more articulate in describing the pertinent difference between psychiatry and cardiac surgery in regard to boundary issues, a direct request by the treating psychiatrist can risk exploitation of the patient. The first option ignores the unique features of the psychiatrist-patient relationship. The remaining options raise only partial truths and ignore counterbalancing considerations.

American Psychiatric Association: Opinions of the Ethics Committee on the Principles of Medical Ethics With Annotations Especially Applicable to Psychiatry. Washington, DC, American Psychiatric Association, 2001 (section 1-Q, p 9)

190

A managed care organization (MCO) is refusing to pay for additional treatment days for a patient in an inpatient psychiatric facility. The attending psychiatrist believes that the additional treatment days may be needed to ensure the patient's safety. Which of the following statements is correct regarding this situation?

- (A) The psychiatrist is legally responsible to abide by the MCO's decision.
- (B) The psychiatrist is responsible for making provisions for continuity of needed care even if additional days are not covered by the MCO.
- (C) As long as the psychiatrist documents that the MCO will not pay, the psychiatrist may discharge the patient.
- (D) The psychiatrist may inform the patient of his or her right to appeal the MCO's decision only if there are no "gag clauses" that limit what the psychiatrist is allowed to say.

The correct response is option **B**: The psychiatrist is responsible for making provisions for continuity of needed care even if additional days are not covered by the MCO

Even if a managed care organization refuses to pay, once a psychiatrist determines that the patient needs further treatment, especially if the issue of safety is still a concern, the psychiatrist is ethically responsible for providing care or arranging for an acceptable alternative method of care. Gag clauses that limit physician disclosure to patients are unethical.

Simon RI: A Concise Guide to Psychiatry and Law for Clinicians, 3rd ed. Washington, DC, American Psychiatric Publishing, 2001, pp 37–38

American Psychiatric Association: Principles of Medical Ethics With Annotations Especially Applicable to Psychiatry. Washington, DC, American Psychiatric Association, 2001 (annotation addendum 1)

191

The parents of a 14-year-old boy bring him to a clinic because he has been refusing to go to school. In elementary and middle school, he was in a special education class for mildly mentally retarded students. When he has been at school, he ruminates about "something really bad" happening to his mother or father. Recently, he has been awakening with nightmares that his parents have been killed. His parents have had to stay with their son in order for him to get back to sleep. His medical history is significant for strabismus and scoliosis. Physical examination reveals a long face with prominent ears and jaw, a high arched palate, hyperextensible finger joints, macroorchidism, and flat feet. This boy's overall presentation is most consistent with:

(A) Angelman syndrome.
(B) fragile X syndrome.
(C) Prader-Willi syndrome.
(D) Sturge-Weber syndrome.
(E) Williams syndrome.

The correct response is option **B**: Fragile X syndrome

This boy's history and physical presentation are classic for fragile X syndrome. Fragile X syndrome is the most common inherited cause of mental retardation. Anxiety disorders are more common in fragile X syndrome than any other form of mental retardation. The key components of this vignette are a mentally retarded boy with specific physical stigmata who has developed an anxiety disorder. This youth is suffering from separation anxiety disorder. Although the typical age at onset is at the start of elementary school, separation anxiety disorder has a bimodal pattern of presentation, with a second peak emerging in adolescence and typically associated with the transition into high school.

Dulcan MK, Martini DR, Lake MB: Concise Guide to Child and Adolescent Psychiatry, 3rd ed. Washington, DC, American Psychiatric Publishing, 2003, pp 63–71, 183–185
Lewis M (ed): Child and Adolescent Psychiatry: A Comprehensive Textbook, 3rd ed. Philadelphia, Lippincott Williams & Wilkins, 2002, pp 14–20, 824–825

192

Which of the following therapies explicitly gives the patient permission to be in the sick role?

(A) Brief psychotherapy
(B) Cognitive behavior therapy
(C) Insight-oriented therapy
(D) Interpersonal psychotherapy
(E) Rational-emotional therapy

The correct response is option **D**: Interpersonal psychotherapy

Interpersonal psychotherapy is a time-limited therapy that focuses on relationships and interpersonal interactions to effect change in symptoms and behavior. One aspect of interpersonal psychotherapy is that the patient is formally given permission to be in the "sick role," in that their feelings are framed in terms of a medical illness. The therapy focuses on the present and on real-life change more than on altering enduring aspects of the personality. Transference and genetic dream interpretations are avoided.

Hales RE, Yudofsky SC (eds): The American Psychiatric Publishing Textbook of Clinical Psychiatry, 4th ed. Washington, DC, American Psychiatric Publishing, 2003, pp 1208–1209
Sadock BJ, Sadock VA (eds): Synopsis of Psychiatry: Behavioral Sciences/Clinical Psychiatry, 9th ed. Philadelphia, Lippincott Williams & Wilkins, 2003, pp 933–935
Markowitz JC: The clinical conduct of interpersonal psychotherapy. FOCUS 2006; 4:179–184 (180)

193

A 29-year-old woman presents to the emergency department complaining of migraine headache. A review of her medical file reveals one brief admission for a transient psychotic episode and depression within the past 3 years. She is noted to be dressed in odd clothing. She insists that she is clairvoyant and telepathic. Her speech is noted to be metaphorical, overelaborate, and stereotyped. She says she has no close friends or confidants other than her mother and father, and that this has been the case since she was a teenager. She is not particularly bothered about her lack of companionship because she has fears of being harmed in relationships. Her presentation is most consistent with which of the following personality disorders?

(A) Avoidant
(B) Histrionic
(C) Paranoid
(D) Schizoid
(E) Schizotypal

The correct response is option **E**: Schizotypal

This vignette includes several features of each of the above personality disorders. Patients with paranoid personality disorder also fear being harmed by others. It is similar to avoidant personality disorder in the lack of close relationships, but the patient's indifference about this rules out this diagnosis. She is overly dramatic in her presentation, which is suggestive of a histrionic personality disorder, which could include options D or E. However, the oddity of her other symptoms suggests that this is unlikely. She seems to best fit into a cluster A personality disorder marked by oddity and eccentricity. Schizotypal personality disorder is distinguished from schizoid personality disorder by the presence of odd beliefs or magical thinking. Also, her comorbid diagnoses of a transient psychotic episode and depression are consistent with the diagnosis.

Sadock BJ, Sadock VA (eds): Kaplan and Sadock's Comprehensive Textbook of Psychiatry, 7th ed. Philadelphia, Lippincott Williams & Wilkins, 2000, pp 1743–1744
American Psychiatric Association: Diagnostic and Statistical Manual of Mental Disorders, Fourth Edition, Text Revision (DSM-IV-TR). Washington, DC, American Psychiatric Association, 2000, p 701

194

Which of the following would be most appropriate as initial pharmacotherapy for a patient with borderline personality disorder who is exhibiting impulsivity and behavioral dyscontrol?

(A) Sertraline
(B) Clozapine
(C) Haloperidol
(D) Naltrexone
(E) Alprazolam

The correct response is option **A**: Sertraline

Various medications have been shown to be effective for specific symptoms or behavior patterns in patients with borderline personality disorder. SSRIs are considered the treatment of choice for impulsive, disinhibited behavior in this patient group. Of the options listed, initial treatment with an SSRI for the symptoms of impulsivity and behavioral dyscontrol in patients with borderline personality disorder has the most empirical support.

Use of antipsychotics is common for patients with borderline personality disorder, but given the potential side effects, these agents should not be used as a first-line therapy for impulsivity and behavioral dyscontrol. Only preliminary support is available to support the use of naltrexone for this cluster of symptoms in borderline personality disorder. Benzodiazepine treatment may be associated with an increase in impulsivity in patients with borderline personality disorder.

Practice Guideline for the Treatment of Patients With Borderline Personality Disorder (2001), in American Psychiatric Association Practice Guidelines for the Treatment of Psychiatric Disorders, Compendium 2004. Washington, DC, APA, pp 773–775

195

A 30-year-old man with schizophrenia has made several significant suicide attempts over the past 10 years in response to auditory command hallucinations. Which of the following has been shown in studies to be most likely to reduce his risk for further suicidal behaviors?

(A) Aripiprazole
(B) Clozapine
(C) Lithium
(D) Olanzapine
(E) Risperidone

The correct response is option **B**: Clozapine

The 2-year International Suicide Prevention Trial (InterSePT) found that suicidal behavior was significantly less common in patients treated with clozapine than in those treated with olanzapine in the high-risk population studied. (The number of completed suicides was low for both patient groups: three for those treated with clozapine, and five for those treated with olanzapine.) While a substantial literature supports an antisuicide effect for lithium, the studies were not with schizophrenia patients.

Meltzer HY, Alphs L, Green AI, Altamura AC, Anand R, Bertoldi A, Bourgeois M, Chouinard G, Islam MZ, Kane J, Krishnan R, Lindenmayer JP, Potkin S; International Suicide Prevention Trial Study Group: Clozapine treatment for suicidality in schizophrenia: International Suicide Prevention Trial (InterSePT). Arch Gen Psychiatry 2003; 60:82–91
Meltzer HY: Suicide in schizophrenia, clozapine, and adoption of evidence-based medicine. J Clin Psychiatry 2005; 66:530–533
Tondo L, Baldessarini RJ, Hennen J, Floris G, Silvetti F, Tohen M: Lithium treatment and risk of suicidal behavior in bipolar disorder patients. J Clin Psychiatry 1998; 59:405–414

196

A 23-year-old patient with chronic schizophrenia complains of a milky discharge from her nipples. Medication-induced antagonism of which of the following receptors is responsible?

(A) Acetylcholine
(B) Dopamine
(C) GABA
(D) Norepinephrine
(E) Serotonin

The correct response is option **B**: Dopamine

The patient has galactorrhea, which is probably due to antipsychotic drug-induced hyperprolactinemia. This is more common with the older, conventional antipsychotics and with risperidone among the newer atypicals. D_2 receptor stimulation by dopamine has an inhibiting effect on prolactin secretion, and drug-induced blockade of this receptor will lead to an increased release of prolactin. Various explanations have been proposed as to why atypical antipsychotics vary considerably with regard to their effect (or lack of effect) on prolactin.

Haddad PM, Wieck A: Antipsychotic-induced hyperprolactinaemia: mechanisms, clinical features, and management. Drugs 2004; 64:2291–2314
Miller KK: Management of hyperprolactinemia in patients receiving antipsychotics. CNS Spectr 2004; 9(suppl 7):28–32
Practice Guideline for the Treatment of Patients With Schizophrenia, 2nd ed (2004), in American Psychiatric Association Practice Guidelines for the Treatment of Psychiatric Disorders, Compendium 2004. Washington, DC, APA, pp 348–351

197

Which of the following statements is most accurate regarding the current status of gene therapy for the clinical treatment of psychiatric disorders?

(A) Gene therapy will be clinically applicable within the next 2 years.
(B) Finding vectors to transfer genes into the nervous system is a challenge.
(C) Neurons are among the easiest cells into which to insert new genes.
(D) Target genes for gene therapy have been clearly defined.
(E) Viral vectors quickly spread novel genes throughout the nervous system.

The correct response is option **B**: Finding vectors to transfer genes into the nervous system is a challenge

The greatest challenge to gene therapy for the treatment of psychiatric disorders is finding vectors to transfer genes into the nervous system. Neurons are fragile, and so are some of the more difficult genes on which to perform gene therapy. Viral vectors tend to infect only a subset of the cells around them. Potential target genes are still being delineated. It will be many years before gene therapy will be clinically applicable.

Sapolsky RM: Gene therapy for psychiatric disorders. Am J Psychiatry 2003; 160:208–220

198

Which of the following agents would be most appropriate for a geriatric patient who has Parkinson's disease and agitation?

(A) Risperidone
(B) Diazepam
(C) Quetiapine
(D) Haloperidol
(E) Lithium

The correct response is option **C**: Quetiapine

If nonpharmacological interventions are ineffective, a trial of an atypical antipsychotic such as quetiapine or olanzapine may be initiated. Atypical antipsychotics that have been studied with the geriatric population are clozapine, risperidone, olanzapine, and quetiapine. A patient with parkinsonism may not be able to tolerate even the minimal extrapyramidal side effects of risperidone.

Cheong JA: An evidence-based approach to the management of agitation in the geriatric patient. FOCUS 2004; 2:197–205
(pp 200–203)

199

A 32-year-old man is brought to the emergency department by his family, who notes that he has been spending a lot of time sitting motionless in his room and appears to be losing weight. In the past, he had been fearful that family members were poisoning his food, but his parents state that he has not expressed those concerns recently. On examination, he is disheveled and poorly groomed, and he sits quietly in his chair except for intermittent grimacing. He has minimally spontaneous speech but will occasionally repeat the last few words of a question posed by the interviewer. His affect is generally restricted in range, and he does not answer questions about his mood, hallucinations, delusions, and suicidal or homicidal ideation. Which of the following subtypes of schizophrenia would best describe this patient's current presentation?

(A) Catatonic
(B) Disorganized
(C) Paranoid
(D) Residual
(E) Undifferentiated

The correct response is option **A**: Catatonic

This patient has had persecutory delusions during previous episodes of illness and is now disorganized in his appearance. However, he is also exhibiting motoric immobility, mutism, echolalia, and grimacing, making his current presentation most consistent with the catatonic subtype of schizophrenia.

American Psychiatric Association: Diagnostic and Statistical Manual of Mental Disorders, Fourth Edition, Text Revision (DSM-IV-TR). Washington, DC, American Psychiatric Association, 2000, pp 313–317

200

Which of the following is most predictive of a favorable response to lithium in bipolar disorder?

(A) Comorbid substance abuse
(B) Depression-mania-euthymia course
(C) Euphoric mania
(D) Psychotic features

The correct response is option **C**: Euphoric mania

A good clinical response to lithium therapy is predicted if the patient has the following features: euphoric mania, nonrapid cycling, full interepisode remission, no comorbidity, lack of psychotic features, few lifetime episodes, and a mania-depression-euthymia clinical course.

Bowden CL: Efficacy of lithium in mania and maintenance therapy of bipolar disorder. J Clin Psychiatry 2000; 61(suppl 9):35–40

Grof P, Alda M, Grof E, Fox D, Cameron P: The challenge of predicting response to stabilising lithium treatment: the importance of patient selection. Br J Psychiatry 1993; 163(suppl 21):16–19
Jefferson JW, Goodnick PJ (eds): Predictors of Treatment Response in Mood Disorders. Washington, DC, American Psychiatric Press, 1996, pp 95–117

201

A female patient reveals during a psychotherapy session that she does not enjoy sexual intercourse. She states that she is aroused by her partner but has sharp pains throughout intercourse. She cannot relax and enjoy sex and has begun to avoid sex because of the anticipation of the pain. What is the most likely diagnosis?

(A) Dyspareunia
(B) Female orgasmic disorder
(C) Sexual masochism
(D) Sexual sadism
(E) Sexual aversion disorder

The correct response is option **A**: Dyspareunia

Sexual pain disorders are not a common chief complaint in mental health settings. However, during psychotherapy a psychiatrist may become aware of the symptoms and should be able to recognize them. This is a classic description of dyspareunia.

American Psychiatric Association: Diagnostic and Statistical Manual of Mental Disorders, Fourth Edition, Text Revision (DSM-IV-TR). Washington, DC, American Psychiatric Association, 2000, pp 554–556
Hales RE, Yudofsky SC (eds): The American Psychiatric Publishing Textbook of Clinical Psychiatry, 4th ed. Washington, DC, American Psychiatric Publishing, 2003, p 757

202

A 25-year-old woman presents with severe anxiety after finding out that her biological mother was recently diagnosed with Huntington's disease. There is no family history of the disease on her father's side. She wishes to know if she is affected. The probability that she is affected is:

(A) 0%.
(B) 25%.
(C) 50%.
(D) 75%.
(E) 100%.

The correct response is option **C**: 50%

Huntington's disease is inherited by an autosomal dominant transmission. With one affected parent and one unaffected parent, by chance, one could expect 50% of offspring would be affected and 50% unaffected, but each individual child has a 50% chance of developing the disease.

Sadock BJ, Sadock VA (eds): Kaplan and Sadock's Comprehensive Textbook of Psychiatry, 8th ed. Philadelphia, Lippincott Williams & Wilkins, 2005, p 237

Stern TA, Herman JB: Massachusetts General Hospital Psychiatry Update and Board Preparation, 2nd ed. New York, McGraw-Hill, 2004, p 499

203

A 9-year-old boy is referred for evaluation because he is having "temper tantrums" in school. He cannot sit still, constantly disrupts the class, runs out in the hall without permission and refuses to obey directives from the teacher. He frequently fights with his peers, and if he does not get what he wants, he yells, screams, throws objects, and flails about on the floor. Educational testing reveals borderline intellectual functioning and significant delays in reading, writing, spelling, and mathematics. On physical examination, the boy is noted to be in the fifth percentile for head circumference. He has short palpebral fissures, a thin upper lip, and a smooth philtrum. The boy was most likely exposed to which of the following drugs in utero?

(A) Alcohol
(B) Cocaine
(C) Marijuana
(D) Nicotine
(E) Opiates

The correct response is option **A**: Alcohol

The teratological effects of prenatal alcohol exposure have been well studied and are described by fetal alcohol syndrome. Alcohol is a direct neuroteratogen that affects not only fetal facial morphology and growth but also brain growth, structure, and function. As a result, children exposed to alcohol have an unusually high prevalence of intellectual impairment and disruptive behavior disorders. This young boy exhibits evidence of several psychiatric disorders in association with specific physical stigmata. His history suggests the presence of oppositional defiant disorder (ODD), Attention deficit hyperactivity disorder (ADHD), and overall impairment in intellectual functioning leading to deficits in academic functioning. In utero exposure to marijuana has been linked to mild problems with attention and impulsivity but has not been found to permanently affect intellectual functioning or cause craniofacial abnormalities. Cocaine may cause a relative state of hypoxia in fetuses that are small for gestational age and have a small head circumference. Some studies have shown attentional problems in children exposed to cocaine in utero, but no specific physical abnormalities have been demonstrated. Prenatal opiate exposure reduces birth weight and head circumference. However, studies have found no differences in early childhood between children who were exposed to opiates in utero and those who were not. In utero effects of nicotine have been linked to ADHD and growth retardation, but no other sequelae.

Lewis M (ed): Child and Adolescent Psychiatry: A Comprehensive Textbook, 3rd ed. Philadelphia, Lippincott Williams & Wilkins, 2002, pp 449–453

204

Which of the following is the most accurate statement regarding psychotherapy for posttraumatic stress disorder (PTSD)?

(A) The therapist should be as nondirective as possible for the psychotherapy to be effective.
(B) Multiple modalities of psychotherapy have proven effective for PTSD.
(C) Psychotherapy must be combined with pharmacotherapy to be effective.
(D) Cognitive behavioral therapy (CBT) is of little value for patients with PTSD.

The correct response is option **B**: Multiple modalities of psychotherapy have proven effective for PTSD

In meta-analyses of controlled trials of psychological treatments of PTSD, multiple forms of psychotherapy, including exposure therapy, cognitive behavioral therapy, and psychodynamic therapy, have been shown to be effective.

Adhead G: Psychological therapies for post-traumatic stress disorder. Br J Psychiatry 2000; 177:144–148

Sherman JJ: Effects of psychotherapeutic treatments for PTSD: a meta-analysis of controlled clinical trials. J Trauma Stress 1998; 11:413–435

Davidson JRT: Effective management strategies for posttraumatic stress disorder. FOCUS 2003; 1:239–243 (p 241)

205

A husband and wife present for treatment because the wife is concerned. Her husband recently told her that he believes he was born a woman. He states that he has always felt this way but can't fight it anymore. He has started wearing dresses around the house after he arrives home from work at the end of the day. He says that he loves his wife and kids but that he needs to be happy as well. What is the most likely diagnosis?

(A) Exhibitionism
(B) Gender identity disorder
(C) Sexual arousal disorder
(D) Transvestic fetishism
(E) Voyeurism

The correct response is option **B**: Gender identity disorder

This is a complicated disorder, but the scenario describes someone who has been struggling with gender identity disorder despite functioning in culturally expected roles for a prolonged period.

American Psychiatric Association: Diagnostic and Statistical Manual of Mental Disorders, Fourth Edition, Text Revision (DSM-IV-TR). Washington, DC, American Psychiatric Association, 2000, pp 576–582

Hales RE, Yudofsky SC (eds): The American Psychiatric Publishing Textbook of Clinical Psychiatry, 4th ed. Washington, DC, American Psychiatric Publishing, 2003, p 745

206

Which of the following describes the pharmacokinetics of children younger than 12 years old?

(A) Children have a smaller volume of distribution than adults.
(B) Children have more efficient renal function than adults.
(C) Children metabolize through hepatic pathways more slowly than adults.
(D) Children absorb medications more slowly than adults.

The correct response is option **B**: Children have more efficient renal function than adults

Children have more efficient renal elimination than adults and therefore will clear drugs using this pathway more quickly.

Martin A, Scahill L, Charney D, Leackman J (eds): Pediatric psychopharmacology principles and practice. New York, Oxford University Press, 2003, pp 48–50

207

A 32-year-old woman develops anorgasmia while taking paroxetine. Switching to which of the following medications is most likely to resolve this problem?

(A) Citalopram
(B) Venlafaxine
(C) Sertraline
(D) Bupropion
(E) Fluoxetine

The correct response is option **D**: Bupropion

A large survey of primary care clinics found that the lowest risk of sexual dysfunction was with bupropion. Double-blind placebo-controlled studies found substantially more orgasm dysfunction with sertraline and with fluoxetine than with bupropion.

Clayton AH, Pradko JF, Croft HA, Montano CB, Leadbetter RA, Bolden-Watson C, Bass KI, Donahue RM, Jamerson BD, Metz A: Prevalence of sexual dysfunction among newer antidepressants. J Clin Psychiatry 2002; 63:357–366

Croft H, Settle E Jr, Houser T, Batey SR, Donahue RM, Ascher JA: A placebo-controlled comparison of the antidepressant efficacy and effects on sexual functioning of sustained-release bupropion and sertraline. Clin Ther 1999; 21:643–658

Coleman CC, King BR, Bolden-Watson C, Book MJ, Segraves RT, Richard N, Ascher J, Batey S, Jamerson B, Metz A: A placebo-controlled comparison of the effects on sexual functioning of bupropion sustained released and fluoxetine. Clin Ther 2001; 23:1040–1058

Schatzberg AF, Nemeroff CB (eds): The American Psychiatric Publishing Textbook of Psychopharmacology, 3rd ed, Washington, DC, American Psychiatric Publishing, 2004, Tables 52–57, p 859

208

A 4-year-old boy is brought to the clinic by his parents with the chief complaint that "he keeps having nightmares." His parents report that for the past month, during the first one-third of the night, the boy awakens from his sleep with a startled scream. When they enter the room, they find that he has broken out in a sweat, is difficult to awaken, and looks "scared to death." The next morning he has no recall of the event. These episodes are most likely occurring during which stage of sleep?

(A) REM
(B) Stage 0 — non-REM
(C) Stage 1 — non-REM
(D) Stage 2 — non-REM
(E) Stage 3 or 4 — non-REM

The correct response is option **E**: Stage 3 or 4 — non-REM

Sleep terror disorder is a parasomnia. It occurs in deep non-REM (i.e., stages 3 or 4) sleep. This stage of sleep occurs predominantly in the first third of the night. Although many parents assume that a child in this state is having nightmares, in fact he has sleep terror disorder. According to DSM-IV-TR, the awakenings from nightmares generally occur during REM sleep.

Sadock BJ, Sadock VA: Kaplan and Sadock's Synopsis of Psychiatry, 9th ed. Philadelphia, Lippincott Williams & Wilkins, 2003, p 775
American Psychiatric Association: Diagnostic and Statistical Manual of Mental Disorders, Fourth Edition, Text Revision (DSM-IV-TR). Washington, DC, American Psychiatric Association, 2000, pp 634–639

209

A 25-year-old male with a history of schizophrenia is hospitalized and treated with haloperidol and benztropine. The patient becomes distressed, has a temperature of 103°F and has labile blood pressure. Physical examination reveals hypertonicity, diaphoresis, and tachycardia. Laboratory studies reveal a creatine kinase of 55,000 IU/L. What is the most likely diagnosis?

(A) Anticholinergic syndrome
(B) CNS infection
(C) Malignant hyperthermia
(D) Neuroleptic malignant syndrome
(E) Serotonin syndrome

The correct response is option **D**: Neuroleptic malignant syndrome

Essential for the diagnosis of neuroleptic malignant syndrome in a patient on antipsychotic medication are rigidity and elevated temperature. Two or more of the following symptoms are also required: diaphoresis, tachycardia, elevated or labile blood pressure, dysphagia, incontinence, tremor, changes in the level of consciousness ranging from confusion to coma, mutism, leukocytosis, laboratory evidence of muscle injury (e.g., elevated creatine kinase).

Sadock BJ, Sadock VA (eds): Kaplan and Sadock's Comprehensive Textbook of Psychiatry, 8th ed. Philadelphia, Lippincott Williams & Wilkins, 2005, p 2714

210

A previously well 24-year-old woman presented with a 4-week history of progressively worsening expansive irritable mood, pressured speech, racing thoughts, grandiosity, and distractibility. More recently she heard the voice of God proclaiming her to be a special messenger. Which of the following is the most likely diagnosis?

(A) Brief psychotic disorder without marked stressor
(B) Bipolar disorder with psychotic features
(C) Schizoaffective disorder, bipolar type
(D) Schizophrenia, catatonic subtype
(E) Schizophreniform disorder

The correct response is option **B**: Bipolar disorder with psychotic features

The patient meets DSM-IV-TR criteria for a manic episode with mood-congruent auditory hallucinations. The psychotic symptoms occurring only in the context of a manic episode make the other diagnoses unlikely.

American Psychiatric Association: Diagnostic and Statistical Manual of Mental Disorders, Fourth Edition, Text Revision (DSM-IV-TR). Washington, DC, American Psychiatric Association, 2000, pp 357–362, 413–415

211

According to the principles of dialectical behavior therapy, the core deficit in borderline personality disorder is in:

(A) regulation of affect.
(B) capacity for attachment.
(C) object constancy.
(D) self-integration.
(E) impulsive aggression.

The correct response is option **A**: Regulation of affect

Dialectical behavior therapy is based on the theory that borderline symptoms primarily reflect dysfunction of the emotion regulation system. Cognitive behavior therapies view the problem as cognitive distortions, and behavior management views the issue as learned behavior. Empirical studies suggest that child abuse, incest, and early trauma may play a large role in development of borderline personality disorder. Options B, C, and D are related to psychological formulations of the disorder, and option E relates more to the biological concepts of serotonergic dysfunction. Early psychodynamic formulations postulated a lack of object constancy and splitting of self and objects into "all good" or "all bad" as core problems in borderline personality disorder.

Phillips KA, Yen S, Gunderson JG: Personality disorders, in The American Psychiatric Publishing Textbook of Clinical Psychiatry, 4th ed. Edited by Hales RE, Yudofsky SC. Washington, DC, American Psychiatric Publishing, 2003, pp 810–825

Moeller FG, Barratt ES, Dougherty DM, Schmitz JM, Swann AC: Psychiatric aspects of impulsivity. Am J Psychiatry 2001; 158:1783–1793

McMain S, Korman LM, Dimeff L: Dialectical behavior therapy and the treatment of emotion dysregulation. J Clin Psychol 2001; 57:183–196

Cloninger CR, Svrakic DM: Personality disorders, in Kaplan and Sadock's Comprehensive Textbook of Psychiatry, 7th ed. Edited by Sadock BJ, Sadock VA. Philadelphia, Lippincott Williams & Wilkins, 2000, p 1757

212

According to the American Psychiatric Association guidelines, which of the following is true regarding a psychiatrist engaging in a sexual relationship with a former patient?

(A) Acceptable provided at least 2 years have passed since the termination of the doctor-patient relationship
(B) Acceptable provided at least 5 years have passed since the termination of the doctor-patient relationship
(C) Acceptable provided the former patient initiates the relationship and it is clear to both parties that no exploitation is taking place
(D) Unethical no matter how long it has been since the termination of the doctor-patient relationship

The correct response is option **D**: Unethical no matter how long it has been since the termination of the doctor-patient relationship

While the issue of sexual relationships with former patients is not without controversy, psychiatrists should be aware of the current position of the American Psychiatric Association, which forbids sex with former patients.

American Psychiatric Association: Principles of Medical Ethics With Annotations Especially Applicable To Psychiatry. Washington, DC, American Psychiatric Association, 2001 (section 2, annotation 1)

213

A patient with schizophrenia begins treatment with clozapine. The baseline white blood cell count (WBC) is 8100 (normal=4500–11,000/mm^3). The absolute neutrophil count (ANC) is 6200 (normal=1500–8000/mm^3). The tests remain normal in weekly monitoring. After 3 months, the patient has had significant clinical improvement, but the WBC drops to 3200, the ANC drops to 2100, and immature cell forms are present on peripheral blood smear. Repeat tests show a WBC of 3100, an ANC of 1900, and no immature cell forms. The physical examination is normal, with no fever, sore throat, or other sign of infection. What would be the best next step in the management of this patient?

(A) Continue current dosage of clozapine and begin twice-weekly monitoring of the WBC and differential.
(B) Immediately and permanently discontinue clozapine.
(C) Interrupt clozapine therapy until the WBC is normal, and then resume treatment.
(D) Reduce the dose of clozapine and begin weekly monitoring of the WBC and differential.
(E) Routinely monitor the WBC and differential unless the patient develops signs and symptoms of infection.

The correct response is option **A**: Continue current dosage of clozapine and begin twice-weekly monitoring of the WBC and differential

A protocol has been established for monitoring the hematologic effects of clozapine. In this vignette, the patient's WBC and ANC have dropped from baseline, but the patient has demonstrated an excellent response to medication and has no signs or symptoms of infection. However, the drop in WBC and ANC are not considered large enough to disrupt treatment. Given the clinical response in a treatment-resistant patient, it is recommended that the patient be continued on the dose of clozapine that is effective and for the clinician to monitor the WBC and differential more frequently. For greater decreases in the WBC or ANC, it may be necessary to interrupt clozapine treatment temporarily until these values return to safer levels or to immediately and permanently discontinue clozapine treatment if there are concomitant signs of infection.

Schatzberg AF, Cole JO, DeBattista C: Manual of Clinical Psychopharmacology. Washington, DC, American Psychiatric Publishing, 2005, p 186

Alvir JMJ, Lieberman JA, Safferman AZ, Schwimmer JL, Schaaf JA: Clozapine-induced agranulocytosis. N Engl J Med 1993; 329:162–167

214

According to DSM-IV-TR, which personality disorder cannot be diagnosed in children and adolescents?

(A) Paranoid
(B) Dependent
(C) Schizotypal
(D) Borderline
(E) Antisocial

The correct response is option **E**: Antisocial

Antisocial personality disorder cannot be diagnosed in individuals under the age of 18 years. The other personality disorders can be diagnosed if the maladaptive personality traits are pervasive, persistent, and unlikely to be limited to a particular developmental stage or episode of an axis I disorder. However, traits of a personality disorder that appear in childhood frequently change in adult life. To diagnose a personality disorder in an individual under age 18, the features must have been present for at least 1 year. The one exception to this is antisocial personality disorder, which cannot be diagnosed in individuals under age 18. This is because until that age, the behaviors associated with antisocial personality disorder are better explained by conduct disorder, a diagnosis of childhood and adolescence.

Cloninger CR, Svrakic DM: Personality disorders, in Kaplan and Sadock's Comprehensive Textbook of Psychiatry, 7th ed. Edited by Sadock BJ, Sadock VA. Philadelphia, Lippincott Williams & Wilkins, 2000, pp 1739–1741

American Psychiatric Association: Diagnostic and Statistical Manual of Mental Disorders, Fourth Edition, Text Revision (DSM-IV-TR). Washington, DC, American Psychiatric Association, 2000, p 687

215

The first-line treatment of choice (determined by expert consensus) for acute posttraumatic stress disorder (PTSD) milder severity is:

(A) low-dose venlafaxine.
(B) psychotherapy.
(C) combination of a mood stabilizer and psychotherapy.
(D) any selective serotonin reuptake inhibitor (SSRI).

The correct response is option **B**: Psychotherapy

The expert panel felt that for milder-severity acute PTSD, psychotherapy first was the treatment of choice, although the preferred first-line treatment for chronic PTSD or for more severe acute PTSD is either psychotherapy first or combined medication and psychotherapy. This recommendation holds true for children, adolescents, adults, and geriatric patients.

Foa EB, Davidson JRT, Frances A: The Expert Consensus Guideline Series: Treatment of Posttraumatic Stress Disorder. J Clin Psychiatry 1999; 60(suppl 16):1–76 (p 12)

216

A 54-year-old woman is hospitalized with hyperthermia, myoclonus, delirium, and autonomic instability. Which of the following medication combinations would be most likely to cause this clinical presentation?

(A) Bupropion and venlafaxine
(B) Desipramine and escitalopram
(C) Duloxetine and fluoxetine
(D) Paroxetine and phenelzine
(E) Sertraline and buspirone

The correct response is option **D**: Paroxetine and phenelzine

The patient's symptoms are consistent with a serotonin syndrome. Monoamine oxidase inhibitors, such as phenelzine, combined with serotonergic antidepressants pose a grave risk; hence, such combinations are contraindicated.

Lane R, Baldwin D: Selective serotonin reuptake inhibitor-induced serotonin syndrome: review. J Clin Psychopharmacol 1997; 17:208–221

Beasley CM Jr, Masica DN, Heiligenstein JH, Wheadon DE, Zerbe RL: Possible monoamine oxidase inhibitor-serotonin uptake inhibitor interaction: fluoxetine clinical data and preclinical findings. J Clin Psychopharmacol 1993; 13:312–320

217

In addition to lithium, which of the following is recommended as a first-line monotherapy for bipolar I disorder, depressed mood, in the revised APA Practice Guideline for the Treatment of Patients With Bipolar Disorder (2002)?

(A) Lamotrigine
(B) Divalproex
(C) Gabapentin
(D) Bupropion

The correct response is option **A**: Lamotrigine

The Practice Guideline recommends the initiation of treatment of bipolar depression with lithium or lamotrigine; it further states that monotherapy with conventional antidepressants is not recommended "given the risk of precipitating a switch into mania." A large double-blind monotherapy study of bipolar I depression found lamotrigine to be more effective than placebo on most outcome measures. There have been no published controlled studies of divalproex or gabapentin.

American Psychiatric Association: Practice Guideline for the Treatment of Patients With Bipolar Disorder (Revision). Am J Psychiatry 2002; 159(April suppl). Reprinted in FOCUS 2003; 1:64–110 (p 65)

Calabrese JR, Bowden CL, Sachs GS, Ascher JA, Monaghan E, Rudd GD (Lamictal 602 Study Group): A double-blind placebo-controlled study of lamotrigine monotherapy in outpatients with bipolar I disorder. J Clin Psychiatry 1999; 60:79–88

218

A 15-year-old African American male high school freshman is referred to a psychiatrist because of increasing oppositional behavior at school. In middle school he was an honor roll student, played soccer, and was on student council, all of which he continued in his first 9 weeks of high school. On the weekends, he volunteers at a local Boys and Girls Club and plays the keyboard at his church. After a couple of sessions, he finally admits that he needed to "prove myself to my boys because they said I was 'acting white'." Which of the following is the most likely reason for his peers' denigration?

(A) Being on student council
(B) Doing volunteer work
(C) Having honor roll grades
(D) Playing soccer
(E) Playing the keyboard

The correct response is option **C**: Having honor roll grades

A subset of African American culture that particularly affects male adolescents devalues academic performance and emphasizes aggressive and "street" behavior. The clinician should be aware of this phenomenon in the African American community and take this into account when assessing a student whose grades and behavior change.

Day-Vines NL, Patton JM, Baytops JL: Counseling African American adolescents: the impact of race, culture, and middle class status. Professional School Counseling 2003; 7:40–51

Day-Vines NL, Day-Hairston BO: Culturally congruent strategies for addressing the behavioral needs of urban African American male adolescents. Professional School Counseling 2005; 8:236–243

219

A 55-year-old man presents with depressed mood, poor concentration, poor appetite, feelings of worthlessness, and insomnia 4 weeks after alcohol cessation. There is no history of mania. Which of the following is the best next step?

(A) Begin an antidepressant.
(B) Begin a sleep aid.
(C) Begin an anticonvulsant.
(D) Begin to phase-advance sleep onset.
(E) Wait 7–10 days, then reassess.

The correct response is option **A**: Begin an antidepressant

The patient has symptoms of a major depressive episode that have persisted for 2 weeks. Rather than addressing insomnia as a symptom in isolation, it is preferable to begin treatment for the depressive disorder. Previous investigations have suggested waiting 30 days after onset of abstinence before making a diagnosis of a mood disorder. However, recent data suggest that persistence of mood symptoms 2 weeks after cessation of drinking merits treatment.

Nunes EV, Levin FR: Treatment of depression in patients with alcohol or other drug dependence. JAMA 2004; 291:1887–1896

Brady KT, Malcolm RJ: Substance use disorders and co-occurring axis I psychiatric disorders, in The American Psychiatric Publishing Textbook of Substance Abuse Treatment, 3rd ed. Edited by Galanter M, Kleber HD. Washington, DC, American Psychiatric Publishing, 2004, pp 529–538

220

A 16-year-old girl with depression has suicidal ideation. Which of the following characteristics is the most strongly associated with a greater risk of completed suicide?

(A) Limited cognitive abilities
(B) Perfectionist characteristics
(C) Previous suicide attempt
(D) Strong religious beliefs
(E) Superficial cutting of forearms

The correct response is option **C**: Previous suicide attempt

A previous suicide attempt is the most potent predictor of suicide in girls.

American Academy of Child and Adolescent Psychiatry: Practice Parameters for the Assessment and Treatment of Children and Adolescents With Suicidal Behavior. J Am Acad Child Adolesc Psychiatry 2001; 40(suppl 7):26S–32S

221

A psychiatrist routinely receives free golf outings, concert tickets, and dinners as gifts from a local pharmaceutical representative. Which of the following statements most adequately describes the ethics of this practice?

    (A) It is ethical if no single gift is worth more than $250.
    (B) Self-monitoring and self-regulation are the most effective ways of minimizing harm from conflicts of interest.
    (C) There is no evidence that pharmaceutical company marketing to physicians influences physicians' behavior.
    (D) This is a conflict of interest for the psychiatrist.

The correct response is option **D**: This is a conflict of interest for the psychiatrist

Self-monitoring and self-regulation actions by the psychiatrist are important but usually are not seen as sufficient to prevent abuse due to conflicts of interest. Pharmaceutical company marketing to physicians affects physicians' behavior.

American Medical Association: Council on Ethical and Judicial Affairs of the American Medical Association, 2000–2001, Opinion 8.061
Wazana A: Physicians and the pharmaceutical industry: is a gift ever just a gift? JAMA 2000; 283:373–380
Thompson DF: Understanding financial conflicts of interest. N Engl J Med 1993; 329:573–576

222

The process of gene mapping, performed to determine whether or not a particular allele occurs more frequently than by chance in affected individuals, is known as which type of study?

    (A) Twin
    (B) Linkage
    (C) Association
    (D) Family
    (E) Segregation analysis

The correct response is option **C**: Association

Association studies can examine whether a particular allele occurs more frequently than by chance by comparing affected and unaffected individuals. Twin and family studies are not gene-mapping studies. Linkage studies, a type of gene-mapping study, examine whether two or more genetic loci are co-inherited more often than expected by chance. A segregation analysis is used to determine mode of inheritance (dominant, recessive, etc.).

Sadock BJ, Sadock VA (eds): Kaplan and Sadock's Comprehensive Textbook of Psychiatry, 8th ed. Philadelphia, Lippincott Williams & Wilkins, 2005, pp 256–257

Yudofsky SC, Hales RE (eds): The American Psychiatric Publishing Textbook of Neuropsychiatry and Clinical Neurosciences, 4th ed. Washington, DC, American Psychiatric Publishing, 2002, pp 326–329
Stern TA, Herman JB: Massachusetts General Hospital Psychiatry Update and Board Preparation, 2nd ed. New York, McGraw-Hill, 2004, p 493
Kendler KS, Eaves LJ (eds): Psychiatric Genetics. Review of Psychiatry, vol 24. Washington, DC, American Psychiatric Publishing, 2005, p 55

223

Which of the following is the most common psychiatric disturbance among adolescents who die by suicide?

    (A) Schizophrenia
    (B) Depressive disorders
    (C) Antisocial behavior/conduct disorder
    (D) Anxiety disorders
    (E) Alcohol dependence

The correct response is option **B**: Depressive disorders

Approximately one-half to two-thirds of adolescent suicide victims have a depressive disorder, with the odds ratio for increased suicide risk in those with an affective disorder ranging, in various studies, from 11 to 27. Substance use and abuse are highly comorbid, particularly in male suicide completers, and conduct disorder has been reported in about one-third of male suicide victims. Few adolescent suicides are related to schizophrenia.

Gould MS, Greenberg T, Velting DM, Shaffer D: Youth suicide risk and preventive interventions: a review of the past 10 years. J Am Acad Child Adolesc Psychiatry 2003; 42:386–405

224

Which of the following is the best medication treatment for premature ejaculation?

    (A) Bupropion
    (B) Lorazepam
    (C) Paroxetine
    (D) Risperidone
    (E) Trazodone

The correct response is option **C**: Paroxetine

Premature ejaculation is the persistent or recurrent onset of orgasm and ejaculation with minimal sexual stimulation before, on, or shortly after penetration and before the person wishes it. Typically it is a problem in young men, who eventually develop behavioral strategies to delay ejaculation. However, some men never develop the ability or lose it because of decreased frequency of sexual activity or performance anxiety or as a component of erectile dysfunction. It can be a problem in recovering substance abusers who have relied on the substances to delay ejaculation. SSRIs have been shown to be a good treatment for premature ejaculation, with paroxetine being the medication that delays ejaculation the most.

American Psychiatric Association: Diagnostic and Statistical Manual of Mental Disorders, Fourth Edition, Text Revision (DSM-IV-TR). Washington, DC, American Psychiatric Association, 2000, pp 552–554

Schatzberg AF, Nemeroff CB (eds): The American Psychiatric Publishing Textbook of Psychopharmacology, 3rd ed, Washington, DC, American Psychiatric Publishing, 2004, pp 238, 272

225

The highest rates of posttraumatic stress disorder (PTSD) have been reported to be induced by:

(A) combat.
(B) sexual assault.
(C) natural disasters.
(D) motor vehicle accidents.

The correct response is option **B**: Sexual assault

Assaultive violence, including sexual assault, produces the highest rates of PTSD, compared with other precipitating traumas (i.e., combat, natural disasters, and motor vehicle accidents).

Breslau N, Kessler RC, Chilcoat HD, Schultz LR, Davis GC, Andreski P: Trauma and posttraumatic stress disorder in the community: the 1996 Detroit Area Survey of Trauma. Arch Gen Psychiatry 1998; 55:626–632

226

Which of the following laboratory test results is elevated in some patients with anorexia nervosa?

(A) Amylase
(B) Magnesium
(C) Phosphate
(D) Potassium
(E) Zinc

The correct response is option **A**: Amylase

Values for the other tests are often decreased in patients with anorexia nervosa.

American Psychiatric Association: Diagnostic and Statistical Manual of Mental Disorders, Fourth Edition, Text Revision (DSM-IV-TR). Washington, DC, American Psychiatric Association, 2000, p 586

227

Which of the following is the most common side effect of cholinesterase inhibitors?

(A) Anorexia
(B) Muscle cramps
(C) Nausea
(D) Somnolence
(E) Syncope

The correct response is option **C**: Nausea

Nausea, reported in 11%–47% of patients, is the most common adverse effect of the cholinesterase inhibitors (donepezil, rivastigmine, and galantamine). Vomiting is the next most common side effect, reported in 10%–31% of patients. Diarrhea was reported in 5%–19% of patients, and anorexia in 4%–17%. Other, less frequent side effects include insomnia, muscle cramps, syncope, fatigue, abnormal dreams, incontinence, and bradycardia.

Cummings JL: Use of cholinesterase inhibitors in clinical practice: evidence-based recommendations. Am J Geriatr Psychiatry 2003; 11:131–145

228

There is accumulating evidence suggesting that all of the following psychotherapies are beneficial in bipolar I disorder EXCEPT:

(A) interpersonal and social rhythm therapy.
(B) cognitive behavioral therapy.
(C) family therapy.
(D) psychoanalysis.

The correct response is option **D**: Psychoanalysis

There is peer-reviewed evidence suggesting that interpersonal and social rhythm therapy, family therapy, and cognitive behavioral therapy may decrease cycling and decrease the severity of bipolar I disorder. There are no controlled studies demonstrating that psychoanalysis decreases the frequency or severity of episodes of mania or depression.

Rapaport MH, Hales D: Relapse prevention and bipolar disorder: a focus on bipolar depression. FOCUS 2003; 1:15–31 (p 21)

Miklowitz DJ, Simoneau TL, George EL, Richards JA, Kalbag A, Sachs-Ericsson N, Suddath R: Family-focused treatment of bipolar disorder: 1-year effects of a psychoeducational program in conjunction with pharmacotherapy. Biol Psychiatry 2000; 48:582–592

Frank E, Novick D: Progress in the psychotherapy of mood disorders: studies from the Western Psychiatric Institute and Clinic. Epidemiol Psichiatr Soc 2001; 120:245–252

A 45-year-old patient with heroin dependence is admitted to the infectious disease service for intravenous antibiotic treatment of bacterial endocarditis. An HIV test is negative. There is no other past psychiatric history. Opiate withdrawal is adequately controlled with oral methadone. On hospital day 3, the patient becomes acutely anxious, has moderate tachycardia, and asks to be discharged from the hospital. A low-grade fever develops, but blood cultures are negative and a complete blood count shows no significant increase or shift in leukocytes. The most likely explanation for the change in the patient's condition is:

(A) an occult infection.
(B) alcohol or sedative-hypnotic withdrawal.
(C) an undiagnosed anxiety disorder.
(D) a medication reaction, most likely to the antibiotic.

The correct response is option **B**: Alcohol or sedative-hypnotic withdrawal

The patient's tachycardia and symptoms of anxiety are consistent with the time frame for alcohol or sedative-hypnotic withdrawal. Multiple drug use is common in patients with substance dependence. Rather than intentionally concealing polydrug use, a patient may be much more focused on a drug-of-choice to the point that abuse of other substances is not acknowledged.

American Psychiatric Association: Practice Guideline for the Treatment of Patients With Substance Use Disorders: Alcohol, Cocaine, Opioids. Am J Psychiatry 1995; 152(Nov suppl)

230

Long-term treatment with which of the following medications has been demonstrated to reduce suicide risk in bipolar disorder?

(A) Carbamazepine
(B) Divalproex
(C) Lithium
(D) Olanzapine

The correct response is option **C**: Lithium

Analyses of the results of many studies support a marked reduction in suicide rates and suicide attempts during long-term lithium treatment.

Tondo L, Hennen J, Baldessarini RJ: Lower suicide risk with long-term lithium treatment in major affective illness: a meta-analysis. Acta Psychiatr Scand 2001; 104:163–172
Baldessarini RJ, Tondo L, Hennen J: Treating the suicide patient with bipolar disorder: reducing suicide risk with lithium. Ann NY Acad Sci 2001; 932:24–38
Jefferson JW: Bipolar disorders: a brief guide to diagnosis and treatment. FOCUS 2003; 1:7–14 (p 12)

A psychiatric referral is requested to evaluate a 25-year-old woman who wishes to undergo a second rhinoplasty because, she states, "the first one left my nose too big." In tears, the patient states that her discomfort about the appearance of her nose prevents her from having an active social life. She pleads with the psychiatrist to render an opinion that will permit the surgery. The patient does not appear psychotic. She does not express any other obsessional thoughts. In the psychiatrist's opinion, the patient's nose is unremarkable. Which of the following disorders is the most likely diagnosis for this patient?

(A) Delusional disorder, somatic type
(B) Obsessive-compulsive disorder
(C) Body dysmorphic disorder
(D) Hypochondriasis
(E) Somatization disorder

The correct response is option **C**: Body dysmorphic disorder

This patient demonstrates the diagnostic criteria for body dysmorphic disorder. She is preoccupied with a perceived defect in her appearance, and this concern affects her adaptation socially. On the basis of the information given, there are no signs or symptoms of a delusional disorder or an obsessive-compulsive disorder. She does not believe she has a serious illness, which usually is associated with hypochondriasis, and she does not have the list of physical complaints that define somatization disorder.

American Psychiatric Association: Diagnostic and Statistical Manual of Mental Disorders, Fourth Edition, Text Revision (DSM-IV-TR). Washington, DC, American Psychiatric Association, 2000, pp 507–511

232

A 50-year-old man is treated with several trials of single antidepressants. His unipolar depression has been only partially responsive. Which of the following agents has the best evidence from randomized controlled trials to support its use in augmenting his antidepressant?

(A) Bupropion
(B) Buspirone
(C) Lithium
(D) Methylphenidate
(E) Triiodothyronine (T$_3$)

The correct response is option **C**: Lithium

Lithium is the best studied augmentation agent in the treatment of unipolar depression. Most studies have been with lithium augmentation of tricyclic antidepressants. Fewer data are available on the effectiveness of T$_3$ or stimulants, although both are used.

Dubovsky SL, Dubovsky AN: Concise Guide to Mood Disorders. Washington, DC, American Psychiatric Publishing, 2002, p 225
Marangell LB, Silver JM, Goff DC, Yudofsky SC: Psychopharmacology and electroconvulsive therapy, in The American Psychiatric Publishing Textbook of Clinical Psychiatry, 4th ed. Edited by Hales RE, Yudofsky SC. Washington, DC, American Psychiatric Publishing, 2003, pp 1070–1072

233

A 65-year-old man seen in the emergency department is agitated, tachycardic, hypertensive, and tremulous. He sees fish swimming on the wall: "It's just like watching television." The most likely diagnosis is:

(A) delirium.
(B) delusional disorder.
(C) depression.
(D) obsessive-compulsive disorder.
(E) schizophrenia.

The correct response is option **A**: Delirium

Visual hallucinations suggest the need to rule out an organic cause related to a delirium. Rarely, patients with schizophrenia, mania, or depression may experience visual hallucinations.

Sadock BJ, Sadock VA (eds): Kaplan and Sadock's Comprehensive Textbook of Psychiatry, 8th ed. Philadelphia, Lippincott Williams & Wilkins, 2005, pp 1061–1063

234

A 42-year-old morbidly obese man is seen for chronic fatigue. Findings on polysomnography indicate obstructive sleep apnea. If the sleep apnea is left untreated over a prolonged period, which of the following conditions is most likely to develop?

(A) Cataplexy
(B) Catalepsy
(C) Pulmonary hypertension
(D) Obstructive pulmonary disease
(E) Sleep paralysis

The correct response is option **C**: Pulmonary hypertension

Long-standing sleep apnea is associated with increased pulmonary blood pressure and eventually increased systemic blood pressure as well. These changes may account for a considerable number of cases in which the diagnosis is essential hypertension.

Sadock BJ, Sadock VA: Kaplan and Sadock's Synopsis of Psychiatry, 9th ed. Philadelphia, Lippincott Williams & Wilkins, 2003, p 770

235

A patient in psychotherapy believes that her therapist wants to help her, she characteristically trusts him with very private material, and she has at times expressed her feeling that they have many things in common and that in many ways she views him as a role model. This patient's alliance is best characterized as:

(A) erotic.
(B) idealized.
(C) positive.
(D) primitive.
(E) mirroring.

The correct response is option **C**: Positive

It is important to recognize an "average expectable" positive transference and not to confuse it with other transference configurations. While positive transference has elements of idealization in it, this is still very different from an idealized transference per se. In order for therapy to proceed most effectively, a positive alliance needs to be in place. Erotic, idealized, primitive, and mirroring transference may all occur in the therapy and be amenable to examination/analysis because of the positive alliance.

Beitman BD, Yue D: Learning Psychotherapy: A Time-Efficient, Research-Based, and Outcome-Measured Psychotherapy Training Program. New York, WW Norton, 1999

236

For which of the anxiety disorders does clonazepam have an FDA indication?

(A) Generalized anxiety disorder
(B) Obsessive-compulsive disorder
(C) Panic disorder
(D) Posttraumatic stress disorder
(E) Social phobia

The correct response is option **C**: Panic disorder

Although clonazepam is often used as a general anxiolytic, its only FDA indications are seizure disorders and panic disorder. For most clinicians clonazepam would be a second-choice agent after the SSRIs for treating panic disorder. Clonazepam, a longer-acting benzodiazepine, is especially useful because it can be given less frequently and is associated with less rebound anxiety.

Stein DJ, Hollander E (eds): American Psychiatric Publishing Textbook of Anxiety Disorders. Washington, DC, American Psychiatric Publishing, 2002, pp 260–263

237

A 22-year-old female presents with symptoms of depression. She is always thinking that the worst will occur in her relationships and employment, and she feels powerless to alter or control these events. She is seeking treatment with a therapist who provides cognitive behavior therapy. What is the most likely focus of the therapy for this patient?

(A) Anger turned inward
(B) Early deprivation
(C) Difficulties in relationships
(D) Self-image
(E) Maladaptive thought patterns

The correct response is option **E**: Maladaptive thought patterns

Depression in cognitive behavior therapy is defined as resulting from distortions of thinking. These include a negative self-image and a tendency to experience the world as negative, demanding, and self-defeating. Depressed patients catastrophize, leaping from one imagined worst-case scenario to the next. The patient will expect failure, punishment, and continued hardship. In order to provide relief from symptoms the therapist will address issues of pessimistic anticipation, which is an example of a maladaptive thought process.

Sadock BJ, Sadock VA (eds): Kaplan and Sadock's Comprehensive Textbook of Psychiatry, 8th ed. Philadelphia, Lippincott Williams & Wilkins, 2005, pp 1607–1609

238

A 36-year-old female graduate student presents with atypical depression that has not responded to selective serotonin reuptake inhibitors (SSRIs). Which of the following medications has the most evidence for efficacy in this situation?

(A) Bupropion
(B) Phenelzine
(C) Valproic acid
(D) Trazodone
(E) Imipramine

The correct response is option **B**: Phenelzine

The available data indicate that monoamine oxidase inhibitors are more effective than tricyclic antidepressants for atypical depression. SSRIs are probably between these two classes in efficacy. Despite widespread use in clinical practice, there are no data supporting the efficacy of trazodone, bupropion, or any anticonvulsants in patients with atypical depression.

Dubovsky SL, Dubovsky AN: Concise Guide to Mood Disorders. Washington, DC, American Psychiatric Publishing, 2002, p 221
Practice Guideline for the Treatment of Patients With Major Depressive Disorder, 2nd ed (2000), in American Psychiatric Association Practice Guidelines for the Treatment of Psychiatric Disorders, Compendium 2004. Washington, DC, APA, 2004, p 469

239

"*Guevodoces*," which translates as "penis at 12," refers to Dominican children with a female appearance at birth, reared as girls, who at puberty develop male secondary sexual characteristics and male-typical sexual urges and behaviors. The genetic condition they have is called:

(A) androgen insensitivity syndrome.
(B) cloacal extrophy.
(C) congenital adrenal hyperplasia.
(D) Klinefelter syndrome.
(E) 5-α reductase deficiency.

The correct response is option **E**: 5-α Reductase deficiency

5-a Reductase is the enzyme that converts testosterone to dihydrotestosterone (DHT), the hormone necessary for fetal masculinization. As testosterone levels rise at puberty in these chromosomal males, predominant maleness emerges.

Panksepp J: Affective Neuroscience: The Foundations of Human and Animal Emotions. New York, Oxford University Press, 1998, p 233
Sadock BJ, Sadock VA (eds): Kaplan and Sadock's Comprehensive Textbook of Psychiatry, 8th ed. Philadelphia, Lippincott Williams & Wilkins, 2005, pp 1990–1991

240

Rapid cycling is LEAST likely to respond to:

(A) divalproex.
(B) carbamazepine.
(C) haloperidol.
(D) lithium.

The correct response is option **C**: Haloperidol

Haloperidol, a conventional antipsychotic, has no indication for the treatment of the rapid cycling subtype of bipolar disorder. In the treatment of bipolar disorder it is used as an adjunct to a mood stabilizer to treat psychotic symptoms. Data support the use of divalproex as the most effective treatment for rapid cycling. Lithium and carbamazepine are much less effective for rapid cycling.

Bowden CL: Valproate: drugs for the treatment of bipolar disorder, in The American Psychiatric Publishing Textbook of Psychopharmacology, 3rd ed. Edited by Schatzberg AF, Nemeroff CB. Washington, DC, American Psychiatric Publishing, 2004, pp 573–574

American Psychiatric Association: Practice Guideline for the Treatment of Patients With Bipolar Disorder (Revision). Am J Psychiatry 2002; 159(April suppl). Reprinted in FOCUS 2003; 1:64–110 (pp 94–97)

241

During an office follow-up visit, a 19-year-old woman with schizophrenia reports no improvement in her symptoms despite being on an appropriate dose of an antipsychotic medication for 3 weeks. The most reasonable initial approach would be to:

(A) add an anticonvulsant medication.
(B) add another antipsychotic medication.
(C) change to another antipsychotic medication.
(D) explore potential nonadherence.
(E) increase the dose of the patient's current medication.

The correct response is option **D**: Explore potential nonadherence

Poor adherence with the antipsychotic medication regimen is a common reason for lack of improvement. Even when adherence is not an issue, 2 to 4 weeks of treatment may be needed to see an initial effect of treatment, and 6 months or more may be needed to obtain a full or optimal response to medication.

Sadock BJ, Sadock VA (eds): Kaplan and Sadock's Comprehensive Textbook of Psychiatry, 8th ed. Philadelphia, Lippincott Williams & Wilkins, 2005, p 1473

American Psychiatric Association: Practice Guideline for the Treatment of Patients With Schizophrenia, 2nd ed. Am J Psychiatry 2004; 161(Feb suppl): 24–25

242

A small-town newspaper's reporter calls a psychiatrist to get "a professional's opinion" on the publicized misbehavior of the district's elected representative, who may or may not have bipolar disorder. The reporter asks the psychiatrist, who has never met the representative, "Why do you think the representative misbehaved, doctor?" The psychiatrist's ethical obligations would lead to which of the following responses?

(A) Inform the public about the representative's bipolar disorder, since this person is a public figure.
(B) Comment on the representative's condition only if the representative has not been a patient.
(C) Comment on either childhood dynamic origins or brain abnormality as the possible cause of the representative's problems, if public records contain information that is consistent with such possibilities.
(D) Comment on the general nature of psychiatric illnesses.

The correct response is option **D**: Comment on the general nature of psychiatric illnesses

A psychiatrist may comment on the general nature of psychiatric illnesses. However, it is unethical for a psychiatrist to publicly render a professional opinion about a person who is not the psychiatrist's own patient, who has not been properly examined by the psychiatrist, and who has not given proper informed consent to the psychiatrist to disclose professional opinions.

American Psychiatric Association: Opinions of the Ethics Committee on the Principles of Medical Ethics With Annotations Especially Applicable to Psychiatry. Washington, DC, American Psychiatric Association, 2001 (section 7-B)

Beauchamp TL, Childress JF: Principles of Biomedical Ethics, 5th ed. New York, Oxford University Press, 2001

243

In psychodynamic psychotherapy, a boundary crossing—unlike a boundary violation—is:

(A) discussed with the patient.
(B) an exploitative break in the therapeutic frame.
(C) generally not examined in the therapy.
(D) harmful to the therapy.
(E) a repeated occurrence.

The correct response is option **A**: Discussed with the patient

A boundary crossing is typically a benign and even helpful break in the therapeutic frame, especially when it is discussed in the therapy and the countertransference action leads to further exploration of the transference. According to Gabbard, boundary crossings usually occur in isolation, they are minor, and they ultimately do not cause harm; an example would be allowing the patient to stay a few extra minutes at the end of a session. Boundary violations, in contradistinction, are exploitative and are often not discussable.

Gabbard GO: Long-Term Psychodynamic Psychotherapy: A Basic Text. Washington, DC, American Psychiatric Publishing, 2004, pp 49–53

244

A male psychiatrist has been conducting weekly psychotherapy for the last 4 months with a female patient. The patient has serious financial problems due to overspending. One day, the patient brings in a gift-wrapped box to the session and, handing the box to the psychiatrist, blurts out, "It's a $100 tie ... I couldn't help myself, it just looked like something you'd wear and I'm so grateful for all of your help. Please accept it!" Which of the following is an appropriate response for the psychiatrist to give to this patient?

(A) Accept the gift but donate it to charity without telling the patient.
(B) Accept the gift but make it clear that the psychiatrist is uncomfortable doing so, given the patient's financial difficulties.
(C) Acknowledge the patient's gratitude, discuss the implications, but state that as a general policy the psychiatrist does not accept gifts from patients.
(D) Decline the gift without further explanation.

The correct response is option **C**: Acknowledge the patient's gratitude, discuss the implications, but state that as a general policy the psychiatrist does not accept gifts from patients

While accepting small gifts from patients may be ethically acceptable at times (when the gift is a genuine token of appreciation and to decline it would harm the therapeutic alliance), in the scenario in this question, accepting the tie is probably unethical for several reasons. First, the gift may represent a financial hardship for this patient. Second, the gift may signify more than a "token" of gratitude described by the patient (e.g., it may indicate the development of romantic transference, or may be more indicative of the patient's mood state). Third, the psychiatrist's acceptance of the gift could send the wrong signal to the patient, that is, that gifts are an accepted and even expected part of the psychiatrist's practice.

American Psychiatric Association: Ethics Primer of the American Psychiatric Association. Washington, DC, American Psychiatric Association, 2001 pp 46–47

245

A consultation is requested for a 16-year-old male who has been in detention for the past 2 months on charges of possession of cocaine. The detention center staff describe the youth as hyperactive, inattentive, impulsive, and easily distracted. A review of his educational history indicates that the youth has been in special education classes since the first grade because of attention deficit hyperactivity disorder and a mixed expressive-receptive language disorder. On examination, there is no evidence of a mood or anxiety disorder or current substance abuse. Which of the following medications would be most appropriate for this patient?

(A) Atomoxetine
(B) Clonidine
(C) Desipramine
(D) Mixed salts of amphetamines
(E) Pemoline

The correct response is option **A**: Atomoxetine

Atomoxetine is a recently approved nonstimulant medication for the treatment of ADHD. The drug is a potent inhibitor of presynaptic norepinephrine transporters with minimal affinity for other receptors or transporters. The most common side effects associated with it, which are generally mild, include sedation, decreased appetite, nausea, vomiting, and dizziness. Because atomoxetine is not known to be abusable, it is an excellent alternative for use with youths who have a history of illicit substance use or abuse and ADHD. Mixed salts of amphetamines is a Schedule II stimulant with a potential for abuse and would not be a good choice for this patient. The other three agents listed are considered second-line agents for ADHD and should be tried only after a failed trial of a first-line agent.

Dulcan MK, Martini DR, Lake MB: Concise Guide to Child and Adolescent Psychiatry, 3rd ed. Washington, DC, American Psychiatric Publishing, 2003, p 277

246

A 78-year-old patient with major depressive disorder is being treated with atorvastatin and metoprolol for cardiovascular disease. Which of the following antidepressants is best used with these two other medications?

(A) Bupropion
(B) Escitalopram
(C) Fluoxetine
(D) Nefazodone
(E) Paroxetine

The correct response is option **B**: Escitalopram

Escitalopram has no clinically meaningful P450 inhibitory effects, although it can cause a minor increase in metoprolol blood levels. Atorvastatin is a substrate for cytochrome P450 3A4. Inhibition of 3A4 by nefazodone could substantially increase atorvastatin blood levels and increase the risk of side effects. Metoprolol is a substrate for CYP 2D6, an enzyme potently inhibited by bupropion, fluoxetine, and paroxetine. Side effects of this beta-blocker could become problematic if there is a considerable increase in its blood level.

Williams D, Feely J: Pharmacokinetic-pharmacodynamic drug interactions with HMG-CoA reductase inhibitors. Clin Pharmacokinet 2002; 41:343–370
Wuttke H, Rau T, Heide R, Bergmann K, Bohm M, Weil J, Werner D, Eschenhagen T: Increased frequency of cytochrome P450 2D6 poor metabolizers among patients with metoprolol-associated adverse effects. Clin Pharmacol Ther 2002; 72:429–437
DeVane CL, Nemeroff CB: 2002 Guide to Psychotropic Drug Interactions. Primary Psychiatry 2002; 9:28–57

247

A 23-year-old woman presents to the clinic with a chief complaint of having sexual problems. She reports that she gets aroused and enjoys intercourse but is unable to have an orgasm. She believes the problem started about a month ago, when her physician prescribed a medication for her "anxiety attacks." The medication was most likely:

(A) bupropion.
(B) buspirone.
(C) citalopram.
(D) mirtazapine.
(E) trazodone.

The correct response is option **C**: Citalopram

Sexual side effects are the most common adverse effect of SSRIs, with an incidence between 50% and 80%. The most common complaints are inhibited orgasm and decreased libido. Impaired ability to achieve an orgasm may occur with other types of anti-depressants but is most likely with the SSRIs. Among the answer choices for this question, none of the medications listed other than the SSRI are likely to be prescribed for the treatment of paroxysmal anxiety.

Sadock BJ, Sadock VA (eds): Kaplan and Sadock's Synopsis of Psychiatry, 9th ed. Philadelphia, Lippincott Williams & Wilkins, 2003, p 1099
Schatzberg AF, Nemeroff CB (eds): The American Psychiatric Publishing Textbook of Psychopharmacology, 3rd ed, Washington, DC, American Psychiatric Publishing, 2004, pp 239, 331, 343, 395–398, 915–917

248

Methylphenidate has its greatest action on which of the following neurotransmitter systems?

(A) Acetylcholine
(B) Dopamine
(C) Gamma-aminobutyric acid
(D) Glutamate
(E) Serotonin

The correct response is option **B**: Dopamine

Methylphenidate's mechanism of action is believed to lie in dopamine presynaptic release and reuptake blockade.

Lewis M (ed): Child and Adolescent Psychiatry: A Comprehensive Textbook, 3rd ed. Philadelphia, Lippincott Williams & Wilkins, 2002, p 959
Martin A, Scahill L, Charney D, Leackman J (eds): Pediatric psychopharmacology principles and practice. New York, Oxford University Press, 2003, appendix

249

Which mental disorder is the most frequent cause of first-onset psychosis after age 60?

(A) Dementia of the Alzheimer's type
(B) Bipolar disorder
(C) Delusional disorder
(D) Major depression
(E) Very late onset schizophrenia

The correct response is option **A**: Dementia of the Alzheimer's type

Several epidemiological studies have established dementia of the Alzheimer's type as the most common cause of late-life psychosis. Late-onset schizophrenia is uncommon. The other disorders listed can cause psychosis in late life but not as commonly as dementia of the Alzheimer's type.

Spar JE, La Rue A: Concise Guide to Geriatric Psychiatry, 3rd ed. Washington, DC, American Psychiatric Publishing, 2002, pp 253–254

250

Psychotic features do NOT occur during which of the following?

(A) Manic episode
(B) Mixed episode
(C) Hypomanic episode
(D) Major depressive episode

The correct response is option **C**: Hypomanic episode

DSM-IV-TR criterion E for hypomanic episode includes ". . . and there are no psychotic features." Psychotic features can be associated with manic, mixed, and major depressive episodes.

American Psychiatric Association: Diagnostic and Statistical Manual of Mental Disorders, Fourth Edition, Text Revision (DSM-IV-TR). Washington, DC, American Psychiatric Association, 2000, pp 365–368

251

The parents of a 7-year-old boy express concern about his bed-wetting. The boy seems well adjusted, and the family has developed a nonstigmatizing system to care for his bed and personal hygiene. He has no medical problems. After explaining the natural history of enuresis, the most reasonable initial approach would be to:

(A) start desmopressin.
(B) start imipramine.
(C) provide observation and follow-up.
(D) order a bell and pad.
(E) start psychotherapy.

The correct response is option **C**: Provide observation and follow-up

The natural history of enuresis is that a substantial number of children remit after age 7. Given that the boy appears to be doing well, a reasonable approach is to wait and see if the enuresis improves with age.

Sadock BJ, Sadock VA (eds): Kaplan and Sadock's Comprehensive Textbook of Psychiatry, 8th ed. Philadelphia, Lippincott Williams & Wilkins, 2005, p 3243

252

A psychiatrist repeatedly and increasingly fantasizes about a sexual relationship with a patient in psychotherapy whom the psychiatrist finds very attractive. The psychiatrist is considering the possibility that the prohibition of sex with patients may not apply in this case because of some extenuating circumstances. Which of the following options would be the most ethical behavior on the part of the psychiatrist?

(A) Keep a diary of the sexual fantasies in order to contain them.
(B) Increase the frequency of therapy sessions in order to make the best use of the intensity of the transference that is developing.
(C) Transfer the patient's care to another psychiatrist.
(D) Because there are important psychodynamic therapeutic implications for the patient, share the fantasies with the patient if the benefits seem to outweigh the risks.

The correct response is option **C**: Transfer the patient's care to another psychiatrist

While termination of psychotherapy is a dramatic step, it is the best choice among the four options in preserving the patient's welfare. All of the other options are based on the impaired judgment of the psychiatrist. Indulging in the fantasies (option A) and increasing interactions with the patient (option B) may gratify the psychiatrist more than the patient and often precede eventual boundary violation by the psychiatrist. Self-disclosure of any kind should be done with caution; a psychiatrist's disclosure of sexual feelings toward the patient often precedes sexual boundary violations.

Simon RI: A Concise Guide to Psychiatry and Law for Clinicians, 3rd ed. Washington, DC, American Psychiatric Publishing, 2001, pp 228–238
Hundert EM, Appelbaum PS: Boundaries in psychotherapy: model guidelines. Psychiatry 1995; 58:345–356

253

Which of the following statements about a defendant's competency to stand trial for a criminal offense is NOT correct?

(A) The defendant must be able to remember what he or she was doing at the time of the offense.
(B) The defendant must be able to communicate with attorneys.
(C) The defendant must be able to understand basic courtroom procedure.
(D) The defendant must be able to understand the nature of various possible pleas and their consequences.

The correct response is option **A**: The defendant must be able to remember what he or she was doing at the time of the offense

Amnesia for the time of the offense usually does not interfere with the defendant's ability to consult with the attorney(s) and construct a valid defense unless the amnesia is part of an ongoing mental process such as dementia. To be competent to stand trial, a defendant must have a "rational as well as factual" understanding of the proceedings against the defendant; be able to communicate with the attorney(s) and assist in the defense; have the capacity to understand the basics of court procedures; and have the capacity to understand the charges and the possible consequences of the charges.

Hales RE, Yudofsky SC (eds): The American Psychiatric Publishing Textbook of Clinical Psychiatry, 4th ed. Washington, DC, American Psychiatric Publishing, 2003, pp 1611–1612

254

A 34-year-old Puerto Rican woman presents in distress at the outpatient clinic. She reports that her grandfather recently died, and since then she has been afflicted by several bouts of *ataque de nervios*. She has these spells only when she is upset. A detailed history should be obtained to distinguish *ataque* from which other axis I diagnosis?

(A) Bipolar disorder
(B) Histrionic personality disorder
(C) Obsessive-compulsive disorder
(D) Panic disorder
(E) Schizophrenia

The correct response is option **D**: Panic disorder

Symptoms of *ataque de nervios* include uncontrollable shouting, attacks of crying, trembling, a sense of heat in the chest that migrates to the head, and verbal and physical aggression, some of which overlap with panic disorder. However, unlike panic disorder, *ataques* are often associated with a specific event and an absence of acute fear.

Lewis-Fernandez R, Garrido-Castillo P, Bennasar MC, Parrilla EM, Laria AJ, Ma G, Petkova E: Dissociation, childhood trauma, and ataque de nervios among Puerto Rican psychiatric outpatients. Am J Psychiatry 2002; 159:1603–1605
American Psychiatric Association: Diagnostic and Statistical Manual of Mental Disorders, Fourth Edition, Text Revision (DSM-IV-TR). Appendix I: Outline for Cultural Formulation and Glossary of Culture-Bound Syndromes. Washington, DC, American Psychiatric Association, 2000, p 899

255

Which of the following signs or symptoms alone would be sufficient to meet criterion A for the active phase of schizophrenia?

(A) Bizarre delusions
(B) Catatonic behavior
(C) Incoherent speech
(D) Negative symptoms
(E) Tactile hallucinations

The correct response is option **A**: Bizarre delusions

In order to meet criterion A for schizophrenia, there has to be at least 1 month of symptoms, or less if successfully treated. The symptoms are two or more out of five items: delusions, hallucinations, disorganized speech, disorganized or catatonic behavior, and negative symptoms. One of the five items could be sufficient to fulfill criterion A if delusions are bizarre or if there is a voice running a commentary on the patient's behavior or thoughts, or two or more voices are conversing with each other.

American Psychiatric Association: Diagnostic and Statistical Manual of Mental Disorders, Fourth Edition, Text Revision (DSM-IV-TR). Washington, DC, American Psychiatric Association, 2000, pp 312–313

256

A 32-year-old woman was unexpectedly terminated from her job. Two months later she presents tearfully with depressed mood and occasional feelings of hopelessness; she still feels stressed by the loss of her job. She has no prior history of depression, is not suicidal, has not had changes in appetite, weight, sleep, or energy level, and still gets pleasure from family and hobbies. Which of the following diagnoses would be the most appropriate?

    (A) Major depressive disorder
    (B) Bipolar II disorder
    (C) Bereavement
    (D) Adjustment disorder
    (E) Dysthymic disorder

The correct response is option **D**: Adjustment disorder

Her symptoms developed in response to an identifiable stressor and appeared within 3 months of the stressor. The symptoms do not meet criteria for a major depressive episode. Bereavement is a reaction to the loss of a loved one. Dysthymic disorder has a 2-year duration criterion in adults.

American Psychiatric Association: Diagnostic and Statistical Manual of Mental Disorders, Fourth Edition, Text Revision (DSM-IV-TR). Washington, DC, American Psychiatric Association, 2000, pp 679–683

257

Which of the following has been approved by the FDA for the treatment of alcohol dependence?

    (A) Buprenorphine
    (B) Levo-alpha-acetylmethadol (LAAM)
    (C) Naloxone
    (D) Naltrexone

The correct response is option **D**: Naltrexone

In 1995 the FDA approved naltrexone, an opioid antagonist, for the treatment of alcohol dependence. Buprenorphine, LAAM, naloxone, and naltrexone are all used in the treatment of opioid dependence or overdose.

Schatzberg AF, Nemeroff CB (eds): The American Psychiatric Publishing Textbook of Psychopharmacology, 3rd ed. Washington, DC, American Psychiatric Publishing, 2004, p 1011
Schuckit MA, Tapert S: Alcohol, in The American Psychiatric Publishing Textbook of Substance Abuse Treatment, 3rd ed. Edited by Galanter M, Kleber HD. Washington, DC, American Psychiatric Publishing, 2004, p 162

258

A psychiatrist maintains private therapy progress notes, in addition to medical record notes, that contain extremely sensitive clinical information. This practice is:

    (A) an acceptable means of enhancing patient confidentiality.
    (B) an acceptable way of preventing court-mandated access to sensitive clinical information.
    (C) not acceptable, because all clinical material should be included in patients' medical records.
    (D) not acceptable, because the risks to the patient outweigh the benefits.

The correct response is option **A**: An acceptable means of enhancing patient confidentiality

Private progress notes can be a useful tool for protecting patient confidentiality, since there is value in maintaining more detailed therapy notes for patient care as well as for teaching purposes. However, private progress notes may be accessed under a court order. Medical record notes should be detailed enough to provide for continuity of patient care as well as for necessary administrative transactions (e.g., third-party payment for services) but should not contain highly sensitive material.

American Psychiatric Association, Committee on Confidentiality: Guidelines on Confidentiality. Am J Psychiatry 1987; 144:1522–1526
American Psychiatric Association: Principles of medical ethics with annotations especially applicable to psychiatry. Washington, DC, American Psychiatric Association, 2001 (section 4)
Gutheil TG, Appelbaum PS: Clinical Handbook of Psychiatry and the Law, 3rd ed. Philadelphia, Lippincott Williams & Wilkins, 2000

259

Which of the following psychosocial treatments is most likely to be effective in the treatment of obsessive-compulsive disorder?

    (A) Cognitive therapy
    (B) Supportive psychotherapy
    (C) Interpersonal therapy
    (D) Behavioral therapy
    (E) Group therapy

The correct response is option **D**: Behavioral therapy

Of the psychosocial treatments listed, the data for effectiveness are strongest for behavior treatment, and especially for treatment with a response-inhibition component. Cognitive therapy is promising, and group therapy is cost effective and helpful for some patients. Interpersonal therapy is not commonly indicated for obsessive-compulsive disorder.

Stein DJ, Hollander E (eds): American Psychiatric Publishing Textbook of Anxiety Disorders. Washington, DC, American Psychiatric Publishing, 2002, pp 221–230

Van Noppen BL, Steketee G: Individual, group, and multifamily cognitive-behavioral treatments, in Current Treatments of Obsessive-Compulsive Disorder, 2nd ed. Edited by Pato MT, Zohar J. Washington, DC, American Psychiatric Publishing, 2001. Reprinted in FOCUS 2004; 2:475–495 (p 475)

260

A 7-year-old boy presents to a clinic on referral from the school with a number of behavior problems, including impaired attention, hyperactivity, and impulsivity. His parents have described him as a "whirling dervish" for years. At age five, he was evaluated by his primary care physician and started on methylphenidate, which produced significant improvement in his behavior. However, he then developed jerky, irregular muscle movements around the eyes and mouth that persisted when he was off the medication. The medication that could address all of his symptoms is:

(A) clonidine.
(B) d,l-amphetamine.
(C) haloperidol.
(D) magnesium pemoline.
(E) pimozide.

The correct response is option **A**: Clonidine

This boy has classic symptoms of attention deficit hyperactivity disorder (ADHD), including impaired attention, hyperactivity, and impulsivity in school and at home, with onset before the age of 7 years. He has had a positive response to the stimulant medication methylphenidate but has developed simple motor tics involving the eyes and mouth. With some youths, the tics go away when stimulant medication is discontinued, but for this boy they have persisted. Therefore, treatment will need to target the symptoms of inattention, hyperactivity, impulsivity, and the motor disorder. Clonidine, an alpha-2 noradrenergic agonist, has been used successfully to treat ADHD and tic disorders and thus is the one single agent that would be most effective.

D,l-amphetamine and pemoline are both stimulants that may be helpful in addressing the ADHD symptoms, but they will not help with the tic disorder, and in fact they would probably make it worse. Haloperidol and pimozide are both antipsychotic medications that are useful in decreasing or eliminating tic-like movements, but they will not have an impact on the inattention, distractibility, and hyperactivity.

Lewis M (ed): Child and Adolescent Psychiatry: A Comprehensive Textbook, 3rd ed. Philadelphia, Lippincott Williams & Wilkins, 2002, pp 952, 956

Dulcan MK, Martini DR, Lake MB: Concise Guide to Child and Adolescent Psychiatry, 3rd ed. Washington, DC, American Psychiatric Publishing, 2003, p 81

261

A 16-year-old girl has been blinking her eyes and clearing her throat on an intermittent basis for years. She has no control of the symptoms and has never been free of them for more than a few days, and they cause significant problems. What medication may be helpful for treating this problem?

(A) Pimozide
(B) Nortriptyline
(C) Paroxetine
(D) Lorazepam
(E) Methylphenidate

The correct response is option **A**: Pimozide

The symptoms are those of Tourette's disorder. Pimozide is a frequently prescribed medication. Pimozide is approved by the FDA for the treatment of Tourette's disorder. D_2 receptor antagonists are thought to be effective because the dopamine system is hypothesized to be involved in the pathogenesis of Tourette's disorder. Drugs that increase dopamine (such as methylphenidate) may make the tics worse.

Sadock BJ, Sadock VA (eds): Kaplan and Sadock's Comprehensive Textbook of Psychiatry, 8th ed. Philadelphia, Lippincott Williams & Wilkins, 2005, p 3232

262

Blocking craving for opiates with subsequent reduction in associated drug use generally requires which of the following daily doses of methadone?

(A) 5 mg
(B) 10 mg
(C) 20 mg
(D) 40 mg
(E) 80 mg

The correct response is option **E**: 80 mg

Most patients require doses greater than 60 mg to block craving for opiates and to reduce subsequent associated drug use. A dose of 40 to 60 mg/day of methadone is usually sufficient to block opioid withdrawal symptoms.

American Psychiatric Association: Practice Guideline for the Treatment of Patients With Substance Use Disorders: Alcohol, Cocaine, Opioids. Am J Psychiatry 1995; 152(Nov suppl)

263

Which of the following is the most important consideration for the treatment plan when performing an initial evaluation of a patient with borderline personality disorder in suicidal crisis?

(A) Safety
(B) Goals
(C) Type
(D) Frame
(E) Outcome

The correct response is option **A**: Safety

Safety should be the priority. Suicidal ideation and suicide attempts are common, and it is essential during an initial assessment to decide whether inpatient treatment is necessary.

Practice Guideline for the Treatment of Patients With Borderline Personality Disorder (2001), in American Psychiatric Association Practice Guidelines for the Treatment of Psychiatric Disorders, Compendium 2004. Washington, DC, APA, 2004, p 753

264

The best documented treatment for posttraumatic stress disorder (PTSD) precipitated by a violent rape includes:

(A) event recall.
(B) martial arts instruction.
(C) prosecution of the rapist.
(D) cognitive-based therapy.

The correct response is option **D**: Cognitive-based therapy

Published reports by Foa and colleagues demonstrate that cognitive-based psychotherapies that facilitate destigmatization and desensitization are particularly effective for rape victims. Bringing the rapist to justice and requiring the victim to be at trial often causes a reliving of the traumatic experience and becomes an emotionally painful event for the victim. There is controversy about whether it is helpful or harmful to the patient's recovery if the victim is encouraged to tell the story in detail. The choice of approaches depends on the needs of the victim. Martial arts training for some victims can be helpful in preventing rape and perhaps providing a victim with some sense of security and protection against a repeated experience. However, many victims would be uncomfortable in having to consider that the event could occur again with such certainty that they must prepare for it by martial arts training.

Hales RE, Yudofsky SC (eds): The American Psychiatric Publishing Textbook of Clinical Psychiatry, 4th ed. Washington, DC, American Psychiatric Publishing, 2003, pp 606–607
Hembree EA, Foa EB: Interventions for trauma-related emotional disturbances in adult victims of crime. J Trauma Stress 2003; 16:187–199
Connor KM, Butterfield MI: Posttraumatic stress disorder. FOCUS 2003; 1:247–262 (p 256)

265

A 40-year-old female comes to the mental health center for the first time. After a thorough assessment, she is told that the best treatment would be a course of brief psychotherapy. She looks concerned and asks if she can be transferred to a doctor of her own race. The appropriate step to take would be to:

(A) attempt to convince her that any doctor is capable.
(B) explore why she feels this is necessary.
(C) grant her request and transfer her.
(D) help her find another clinic that will suit her.
(E) switch to medication management only.

The correct response is option **B**: Explore why she feels this is necessary

Although the patient may ultimately be transferred to another clinician, one should still make an attempt to find out the reasoning behind her request.

Tseng W, Streltzer J: Culture and Psychotherapy. Washington, DC, American Psychiatric Publishing, 2001, pp 146–147

266

DSM-IV-TR cultural formulation for a patient from a culture different than the psychiatrist's requires:

(A) a history of the patient's education and occupational training.
(B) independent information from a cultural consultant.
(C) an understanding of the neurobiology of the patient's disorder.
(D) an understanding of the effect of the psychiatrist's own culture on treatment variables.
(E) use of an interpreter from or assimilated in the patient's culture.

The correct response is option **D**: An understanding of the effect of the psychiatrist's own culture on treatment variables

According to DSM-IV-TR, the cultural formulation provides a systematic review of the individual's cultural background, the role of the cultural context in the expression and evaluation of symptoms and dysfunction, and the effect that cultural differences may have on the relationship between the individual and the clinician. One of the components of a cultural formulation is a summary of the cultural elements of the relationship between the individual and the clinician, such as differences in culture and social status. This requires that the psychiatrist be knowledgeable about his or her own culture.

Interpreters would be used only in cases where the psychiatrist and the patient were not fluent in the same language. The educational history per se is not a required component of the formulation. Since the neurobiology of a number of psychiatric disorders remains to be elucidated, this could not be a formulation component.

American Psychiatric Association: Diagnostic and Statistical Manual of Mental Disorders, Fourth Edition, Text Revision (DSM-IV-TR) Appendix I: Outline for Cultural Formulation and Glossary of Culture-Bound Syndromes. Washington, DC, American Psychiatric Association, 2000

267

A 20-year-old male college student presents in the emergency department with confusion and agitation. He is distracted and talks in a rambling manner. During the interview, he reports seeing an angel who is telling him about his mission. His roommate states that the student has been having problems for months, with worsening grades, not sleeping, and withdrawal from friends. In establishing a diagnosis and preparing to initiate treatment, the most appropriate laboratory test to obtain at this point would be:

(A) a complete blood count, including a platelet count.
(B) an electrocardiogram.
(C) hepatic function tests.
(D) thyroid function tests.
(E) a toxicology screen.

The correct response is option **E**: A toxicology screen

Substance use is a common cause of psychotic symptoms and should be eliminated before diagnosis and treatment of other psychiatric disorders.

Sadock BJ, Sadock VA (eds): Kaplan and Sadock's Comprehensive Textbook of Psychiatry, 8th ed. Philadelphia, Lippincott Williams & Wilkins, 2005, p 1124
American Psychiatric Association: Practice Guideline for the Treatment of Patients With Schizophrenia, 2nd ed. Am J Psychiatry 2004; 161(Feb suppl):1–56

268

A 60-year-old woman presents with daytime fatigue, morning headache, and poor memory. Findings from her physical examination and blood studies are all within normal limits, and she reports that her mood is normal. On further questioning she reports that her husband sleeps in a separate room because of her snoring and thrashing. The most effective treatment for this condition is:

(A) fluoxetine.
(B) continuous positive airway pressure.
(C) lorazepam.
(D) methylphenidate.
(E) relaxation therapy.

The correct response is option **B**: Continuous positive airway pressure

The patient likely has sleep apnea. The best treatment is continuous positive airway pressure (CPAP). Other measures are also helpful, such as weight loss and sleep-position training.

Hales RE, Yudofsky SC (eds): The American Psychiatric Publishing Textbook of Clinical Psychiatry, 4th ed. Washington, DC, American Psychiatric Publishing, 2003, p 984
Krahn LE, Richardson JW: Sleep disorders, in The American Psychiatric Publishing Textbook of Psychosomatic Medicine. Edited by Levenson JL. Washington, DC, American Psychiatric Publishing, 2005, pp 342–344

269

Which of the following best describes a characteristic of the assertive community treatment (ACT) model for management of schizophrenia?

(A) Clinic-based services
(B) Focus on symptom resolution
(C) Hospital-based services
(D) Psychiatrist-led treatment team
(E) 24-hour availability of services

The correct response is option **E**: 24-hour availability of services

In the ACT model, some level of case management is typically available around the clock. The ACT model emphasizes a flexible, horizontally organized treatment team that delivers services in the community, where the client lives, rather than in a clinic setting. Symptom recurrence is handled by increasing the intensity of outpatient services rather than relying on inpatient services. Improved community functioning, often based on treatment goals negotiated with the client, is the desired outcome, not necessarily the elimination of the symptoms of the disorder.

Phillips SD, Burns BJ, Edgar ER, Mueser KT, Linkins KW, Rosenheck RA, Drake RE, McDonel Herr EC: Moving assertive community treatment into standard practice. Psychiatr Serv 2001; 52:771–779
Dixon L: Assertive community treatment: twenty-five years of gold. Psychiatr Serv 2000; 51:759–765

270

The strong association between physical illness and suicide has been demonstrated for which of the following conditions?

(A) Amyotrophic lateral sclerosis
(B) Blindness
(C) Epilepsy
(D) Hypertension
(E) Diabetes mellitus

The correct response is option **C**: Epilepsy

An association between seizure disorders and increased suicide risk has been found in many studies. Temporal lobe epilepsy in particular is associated with a higher suicide risk, perhaps because of its impulsivity, presence of mood disorders, and psychosis. Studies have not demonstrated an increased suicide risk with the other conditions listed.

Practice Guideline for the Assessment and Treatment of Patients With Suicidal Behaviors (2003), in Practice Guidelines for the Treatment of Psychiatric Disorders, Compendium 2004. Washington, DC, APA, 2004, pp 875–876

271

A 32-year-old man sees his primary care physician because of a recurrent productive cough. The physician recommends blood work and a chest X-ray. When the patient enters the phlebotomy suite, his heart begins to race, he perspires, and his muscles tense. When he sits in the phlebotomy chair and a tourniquet is applied, his symptoms worsen. In addition, he becomes short of breath, begins to hyperventilate, and feels numbness and tingling in his hands and feet and around his mouth. When the phlebotomist uncaps the needle, the patient passes out. He awakens shortly after an ammonia capsule is broken under his nose. He apologizes for his behavior and says, "I always get this way when I see a needle." This presentation is most consistent with:

(A) agoraphobia.
(B) generalized anxiety disorder.
(C) panic disorder.
(D) social phobia.
(E) specific phobia.

The correct response is option **E**: Specific phobia

The essential feature of a specific phobia is marked and persistent fear of a specific object or situation. Exposure to the phobic stimulus provokes an immediate anxiety response that may appear as panic. However, unlike in panic disorder, the anxiety response in specific phobia is situationally bound. In this case, the phobia is related to the fear of needles.

American Psychiatric Association: Diagnostic and Statistical Manual of Mental Disorders, Fourth Edition, Text Revision (DSM-IV-TR). Washington, DC, American Psychiatric Association, 2000, pp 443–450

272

Which of the following symptoms is significantly more likely to be associated with posttraumatic stress disorder (PTSD) than with normal bereavement?

(A) Initial shock
(B) Depressive symptoms
(C) Numbing
(D) Avoidance of reminders
(E) Sleep disturbance

The correct response is option **C**: Numbing

Restricted range of affect, often called numbing, is more likely to be associated with PTSD than with normal bereavement. Numbing, a decrease in general responsiveness, is a mechanism for avoiding stimuli that may be associated with the trauma. Initial shock, depressive symptoms, and avoidance of reminders of the traumatic event or loved one are common to both PTSD and to normal bereavement.

American Psychiatric Association: Diagnostic and Statistical Manual of Mental Disorders, Fourth Edition, Text Revision (DSM-IV-TR). Washington, DC, American Psychiatric Association, 2000, pp 463–468, 740–741

Shalev AY: What is posttraumatic stress disorder? J Clin Psychiatry 2001; 62(suppl 17):4–10

273

A patient with schizophrenia is in the midst of a severe exacerbation but refuses treatment. The patient is able to paraphrase what the psychiatrist has said about the diagnosis, the prognosis, and the reasons for the proposed treatment with medications. Which of the following statements by the patient is the clearest example of an impaired ability to "appreciate or understand"?

   (A) "I have tried all those antipsychotics before. None of them work that well for me so why try again."
   (B) "Your office is bugged, but the reason why I do not want to take the medication is that I am really afraid of gaining more weight."
   (C) "The space aliens living in my stomach would be injured if I took those pills."
   (D) "I am a Christian Scientist and I do not believe that I have a disease."

The correct response is option **C**: "The space aliens living in my stomach would be injured if I took those pills."

In option C, the patient's delusion is the causal factor leading to the false belief. The appreciation standard focuses on whether the patient is able to apply facts to his or her own medical situation. Often this means that the patient has a contrary, false belief regarding some medical fact. A delusional belief can impair appreciation if it directly causes the patient to fail to apply important facts to his or her own case. Thus, in option B, the delusion cannot be said to directly cause the false belief. Skepticism based on potentially realistic experiences or on established religious beliefs also does not constitute delusional beliefs that directly affect appreciation.

Grisso T, Appelbaum PS: Assessing Competence to Consent to Treatment: A Guide for Physicians and Other Health Professionals. New York, Oxford University Press, 1998

274

A 42-year-old woman with generalized anxiety disorder has responded favorably to 60 mg/day of buspirone. To avoid substantially increasing the blood level of the medication and producing side effects, you caution her to avoid regular consumption of which of the following beverages?

   (A) Apple juice
   (B) Coffee
   (C) Grapefruit juice
   (D) Milk
   (E) Red wine

The correct response is option **C**: Grapefruit juice

Grapefruit juice is a potent inhibitor of intestinal cytochrome P450 3A4. In addition, it inhibits P-glyco-protein (a transmembrane efflux pump protein). Even a single glass of grapefruit juice will have strong inhibitory effects for as long as 24 hours on the metabolism of various drugs, including some calcium channel blockers, benzodiazepines, statins, and cyclosporine. Similar effects have been noted with Seville (sour) orange juice but not with sweet (regular) orange juice. In a study with healthy volunteers, grapefruit juice caused a 4.3-fold increase in the peak blood level of buspirone and a 9.2-fold increase in extent of absorption (area under the curve).

Lilja JJ, Kivisto KT, Backman JT, Lamberg TS, Neuvonen PJ: Grapefruit juice substantially increases plasma concentrations of buspirone. Clin Pharmacol Ther 1998; 64:655–660

Malhotra S, Bailey DG, Paine MF, Watkins PB: Seville orange juice-felodipine interaction: comparison with dilute grapefruit juice and involvement of furocoumarins. Clin Pharmacol Ther 2001; 69:14–23

Marangell LB, Silver JM, Goff DC, Yudofsky SC: Psychopharmacology and electroconvulsive therapy, in The American Psychiatric Publishing Textbook of Clinical Psychiatry, 4th ed. Edited by Hales RE, Yudofsky SC. Washington, DC, American Psychiatric Publishing, 2003, table 24-24, Drug Interactions, p 1117

Lown KS: Grapefruit juice increases felodipine oral availability in humans by decreasing intestinal CYP3A protein expression. J Clin Invest 1997; 99:2545–2553

275

Which of the following therapies has the best evidence for effectiveness in the treatment of posttraumatic stress disorder?

(A) Present-centered group therapy
(B) Psychological debriefings
(C) Single-session techniques
(D) Cognitive behavior therapy
(E) Trauma-focused group therapy

The correct response is option **D**: Cognitive behavior therapy

Evidence has shown a variety of psychotherapeutic approaches to be highly efficacious in reducing the symptoms of posttraumatic stress disorder. Exposure and other cognitive behavior therapy approaches as well as eye movement desensitization and reprocessing (EMDR) have been shown to reduce symptoms. There is far less evidence to support the use of present-centered or trauma-focused group therapies and no evidence to support the use of psychological debriefings or single-session techniques. Early supportive interventions, psychoeducation, and case management also appear to be helpful for acutely traumatized individuals and may facilitate their entry into evidence-based psychotherapeutic and psychopharmacological treatments.

Bradley R, Greene J, Russ E, Dutra L, Westen D: A multidimensional meta-analysis of psychotherapy for PTSD. Am J Psychiatry 2005; 162:214–227
American Psychiatric Association: Practice Guideline for the Treatment of Patients With Acute Stress Disorder and Posttraumatic Stress Disorder. Am J Psychiatry 2004; 161(Nov suppl)

276

Linkage analysis can be defined as:

(A) a test to identify which of several genes in a chromosomal region is involved in the disorder in question.
(B) a test to determine the chromosomal region where a disorder resides by searching for co-segregation of a genetic marker with the disorder locus.
(C) a study that requires the cause of the disorder to be a common risk variant.
(D) an analysis that is not sensitive to a genetic model.

The correct response is option **B**: A test to determine the chromosomal region where a disorder resides by searching for co-segregation of a genetic marker with the disorder locus

In linkage analysis, geneticists use genetic markers to determine the chromosomal location of the gene for a disorder. Options C and D are features of association study. In comparison, linkage analysis allows many different rare mutations in the linked genes and requires a genetic model.

Burmeister M: Genetics of psychiatric disorders: a primer. FOCUS 2006; in press

277

Which of the following is true regarding adolescents with attention deficit hyperactivity disorder (ADHD) who are treated with methylphenidate?

(A) Significantly reduced risk of substance abuse in later life
(B) Higher level of all substance abuse in adulthood
(C) Increased alcohol abuse in adulthood
(D) Increased cannabis abuse in adulthood

The correct response is option **A**: Significantly reduced risk of substance abuse in later life

In a long-term study of pediatrically and psychiatrically referred ADHD and non-ADHD youth, pharmacotherapy for ADHD did not predict a greater risk of substance use disorder. Subjects with ADHD who did not receive pharmacologic treatment were at a significantly increased risk of substance use disorder, suggesting that pharmacotherapy may protect children with ADHD from this risk.

Biederman J, Wilens T, Mick E, Spencer T, Faraone SV: Pharmacotherapy of attention-deficit/hyperactivity disorder reduces risk for substance use disorder. Pediatrics 1999; 104:e20
Hales RE, Yudofsky SC (eds): The American Psychiatric Publishing Textbook of Clinical Psychiatry, 4th ed. Washington, DC, American Psychiatric Publishing, 2003, p 368

278

Elements of an individual's ability to make decisions about undergoing treatment or participating in research include all of the following EXCEPT:

(A) understanding the information provided.
(B) reasoning with the information or weighing options.
(C) repeating the outlined risks and benefits without prompting.
(D) appreciating the significance of the information for the individual's own situation.

The correct response is option **C**: Repeating the outlined risks and benefits without prompting

An individual is not required to memorize or recite the risks and benefits of a recommended procedure without prompting in order to be able to make a decision about treatment or research. Options A, B, and D in this question are considered by most experts to be crucial elements of decision-making capacity, along with communication of a choice. The individual's choice need not be in accord with what the physician recommends. Only a careful evaluation of capacity-related abilities, in the context of a patient's illness or situation, can lead to a determination of capacity status.

Simon RI: A Concise Guide to Psychiatry and Law for Clinicians, 3rd ed. Washington, DC, American Psychiatric Publishing, 2001, pp 64–65

Grisso T, Appelbaum PS: Assessing Competence to Consent to Treatment: A Guide for Physicians and Other Health Professionals. New York, Oxford University Press, 1998

279

A school guidance counselor refers a 5-year-old girl who will not speak. The girl has been enrolled in school for 3 months. During this time, she has been noted to make hand gestures or nod in response to her teacher or peers. The guidance counselor has been meeting with the girl regularly, and recently the child has begun to whisper. However, she will not use a normal voice. The girl's parents report that the child has no problems speaking at home. The girl plays with her peers, makes appropriate eye contact when spoken to, seems interested in others, and has no unusual movements. There have been no delays or abnormalities in development. As an adult, this child is at high risk of developing:

(A) major depressive disorder.
(B) obsessive-compulsive disorder.
(C) posttraumatic stress disorder.
(D) schizophrenia.
(E) social phobia.

The correct response is option **E**: Social phobia

This young girl is suffering from selective mutism. Although the disorder is fairly rare (a prevalence of less than 1% of children seen in mental health settings), the most common manifestations are a refusal to speak in school and to adults outside of the home despite speaking normally within the home environment. Although these children do not speak, they appear to be interested in their surroundings, as evidenced by interaction, head nodding, gesturing, and so on. Many of these children are shy, anxious, and overly dependent. Recent studies have identified a link between selective mutism in children and social phobia in adulthood.

Lewis M (ed): Child and Adolescent Psychiatry: A Comprehensive Textbook, 3rd ed. Philadelphia, Lippincott Williams & Wilkins, 2002, pp 616–617

Dulcan MK, Martini DR, Lake MB: Concise Guide to Child and Adolescent Psychiatry, 3rd ed. Washington, DC, American Psychiatric Publishing, 2003, pp 91–94

280

A 10-year-old boy is brought for consultation for "bed-wetting." His parents report that he began using the toilet and staying dry during the day when he was 3 years old. However, he has never consistently been able to control his bladder during sleep. Physical examination and laboratory studies have demonstrated no abnormalities. His father reports that he also wet the bed as a child but stopped when he was about 12 years old. The intervention that is most likely to have long-term effectiveness with this boy is:

(A) hypnotherapy.
(B) low-dose tricyclic antidepressants.
(C) oral desmopressin.
(D) psychotherapy.
(E) urine alarm (bell and pad).

The correct response is option **E**: Urine alarm (bell and pad)

Primary enuresis is diagnosed when a child has never attained bladder control. With nocturnal enuresis, there is usually a positive family history and no demonstrable physical abnormalities to explain the bladder incontinence. Behavioral interventions such as the urine alarm—the "bell and pad"—have been demonstrated to be the most innocuous and to have the greatest efficacy in permanently eliminating nocturnal enuresis. Hypnotherapy has not been proven as a reliable intervention for this disorder. Psychotherapy may be helpful in managing the emotional impact of bed-wetting, but does not help with continence.

The mechanism by which tricyclic antidepressants, such as imipramine, are helpful in this disorder is unknown. Desmopressin, an analogue of antidiuretic hormone, is available in a nasal spray and tablets. Desmopressin is as effective as the tricyclic antidepressants in the treatment of primary enuresis and has fewer side effects, but it is much more expensive. Both the tricyclics and desmopressin have limited, short-term efficacy in attaining bladder control but have not proven to be effective in long-term management.

Lewis M (ed): Child and Adolescent Psychiatry: A Comprehensive Textbook, 3rd ed. Philadelphia, Lippincott Williams & Wilkins, 2002, pp 702–705

281

A 58-year-old man has a history of ingesting 1 to 2 pints of vodka on a daily basis over the past 20 years. He presents to the emergency department after a minor motor vehicle accident and appears disorganized. A computerized tomography scan of his head is most likely to show which of the following?

(A) Acoustic neuroma
(B) Caudate calcification
(C) Cerebellar degeneration
(D) Frontal lobe tumor
(E) Prolactinoma

The correct response is option **C**: Cerebellar degeneration

Chronic alcoholism is associated with several neurologic findings: cerebellar anterior lobe degeneration, retrobulbar optic neuropathy, Wernicke's encephalopathy, and amnestic disorder (Korsakoff's syndrome). Cerebellar degeneration is characterized by unsteadiness of gait, problems with standing, and mild nystagmus. Cerebellar degeneration is probably caused by a combination of the effects of ethanol and acetaldehyde along with vitamin deficiencies.

Sadock BJ, Sadock VA (eds): Kaplan and Sadock's Comprehensive Textbook of Psychiatry, 8th ed. Philadelphia, Lippincott Williams & Wilkins, 2005, p 1172
Mack AH, Franklin JE, Frances RJ: Substance use disorders, in The American Psychiatric Publishing Textbook of Clinical Psychiatry, 4th ed. Edited by Hales RE, Yudofsky SC. Washington, DC, American Psychiatric Publishing, 2003, pp 329–330

282

Symptoms of obsessive-compulsive disorder respond best to which of the following tricyclic antidepressants?

(A) Imipramine
(B) Amitriptyline
(C) Doxepin
(D) Clomipramine
(E) Desipramine

The correct response is option **D**: Clomipramine

Clomipramine, which blocks the neuronal reuptake of serotonin, improves the symptoms of obsessive-compulsive disorder in a manner similar to the newer SSRIs. Clomipramine was the first drug approved by the FDA for the treatment of obsessive-compulsive disorder.

Stein DJ, Hollander E (eds): American Psychiatric Publishing Textbook of Anxiety Disorders. Washington, DC, American Psychiatric Publishing, 2002, p 207

283

A 23-year-old woman presented with a 2-week history of difficulty sleeping, hearing voices, and problems with thinking. She was fearful and suspicious, and talked about evil alien forces out in the world. Some of her relatives have had "nervous breakdowns" requiring hospitalization. Further evaluation revealed that the woman had been raped about 3 weeks earlier. However, she has no recollection of the event. One week after initial presentation, her symptoms have disappeared and she has returned to normal functioning. The most likely diagnosis at this time is:

(A) acute stress disorder.
(B) brief psychotic disorder.
(C) schizoaffective disorder.
(D) posttraumatic stress disorder.
(E) schizophreniform disorder.

The correct response is option **B**: Brief psychotic disorder

Given the recent trauma and short duration of symptoms, brief psychotic disorder is the most reasonable diagnosis. Acute stress disorder and PTSD require the presence of avoidance, increased arousal and reexperiencing the event. PTSD and schizophreniform disorder both require the presence of symptoms for at least 4 weeks.

Sadock BJ, Sadock VA (eds): Kaplan and Sadock's Comprehensive Textbook of Psychiatry, 8th ed. Philadelphia, Lippincott Williams & Wilkins, 2005, pp 1520–1521
American Psychiatric Association: Diagnostic and Statistical Manual of Mental Disorders, Fourth Edition, Text Revision (DSM-IV-TR). Washington, DC, American Psychiatric Association, 2000, pp 329–332

284

Which of the following medications is most likely to be associated with polycystic ovary syndrome?

(A) Carbamazepine
(B) Gabapentin
(C) Lithium
(D) Topiramate
(E) Valproate

The correct response is option **E**: Valproate

Among women who started valproate before age 20, 80% have polycystic ovaries. Since over 50% of women on valproate are also obese and because obesity is associated with polycystic ovary syndrome, it is unclear whether valproate's effects on the high rate of polycystic ovaries are a direct result of the drug or an indirect effect of contributing to obesity.

Schatzberg AF, Cole JO, DeBattista C: Manual of Clinical Psychopharmacology. Washington, DC, American Psychiatric Publishing, 2005, p 271

285

In the National Institute of Mental Health's Epidemiologic Catchment Area study, the ethnic differences in the 1-month prevalence of mental health disorders dropped after which of the following factors was controlled for?

(A) Age
(B) Education
(C) Gender
(D) Literacy rate
(E) Socioeconomic status

The correct response is option **E**: Socioeconomic status

Age, socioeconomic status, and education have been confounders in various studies comparing mental illness prevalences among different races. However, the Epidemiologic Catchment Area study specifically controlled for socioeconomic status.

Sadock BJ, Sadock VA (eds): Kaplan and Sadock's Comprehensive Textbook of Psychiatry, 8th ed. Philadelphia, Lippincott Williams & Wilkins, 2005, pp 2285–2286

Regier DA, Farmer ME, Rae DS, Myers JK, Kramer M, Robins LN, George LK, Karno M, Locke BZ: One-month prevalence of mental disorders in the United States and sociodemographic characteristics: the Epidemiologic Catchment Area study. Acta Psychiatr Scand 1993; 88:35–47

286

A patient has not responded to phenelzine after 10 weeks of treatment, and a switch to fluoxetine is planned. What is the recommended minimum interval between stopping phenelzine and starting fluoxetine?

(A) 1 week
(B) 2 weeks
(C) 4 weeks
(D) 6 weeks
(E) 8 weeks

The correct response is option **B**: 2 weeks

Phenelzine is an irreversible inhibitor of monoamine oxidase. Once discontinued, a period of 2 weeks is required for new enzymes to be synthesized. Thus, the switch from phenelzine to fluoxetine would require a 2-week washout period. Without a washout of sufficient length, a fatal serotonin syndrome could occur. By contrast, because fluoxetine has an extremely long half-life, a washout of at least 5 weeks is advised if a switch is to be made from a monoamine oxidase inhibitor to fluoxetine.

Gadde KM, Krishman KR: Current status of monoamine oxidase inhibitors in psychiatric practice. Essent Psychopharmacol 1997; 1:255–272

Feighner JP, Boyer WF, Tyler DL, Neborsky RJ: Adverse consequences of fluoxetine-MAOI combination therapy. J Clin Psychiatry 1990; 51:222–225

Schatzberg AF, Nemeroff CB (eds): The American Psychiatric Publishing Textbook of Psychopharmacology, 3rd ed, Washington, DC, American Psychiatric Publishing, 2004, p 309 (Table 18-4)

287

The single most effective treatment for major depression in elderly patients is:

(A) bupropion.
(B) citalopram.
(C) ECT.
(D) nortriptyline.
(E) venlafaxine.

The correct response is option **C**: ECT

Remission rates for ECT are 90% or higher among elderly patients. ECT is especially indicated when an elderly patient is actively suicidal, anorexic, noncompliant with medication, or unable to tolerate medication.

Spar JE, La Rue A: Concise Guide to Geriatric Psychiatry, 3rd ed. Washington, DC, American Psychiatric Publishing, 2002, p 143

288

A 30-year-old athletic man presents for evaluation of several syncopal episodes over the past month. He has been treated for hypertension during the past year and has responded nicely to 50 mg/day of metoprolol XR and 25 mg/day of hydrochlorothiazide. Three months ago his primary care physician started him on 20 mg/day of fluoxetine and 0.5 mg/day of lorazepam t.i.d. for mixed anxiety and depression. On examination the patient seems mildly anxious and demonstrates orthostatic hypotension. His ECG is unremarkable except for mild sinus bradycardia. What is the most likely explanation?

(A) Transient ischemic attacks
(B) Fluoxetine–metoprolol interaction
(C) Overdiuresis
(D) Benzodiazepine intoxication
(E) Psychogenic syncope

The correct response is option **B**: Fluoxetine–metoprolol interaction

Fluoxetine is a powerful inhibitor of the cytochrome P450 2D6 isoenzyme, which metabolizes beta-blockers, including metoprolol. This can lead to increased serum levels of the beta-blocker, causing orthostatic hypotension, bradycardia, and often syncope.

Ereshefsky L: Drug interactions of antidepressants. Psychiatr Ann 1996; 26:342–350
Robinson MJ, Owen JA: Psychopharmacology, in The American Psychiatric Publishing Textbook of Psychosomatic Medicine. Edited by Levenson JL. Washington, DC, American Psychiatric Publishing, 2005, pp 872–874, Table 37-2, pp 876–879

289

Attention deficit hyperactivity disorder (ADHD) appears to be most strongly associated with prenatal exposure to:

(A) caffeine.
(B) lithium.
(C) nicotine.
(D) SSRIs.
(E) valproic acid.

The correct response is option **C**: Nicotine

Of the pharmacological agents and substances listed, the only one for which prenatal exposure has been associated with ADHD in a number of case-control studies is nicotine.

Sadock BJ, Sadock VA (eds): Kaplan and Sadock's Comprehensive Textbook of Psychiatry, 8th ed. Philadelphia, Lippincott Williams & Wilkins, 2005, p 3186

Linnet KM, Dalsgaard S, Obel C, Wisborg K, Henriksen TB, Rodriguez A, Kotimaa A, Moilanen I, Thomsen PH, Olsen J, Jarvelin MR: Maternal lifestyle factors in pregnancy risk of attention deficit hyperactivity disorder and associated behaviors: review of the current evidence. Am J Psychiatry 2003; 160:1028–1040

290

Compared with Caucasian Americans, African Americans are more likely to receive a diagnosis of:

(A) bipolar disorder, depressed.
(B) bipolar disorder, manic.
(C) major depression.
(D) schizophrenia.
(E) substance-induced psychosis.

The correct response is option **D**: Schizophrenia

Probably because of multiple factors, such as differential health care utilization patterns, differential symptom presentations, mismatch of provider and patient race, and bias, African Americans are more likely than Caucasians to receive a diagnosis of schizophrenia. African Americans have been underdiagnosed with bipolar and other mood disorders.

Snowden L: Bias in mental health assessment and intervention: theory and evidence. Am J Public Health 2003; 93:239–243
Sadock BJ, Sadock VA (eds): Kaplan and Sadock's Comprehensive Textbook of Psychiatry, 8th ed. Philadelphia, Lippincott Williams & Wilkins, 2005, p 2284
West JC, Herbeck DM, Bell CC, Colquitt WL, Duffy FF, Fitek DJ, Rae D, Stipec MR, Snowden L, Zarin DA, Narrow WE: Race/ethnicity among psychiatric patients: variations in diagnostic and clinical characteristics reported by practicing clinicians. FOCUS 2006; 4:48–56

291

The clinical sign that best differentiates delirium from dementia is:

(A) agitation.
(B) confusion.
(C) fluctuating consciousness.
(D) poor attention span.
(E) psychosis.

The correct response is option **C**: Fluctuating consciousness

Distinguishing delirium from dementia is a frequent clinical challenge. Patients with dementia may exhibit psychosis, agitation, poor attention, and confusion. However, an altered or fluctuating level of consciousness is the hallmark of delirium. Several methods for identifying delirium and rating its severity have been described, including the Delirium Rating Scale and the Confusion Assessment Method. These can assist the clinician in diagnosing and following delirium.

Spar JE, La Rue A: Concise Guide to Geriatric Psychiatry, 3rd ed. Washington, DC, American Psychiatric Publishing, 2002, pp 220–226

American Psychiatric Association: Diagnostic and Statistical Manual of Mental Disorders, Fourth Edition, Text Revision (DSM-IV-TR). Washington, DC, American Psychiatric Association, 2000, p 143

Trepacz PT, Baker RW, Greenhouse J: A symptom rating scale for delirium. Psychiatry Res 1988; 23:89–97

Inouye SK, van Dyck CH, Alessi CA, Balkin S, Siegal AP, Horwitz RI: Clarifying confusion: the confusion assessment method: a new method for detection of delirium. Ann Intern Med 1990; 113:941–948

292

Gabapentin has FDA approval as an indication for which of the following?

(A) Postmenopausal hot flashes
(B) Posttraumatic stress disorder (PTSD)
(C) Postherpetic neuralgia
(D) Cocaine dependence

The correct response is option **C**: Postherpetic neuralgia

Gabapentin is approved by the Food and Drug Administration for adjunctive treatment of partial epilepsy and management of postherpetic neuralgia. Gabapentin, which has a low level of toxicity and renal excretion, was originally indicated as an adjunct antiepileptic medication. As suggested by the other options in the question, the drug has been studied with some promise in the treatment of hot flashes, cocaine addiction, and PTSD.

Physician's Desk Reference. Montvale, NJ, Medical Economics Company, 2003, pp 2563–2564

Jeffery S, Pepe J, Popovich L, Vitagliano G: Gabapentin for hot flashes in prostate cancer. Annals of Pharmacotherapy 2002; 36:433–435

Myrick H, Henderson S, Brady K, Malcolm R: Gabapentin in the treatment of cocaine dependence: a case series. J Clinical Psychiatry 2001; 62:19–23

Hamner M, Brodrick P, Labbate L: Gabapentin in PTSD: a retrospective clinical series of adjunctive therapy. Annals of Clinical Psychiatry 2001; 13:141–146

293

A patient with a first episode of a nonpsychotic major depression has responded well to the acute phase medication treatment. What is the typical duration of the continuation phase?

(A) 3 months
(B) 4 to 9 months
(C) 10 to 15 months
(D) 2 years
(E) Lifelong

The correct response is option **B**: 4 to 9 months

Continuation treatment typically lasts 4 to 9 months for patients with first-episode nonpsychotic depression. For those with psychotic depressions, follow-up studies 1 year after acute phase treatment indicate a poorer prognosis than for those with nonpsychotic depression. Thus, continuation phase treatment for psychotic depressions should be longer.

Sadock BJ, Sadock VA (eds): Kaplan and Sadock's Comprehensive Textbook of Psychiatry, 8th ed. Philadelphia, Lippincott Williams & Wilkins, 2005, p 1659

294

A 40-year-old woman consults a psychiatrist with a chief complaint of anxiety, insomnia with nightmares, loss of appetite, and chest pain. Tearfully, the patient reports that 2 weeks ago her husband left her for another woman. The husband told the patient, "I need someone more adventuresome." She suspected that her husband was having an affair, but she was unprepared for his leaving. She avoids walking by his office in their home because when she sees his litter, still on the desk, she feels chest pain. She reports fear of being alone. She continually daydreams about their life together. She can "barely function" in her job as a hospital administrator. The most likely preliminary diagnosis is:

(A) acute stress disorder.
(B) adjustment disorder with anxiety.
(C) pathological bereavement.
(D) posttraumatic stress disorder.
(E) social phobia.

The correct response is option **B**: Adjustment disorder with anxiety

Adjustment disorder with anxiety is the best working diagnosis. The patient's loss, although painful, is not the kind of life-threatening event that acute stress and posttraumatic stress disorders require for a diagnosis. The clinical material offers little evidence for pathological bereavement, especially because the husband left only 2 weeks ago. Finally, not being "adventurous" and dreading the idea of meeting new people are inadequate data to consider social phobia at this point.

Stein DJ, Hollander E (eds): American Psychiatric Publishing Textbook of Anxiety Disorders. Washington, DC, American Psychiatric Publishing, 2002, pp 374–375

295

A 74-year-old man falls on an ice patch and bumps his head. During the next 4 weeks, his wife notices that he seems more forgetful and that at night he is disoriented. He also develops a persistent headache. Which of the following diagnoses is most likely to be causing this presentation?

(A) Cerebellar tumor
(B) Multi-infarct dementia
(C) Occipital tumor
(D) Subdural hematoma
(E) Wernicke's encephalopathy

The correct response is option **D**: Subdural hematoma

This may be a reversible dementia caused by a chronic subdural hematoma. It frequently follows head trauma, such as those that occur in falls, when the veins of the subdural space are torn. The most common symptoms of subdural hematoma are headache, memory loss, apathy, inattention, and confusion. There can be associated hemiparesis, hemianopsia, and cranial nerve abnormalities, but these are less common.

Sadock BJ, Sadock VA (eds): Kaplan and Sadock's Comprehensive Textbook of Psychiatry, 8th ed, Philadelphia, Lippincott Williams & Wilkins, 2005, pp 368, 482, 1092

296

What proportion of people with dysthymic disorder experience an episode of major depression in their lifetime?

(A) 5%–10%
(B) 20%–30%
(C) 40%–50%
(D) 70%–80%
(E) 100%

The correct response is option **D**: 70%–80%

Some 70%–80% of people with dysthymia have a lifetime diagnosis of major depression, and many seek treatment when they develop major depression superimposed on their dysthymia. In clinical settings, up to 75% of individuals with dysthymic disorder will develop major depressive disorder within 5 years.

Dubovsky SL, Dubovsky AN: Concise Guide to Mood Disorders. Washington, DC, American Psychiatric Publishing, 2002, p 19
American Psychiatric Association: Diagnostic and Statistical Manual of Mental Disorders, Fourth Edition, Text Revision (DSM-IV-TR). Washington, DC, American Psychiatric Association, 2000, p 378

297

Currently, the efficacy of a psychotherapy for treatment of a particular disorder is best judged by:

(A) cohort study.
(B) individual case outcomes.
(C) number needed to treat to number needed to harm ratio.
(D) relative risk reduction measure.
(E) systematic review of controlled studies.

The correct response is option **E**: Systematic review of controlled studies

Systematic reviews and meta-analysis along with randomized controlled trials provide level 1 evidence for treatment strategies. Relative risk is the ratio of the incidence of the disease among persons exposed to the risk factor to the incidence among those not exposed. The number needed to treat is the number of patients who need to receive the experimental treatment in order to prevent one additional bad outcome. The number needed to harm is the number of patients who need to receive the experimental treatment in order to lead to an additional bad outcome.

Sackett DL, Richardson WS, Rosenberg W, Haynes RB: Evidence-Based Medicine: How to Practice and Teach EBM. New York, Churchill Livingstone, 1997, p 15

298

A 25-year-old woman is diagnosed with bipolar I disorder. She has a previous history of several suicide attempts. Of the following medications, which would be the most likely to decrease her risk for suicide if administered on a long-term basis?

(A) Carbamazepine
(B) Lamotrigine
(C) Lithium
(D) Risperidone
(E) Verapamil

The correct response is option **C**: Lithium

Lithium has been shown in naturalistic studies of bipolar disorder to reduce the risk of suicidal behavior. No other medication has been shown to have this effect.

Schatzberg AF, Nemeroff CB (eds): The American Psychiatric Publishing Textbook of Psychopharmacology, 3rd ed. Washington, DC, American Psychiatric Publishing, 2004, p 551
Cipriani A, Pretty H, Hawton K, Geddes JR: Lithium in the prevention of suicidal behavior and all-cause mortality in patients with mood disorders: a systematic review of randomized trials. Am J Psychiatry 2005; 162:1805–1819
Jefferson JW: Bipolar disorders: a brief guide to diagnosis and treatment. FOCUS 2003; 1:7–14 (p 12)

299

A 29-year-old man has severe panic attacks cued by public speaking. He has developed marked avoidance of such situations, which has greatly compromised his career development. Which of the following is the most appropriate diagnosis?

(A) Agoraphobia without panic disorder
(B) Acute stress disorder
(C) Panic disorder with agoraphobia
(D) Social phobia
(E) Specific phobia

The correct response is option **D**: Social phobia

Social phobia is a marked and persistent fear of social and performance situations in which embarrassment may occur. Exposure to the social or performance situation evokes an anxiety response, which may take the form of a panic attack. The situationally bound (cued) panic attacks occurring only in the context of public speaking are consistent with a diagnosis of Social Phobia. According to DSM-IV-TR, panic attacks can occur in the context of many mental disorders. A diagnosis of panic disorder requires unexpected (uncued) panic attacks. Because the fear and avoidance are restricted to a social situation, diagnosis of agoraphobia or specific phobia is not appropriate. Acute stress disorder requires exposure to an extreme trauma.

American Psychiatric Association: Diagnostic and Statistical Manual of Mental Disorders, Fourth Edition, Text Revision (DSM-IV-TR). Washington, DC, American Psychiatric Association, 2000, pp 430–432, 469

300

A patient whose depression has responded well to an SSRI now reports symptoms of erectile dysfunction associated with the SSRI antidepressant therapy. This dysfunction has persisted for more than a month. The best initial approach would be to:

(A) add bupropion.
(B) take a drug holiday.
(C) reduce the dose of the antidepressant.
(D) switch to a different SSRI.
(E) continue treatment until the patient develops tolerance to the side effect.

The correct response is option **C**: Reduce the dose of the antidepressant

When a decrease in libido or a sexual dysfunction persists despite improvement in mood with an SSRI, the best approach is to attempt to lower the dose to see if the side effect will remit without loss of efficacy. This often works, but if the side effect persists, then switching to another antidepressant or adding an antidote drug should be considered.

Labbate LA, Croft HA, Oleshansky MA: Antidepressant-related erectile dysfunction: management via avoidance, switching antidepressants, antidotes, and adaptation. J Clin Psychiatry 2003; 64(suppl 10):11–19

Hales RE, Yudofsky SC (eds): The American Psychiatric Publishing Textbook of Clinical Psychiatry, 4th ed. Washington, DC, American Psychiatric Publishing, 2003, p 1058

301

A patient with a 10-year history of alcohol dependence requests outpatient detoxification. In determining whether outpatient detoxification is an appropriate treatment setting for this patient, the most important variable is:

(A) length of history of alcohol dependence.
(B) support of spouse or significant other.
(C) type of alcohol consumed.
(D) prior history of delirium tremens.

The correct response is option **D**: Prior history of delirium tremens

Patients with a past history of a complicated withdrawal syndrome, especially those with a history of delirium tremens, would not be good candidates for an outpatient treatment setting. Some outpatient treatment settings can accommodate outpatient detoxification that includes frequent clinical assessment.

American Psychiatric Association: Practice Guideline for the Treatment of Patients With Substance Use Disorders: Alcohol, Cocaine, Opioids. Am J Psychiatry 1995; 152(Nov suppl)

302

During the sexual history, a married 35-year-old male reveals that he considers himself to be "on the down low." Regarding his sexual orientation and partners, he would most likely consider himself to be:

(A) bisexual, and has sex equally with men and women.
(B) heterosexual, and exclusively has sex with women.
(C) heterosexual, but also secretly has sex with men.
(D) homosexual, but also has sex with women.
(E) homosexual, and exclusively has sex with men.

The correct response is option **C**: Heterosexual, but also secretly has sex with men

"Down low" generally refers to something that is done in secret. It has also been used to describe men who do not identify themselves as either gay or bisexual but who have sex with women and with men.

Centers for Disease Control and Prevention: Men on the down low. HIV/AIDS Prevention, Questions and Answers. Available at http://www.cdc.gov/hiv/PUBS/faq/Downlow.htm

303

In order for a patient to meet the diagnostic criteria for substance abuse, which of the following must be present?

(A) Physiologic tolerance to the substance
(B) Physiologic withdrawal from the substance
(C) Failure to attend to expected cultural role as a result of the substance
(D) Positron emission tomography findings of mesolimbic tract hyperactivity
(E) Family history of addiction

The correct response is option **C**: Failure to attend to expected cultural role as a result of the substance

The essential feature of substance abuse is a maladaptive pattern of substance use manifested by recurrent and significant adverse consequences. Unlike the criteria for dependence, the criteria for substance abuse do not include tolerance, withdrawal, or a pattern of compulsive use and instead include only the harmful consequences of repeated use.

Mack AH, Frances RJ: Substance-related disorders. FOCUS 2003; 1:125–146 (p 121)
American Psychiatric Association: Diagnostic and Statistical Manual of Mental Disorders, Fourth Edition, Text Revision (DSM-IV-TR). Washington, DC, American Psychiatric Association, 2000, pp 198-199

304

Among patients with major depressive disorder, women have which of the following characteristics compared with men?

(A) Earlier age at onset
(B) Shorter episode duration
(C) Higher rates of comorbid drug abuse
(D) Lower rates of comorbid generalized anxiety
(E) Fewer suicide attempts

The correct response is option **A**: Earlier age at onset

Compared with depressed men, depressed women have an earlier age at onset, longer duration of illness, lower rates of comorbid drug use, higher rates of comorbid anxiety, and more suicide attempts.

Marcus SM, Young EA, Kerber KB, Kornstein S, Farabaugh AH, Mitchell J, Wisniewski SR, Balasubramani GK, Trivedi MH, Rush AJ: Gender differences in depression: findings from the STAR*D study. J Affect Disord 2005; 87:141–150

305

In order to determine the genomic location of a susceptibility gene for panic disorder, which of the following approaches would be most appropriate?

(A) Family risk studies
(B) Genetic epidemiology
(C) Gene finding
(D) Molecular genetics
(E) Twin studies

The correct response is option **C**: Gene finding

Current psychiatric genetics can be organized into four paradigms of inquiry: basic genetic epidemiology, which is used to quantify the degree of familial aggregation and/or heritability; advanced genetic epidemiology, which explores the nature and mode of action of genetic risk factors; gene finding, which attempts to determine the genomic location and identity of susceptibility genes; and molecular genetics, which uses critical DNA variants to trace the biological pathways from DNA to disorder.

Hales RE, Yudofsky SC (eds): The American Psychiatric Publishing Textbook of Clinical Psychiatry, 4th ed. Washington, DC, American Psychiatric Publishing, 2003, pp 3–15
Kendler KS: Psychiatric genetics: a methodologic critique. Am J Psychiatry 2005; 162:3–11

306

During treatment, a female patient reports sexual encounters with a prior therapist in a state that mandates the reporting of sexual abuse by therapists. In the interest of preserving the confidentiality of the doctor-patient relationship, which of the following is the best response of the therapist?

(A) Refer the patient to another physician for consultation, specifically for the role of advocacy.
(B) Request court immunity from the statute to protect the doctor-patient relationship.
(C) Convince the patient to report the matter herself.
(D) Explore the allegation with the patient to determine whether it actually occurred.

The correct response is option **A**: Refer the patient to another physician for consultation, specifically for the role of advocacy

Separating the roles of advocate (one who reports the incident) and therapist (one who treats the patient) is a useful solution in this situation. A therapist must comply with the state statute that requires reporting a sexual abuse incident. However, such reporting may interfere with transference in that the patient may be inhibited from revealing other issues that she may want to be confidential but would hesitate to discuss because she fears her doctor would have to report the information. Either the first therapist who sees the patient reports the incident and then refers the patient to another therapist for treatment or the first therapist sends the patient to another psychiatrist for the role of advocate to report the incident. The patient then returns to the first therapist for further treatment.

Bloom JD, Nadelson CC, Notman MT: Physician Sexual Misconduct. Washington, DC, American Psychiatric Press, 1999, pp 259–261
Simon RI: Therapist-patient sex: maintaining treatment boundaries, in Concise Guide to Psychiatry and Law for Clinicians, 3rd ed. Washington, DC, American Psychiatric Publishing, 2001, p 342

307

Which of the following medications has been shown to be most effective in reducing suicidal behaviors in patients with schizophrenia or schizoaffective disorder?

(A) Clozapine
(B) Haloperidol
(C) Lithium
(D) Olanzapine
(E) Ziprasidone

The correct response is option **A**: Clozapine

In individuals with schizophrenia or schizoaffective disorder, several lines of evidence suggest that rates of suicidal behaviors, including suicide, are diminished by clozapine treatment. For example, analyses of data from the clozapine national registry show decreased rates of suicide compared with expected rates for individuals with schizophrenia. In addition, the International Suicide Prevention Trial (InterSePT) compared clozapine and olanzapine in 980 patients over a 2-year period and found that the clozapine group had substantially fewer suicide attempts and fewer hospitalizations related to suicidality. Lithium maintenance treatment is associated with a substantial decrease in rates of suicide among individuals with mood disorders, particularly bipolar disorder, but it has not been adequately studied in terms of suicidal behaviors in individuals with schizophrenia.

Meltzer HY, Alphs L, Green AI, Altamura AC, Anand R, Bertoldi A, Bourgeois M, Chouinard G, Islam MZ, Kane J, Krishnan R, Lindenmayer JP, Potkin S; International Suicide Prevention Trial Study Group: Clozapine treatment for suicidality in schizophrenia: International Suicide Prevention Trial (InterSePT). Arch Gen Psychiatry 2003; 60:82–91
Reid WH, Mason M, Hogan T: Suicide prevention effects associated with clozapine therapy in schizophrenia and schizoaffective disorder. Psychiatr Serv 1998; 49:1029–1033
American Psychiatric Association: Practice Guideline for the Assessment and Treatment of Patients With Suicidal Behaviors. Am J Psychiatry 2003; 160(Nov suppl):1–60

308

Which of the following diagnostic criteria most clearly distinguishes paranoid personality disorder from paranoid schizophrenia, delusional disorder, and mood disorder with psychotic features?

(A) Absence of positive psychotic symptoms
(B) Age at onset
(C) Degree of impairment in interpersonal relationships
(D) Duration of symptoms
(E) Pervasive nature of symptoms

The correct response is option **A**: Absence of positive psychotic symptoms

Paranoid personality disorder is marked by pervasive distrust and suspiciousness of others. This may be present in paranoid schizophrenia, a delusional disorder, or a mood disorder with psychotic features. The age at onset of symptoms, degree of impairment, duration of symptoms, or pervasive nature of the symptoms may be of little help in differentiating paranoid personality disorder from the other disorders listed. However, in paranoid personality disorder, positive psychotic symptoms should not be present, whereas they are key diagnostic criteria for each of the other disorders.

Sadock BJ, Sadock VA (eds): Kaplan and Sadock's Comprehensive Textbook of Psychiatry, 7th ed. Philadelphia, Lippincott Williams & Wilkins, 2000, pp 1742–1743

309

A 19-year-old exchange student from Malaysia is brought to the emergency department by his host parents after he became violent at home and threatened to kill them. The parents report that he seemed fine until they commented to him that he had left the faucet running in the bathroom. Initially, he went to his room and seemed sullen. He then began "ranting and raving" about how he is not an irresponsible person, accused the host parents of spying on him, threatened them, threw objects about, and collapsed on the floor in exhaustion. In the emergency department, the student is calm and cooperative. Mental status examination is unremarkable. The student denies any recall of the episode. This presentation is most consistent with which culture-bound syndrome?

(A) Amok
(B) Dhat
(C) Koro
(D) Locura
(E) Rootwork

The correct response is option **A**: Amok

Culture-bound syndromes are culturally based signs and symptoms of mental distress or maladaptive behavior that are prominent in folk belief and practice. Amok is a dissociative episode characterized by a period of brooding followed by an outburst of violent, aggressive, or homicidal behaviors directed at persons or objects. The episode tends to be precipitated by a perceived slight or insult and seems to be prevalent only among men. The episode is often accompanied by persecutory ideation, automatism, amnesia, exhaustion, and a return to premorbid state after the episode. The original reports that used this term were from Malaysia.

Sadock BJ, Sadock VA (eds): Kaplan and Sadock's Synopsis of Psychiatry: Behavioral Sciences/Clinical Psychiatry, 9th ed. Philadelphia, Lippincott Williams & Wilkins, 2003, pp 529–530
Griffith EE, Gonzalez CA, Blue HC: Introduction to cultural psychiatry, in The American Psychiatric Publishing Textbook of Clinical Psychiatry, 4th ed. Edited by Hales RE, Yudofsky SC. Washington, DC, American Psychiatric Publishing, 2003, p 1567

310

What is the most common comorbid condition in children with autistic disorder?

(A) Attention deficit hyperactivity disorder
(B) Major depression
(C) Mental retardation
(D) Schizophrenia
(E) Social phobia

The correct response is option **C**: Mental retardation

Approximately 80% of children with autistic disorder are mentally retarded. Psychotic symptoms exclude the diagnosis of autistic disorder. ADHD, major depressive disorder, and social phobia may occur but are less frequent than mental retardation.

Dulcan MK, Martini DR, Lake MB: Concise Guide to Child and Adolescent Psychiatry, 3rd ed. Washington, DC, American Psychiatric Publishing, 2003, p 190

311

A 65-year-old patient is admitted to the surgical inpatient service for a hernia repair. The family reported that over the past few months the patient has had episodes of confusion. While on the ward, the patient began to have prominent visual hallucinations. The staff administered 1 mg of haloperidol orally. A second dose was given 3 hours later. Soon after receiving the second dose of haloperidol, the patient had a severe extrapyramidal response. Which of the following is the most likely diagnosis?

(A) Delirium with preexisting dementia
(B) Parkinson's dementia
(C) Lewy body dementia
(D) Major depressive disorder with psychosis
(E) Alcohol withdrawal

The correct response is option **C**: Lewy body dementia

Lewy body dementia is characterized by the appearance of visual hallucinations and other psychotic symptoms early and sensitivity to extrapyramidal side effects of antipsychotics. It also responds with remarkable sensitivity to antipsychotic medication. The disorder has some Parkinsonian features. These perhaps account for the sensitivity to antipsychotics. The course of this dementia follows a rapid evolution. The combination of "memory problems," visual hallucinations, and sensitivity to haloperidol make the choice of Lewy body dementia the most compelling option for this question.

Practice Guideline for the Treatment of Patients With Alzheimer's Disease and Other Dementias of Late Life (1997), in American Psychiatric Association Practice Guidelines for the Treatment of Psychiatric Disorders, Compendium 2004. Washington, DC, APA, 2004, p 82

312

Which of the following is most likely to be preserved in the early stages of frontotemporal dementia?

(A) Judgment
(B) Personality
(C) Verbal output
(D) Visuospatial skills
(E) Sociability or social involvement

The correct response is option **D**: Visuospatial skills

Unlike in dementia of the Alzheimer's type, visuospatial skills are usually preserved in the early to middle stages of frontotemporal dementia. Common early symptoms of frontotemporal dementia include personality changes (particularly social withdrawal and apathy), loss of judgment and insight, disinhibition, and changes in oral behaviors. Compulsions and cravings are frequently seen (e.g., carbohydrate cravings and hyperorality). Verbal output may be diminished, and semantic anomia, a specific form of anomia, is common.

Coffey CE, Cummings JL: American Psychiatric Press Textbook of Geriatric Neuropsychiatry, 2nd ed. Washington, DC, American Psychiatric Press, 2000, pp 518–519

313

Of the following disorders, which has the greatest genetic contribution or heritability?

(A) Major depressive disorder
(B) Alcoholism
(C) Obsessive-compulsive disorder
(D) Schizophrenia
(E) Panic disorder

The correct response is option **D**: Schizophrenia

The proportion of phenotypic differences among individuals that can be attributed to genetic factors, or heritability, is 70% to 89% for schizophrenia, around 60% for obsessive-compulsive disorder, 40% to 60% for alcohol dependence, and 40% to 45% for major depression and panic disorder.

Knowles JA: Genetics, in The American Psychiatric Publishing Textbook of Clinical Psychiatry, 4th ed. Edited by Hales RE, Yudofsky SC. Washington, DC, American Psychiatric Publishing, 2003, pp 17–34
Sadock BJ, Sadock VA (eds): Kaplan and Sadock's Comprehensive Textbook of Psychiatry, 8th ed. Philadelphia, Lippincott Williams & Wilkins, 2005, p 240

314

A 25-year-old man collects women's bras and underpants from public laundries and uses the objects to become sexually aroused. This description is most consistent with which of the following DSM-IV-TR diagnoses?

(A) Exhibitionism
(B) Fetishism
(C) Frotteurism
(D) Sexual masochism
(E) Kleptomania

The correct response is option **B**: Fetishism

Fetishism involves nonliving objects (other than articles of clothing used for cross-dressing or devices designed for tactile genital stimulation) that result in recurrent, intense, sexually arousing fantasies, sexual urges, or behaviors involving the objects. Exhibitionism is the exposure of one's genitals to an unsuspecting stranger. Frotteurism is the rubbing of one's genitals against unsuspecting, nonconsenting persons. Sexual masochism involves sexual fantasies, urges, or behaviors involving the real act of being humiliated, beaten, bound, or otherwise made to suffer.

American Psychiatric Association: Diagnostic and Statistical Manual of Mental Disorders, Fourth Edition, Text Revision (DSM-IV-TR). Washington, DC, American Psychiatric Association, 2000, pp 569–570

315

A 24-year-old man comes for an evaluation because he cannot relax. He reports that he constantly is thinking about whether his car will break down, his bills will get paid, and if his school performance is adequate. For over a year, he often is tired, irritable, and on edge. Upon reflection, the student is unable to identify any aspect of his life that is going so well that it does not generate concern. The most likely diagnosis is:

(A) depressive disorder not otherwise specified.
(B) generalized anxiety disorder.
(C) obsessive-compulsive disorder.
(D) panic disorder.
(E) social phobia.

The correct response is option **B**: Generalized anxiety disorder

Generalized anxiety disorder is the diagnosis that best explains the student's symptoms. A person with generalized anxiety disorder finds it difficult to control the worry, often about everyday routine life circumstances. The worry is associated with symptoms such as fatigue, difficulty concentrating, and sleep disturbance.

Sadock BJ, Sadock VA (eds): Kaplan and Sadock's Comprehensive Textbook of Psychiatry, 8th ed. Philadelphia, Lippincott Williams & Wilkins, 2005, p 1778
American Psychiatric Association: Diagnostic and Statistical Manual of Mental Disorders, Fourth Edition, Text Revision (DSM-IV-TR). Washington, DC, American Psychiatric Association, 2000, pp 472–476

316

The side effect of pancreatitis is linked most closely to which of the following?

(A) Divalproex
(B) Oxcarbazepine
(C) Lamotrigine
(D) Topiramate

The correct response is option **A**: Divalproex

In 2000, a black box warning about cases of life-threatening pancreatitis was added to the valproate package insert. Although routine monitoring of pancreatic function is not necessary, clinical manifestations consistent with pancreatitis should be promptly and fully evaluated.

Asconapé JJ, Penry JK, Dreifuss FE, Riela A, Mirza W: Valproate-associated pancreatitis. Epilepsia 1993; 34:177–183
Pizzuti DJ: Dear health care professional. Abbott laboratories, July 2000
McArthur KE: Review article: drug-induced pancreatitis. Aliment Pharmacol Ther 1996; 10:23–38

317

Which of the following is a technique of supportive dynamic psychotherapy?

(A) Transference interpretation
(B) Promoting therapeutic regression
(C) Extreme passivity of therapist
(D) Problem-solving focus
(E) Frequent genetic reconstruction

The correct response is option **D**: Problem-solving focus

Problem solving is an important technique and goal of supportive treatment that augments certain weaknesses or deficits in the patient's psychological functioning and provides a sense of mastery. Transference, although of great help in understanding a patient receiving supportive psychotherapy, is rarely addressed because it can often promote disorganization from intense feelings outside the patient's awareness. Although promoting a therapeutic regression is a hallmark of psychoanalysis, patients in supportive psychotherapy often lack the strength (emotionally and cognitively) to recover from a therapeutic regression both within the hour and after its conclusion. Extreme passivity can often raise a patient's level of anxiety to an unhelpful level and lead to discomfort and leaving treatment. The exploration of potentially significant early life experiences is often accompanied by high levels of anxiety and dysphoria, which can compromise a patient's level of functioning.

Kay J: The essentials of psychodynamic psychotherapy. FOCUS 2006; 4:167–172 (171)
Kay J, Kay RL: Individual psychoanalytic psychotherapy, in Psychiatry. Edited by Tasman A, Kay J, Lieberman JA. Philadelphia, WB Saunders, 1997, p 1384

318

The most effective behavior therapy technique used in the treatment of compulsions of obsessive-compulsive disorder is:

(A) exposure and response prevention.
(B) negative reinforcement.
(C) positive reinforcement.
(D) punishment.
(E) systematic desensitization.

The correct response is option **A**: Exposure and response prevention

The compulsions of obsessive-compulsive disorder may be treated by exposing the patient to stimuli that evoke obsessive worries (exposure). Then the patient is not allowed to respond to his/her worries by performing compulsions (response prevention).

Stein DJ, Hollander E (eds): American Psychiatric Publishing Textbook of Anxiety Disorders. Washington, DC, American Psychiatric Publishing, 2002, p 222

319

A man who is receiving cognitive behavior therapy for depression feels guilty for massive layoffs at his workplace, even though he was not involved in the management decision. Which of the following types of cognitive error is most consistent with this patient's feeling?

(A) Arbitrary inference
(B) Absolutist thinking
(C) Catastrophic thinking
(D) Magnification and minimization
(E) Personalization

The correct response is option **E**: Personalization

Personalization (assuming personal causality) is the linking of external occurrences to oneself. Arbitrary inference is the process of coming to a conclusion without adequate supporting evidence or despite contradictory evidence. Absolutist thinking is categorizing oneself into rigid dichotomies. Catastrophic thinking is predicting the worst possible outcome while ignoring more likely eventualities. Magnification and minimization entail over- or undervaluing the significance of a personal attribute, a life event, or a future possibility.

Hales RE, Yudofsky SC (eds): The American Psychiatric Publishing Textbook of Clinical Psychiatry, 4th ed. Washington, DC, American Psychiatric Publishing, 2003, p 1248

320

An actor has received repeated complaints from colleagues about his behavior in professional situations. He has just started rehearsals for a play. The problematic behavior consists of excessive demands for special treatment and outbursts when special treatment is not granted. He is diagnosed as having narcissistic personality disorder. He has been in treatment for several months; treatment has been going well, and there have been fewer demands and outbursts at work. Which of the following is the patient most likely to do next?

(A) Generalize this behavior to his home environment
(B) Demand new concessions from the play's director
(C) Show a new understanding of his behavior
(D) Continue to show appropriate behavior at work
(E) Discuss his feelings about the therapist

The correct response is option **B**: Demand new concessions from the play's director

Patients with narcissistic personality disorder struggle and often cannot tolerate feeling and doing better because that would imply that the therapist has helped them. In psychodynamic therapy, patients with narcissistic personality disorder find it difficult to improve because of this. Improvement means that the therapist can "give" them help, that is, that the therapist has something the patient does not.

Cloninger CR, Svrakic DM: Personality disorders, in Kaplan and Sadock's Comprehensive Textbook of Psychiatry, 7th ed. Edited by Sadock BJ, Sadock VA. Philadelphia, Lippincott Williams & Wilkins, 2000, pp 1757–1758
Gabbard GO: Psychodynamic Psychiatry in Clinical Practice, 4th ed. Washington, DC, American Psychiatric Publishing, 2005, pp 508–509

321

Of the following, which is the best definition of ethnicity? Human groups that:

(A) share a sociopolitical designation.
(B) share common values, beliefs, history, and customs.
(C) have common identities, ancestries, and histories.
(D) share distinct identifying phenotypic characteristics.
(E) are living together in the same location.

The correct response is option **C**: Have common identities, ancestries, and histories

Cultural groups share common values, beliefs, history, and customs, while ethnic groups have common identities, ancestries, and histories. Phenotypic characteristics are often mistakenly used as indicators of race.

Sadock BJ, Sadock VA (eds): Kaplan and Sadock's Synopsis of Psychiatry: Behavioral Sciences/Clinical Psychiatry, 9th ed. Philadelphia, Lippincott Williams & Wilkins, 2003, p 169
Tseng WS, Streltzer J: Culture and Psychotherapy: A Guide to Clinical Practice. Washington, DC, American Psychiatric Publishing, 2001, pp 4–6
Hales RE, Yudofsky SC (eds): The American Psychiatric Publishing Textbook of Clinical Psychiatry, 4th ed. Washington, DC, American Psychiatric Publishing, 2003, p 1552
Levine BH, Albucher RC: Patient management exercise for gender, race, and culture. FOCUS 2006; 4:14–22 (p 20)

322

Which of the following psychotherapeutic approaches provides the primary framework for dialectical behavior therapy for borderline personality disorder?

(A) Cognitive behavior therapy
(B) Interpersonal psychotherapy
(C) Psychodynamic psychotherapy
(D) Family systems therapy
(E) Supportive psychotherapy

The correct response is option **A**: Cognitive behavior therapy

Linehan's dialectical behavior therapy is a cognitive behavior therapy–based approach to borderline personality disorder that includes a mix of individual therapy and intensive skills training.

Linehan MM: Cognitive-Behavioral Treatment of Borderline Personality Disorder. New York, Guilford, 1993, pp 37–41
Practice Guideline for the Treatment of Patients With Borderline Personality Disorder (2001), in Practice Guidelines for the Treatment of Psychiatric Disorders, Compendium 2004. Washington, DC, APA, 2004, p 799

323

The most common DSM-IV axis II personality disorder demonstrated among persons with substance use disorders is:

(A) borderline personality disorder.
(B) narcissistic personality disorder.
(C) dependent personality disorder.
(D) antisocial personality disorder.

The correct response is option **D**: Antisocial personality disorder

In epidemiological studies, antisocial personality disorder has been found to be the most common axis II personality disorder comorbid with substance use disorders.

Regier DA, Farmer ME, Rae DS, Locke BZ, Keith SJ, Judd LL, Goodwin FK: Comorbidity of mental disorders with alcohol and other drug abuse. Results from the Epidemiologic Catchment Area (ECA) Study. JAMA 1990; 264:2511–2518
Skodol AE, Oldham JM, Gallaher PE: Axis II comorbidity of substance use disorders among patients referred for treatment of personality disorders. Am J Psychiatry 1999; 156:733–738

324

A 72-year-old woman is hospitalized with findings of dementia, ataxia, and macrocytic anemia. The most likely diagnosis is:

(A) dementia of the Alzheimer's type.
(B) vascular dementia.
(C) vitamin B_{12} deficiency.
(D) Huntington's disease.
(E) pellagra.

The correct response is option **C**: Vitamin B_{12} deficiency

Vitamin B_{12} deficiency can present with cerebral, spinal cord, and peripheral nerve involvement as well as defective hematopoiesis in the form of a macrocytic or megaloblastic anemia. Pernicious anemia is the most common cause. Pellegra is caused by a deficiency of niacin (vitamin B_3) and is characterized classically by findings of dementia, diarrhea, and dermatitis.

Moore DP, Jefferson JW: Vitamin B_{12} deficiency, in Handbook of Medical Psychiatry, 2nd ed. Philadelphia, Elsevier Mosby, 2004, pp 401–403

325

A 20-year-old woman describes a 6-month history of frequent binge eating followed by self-induced vomiting and laxative use to maintain normal body weight. Which of the following medications is FDA-approved for her disorder?

(A) Bupropion
(B) Citalopram
(C) Escitalopram
(D) Fluoxetine
(E) Venlafaxine

The correct response is option **D**: Fluoxetine

The patient's history is consistent with a diagnosis of bulimia nervosa. The only FDA-approved medication for this disorder is fluoxetine, based on two 8-week and one 16-week placebo-controlled studies. Fluoxetine was also shown to be more effective than placebo in a 1-year relapse prevention study. The FDA approves a medication after evidence of its effectiveness from more than one double-blind, placebo-controlled study. Once a drug has been FDA approved, it can be used for the treatment of other illnesses.

Becker AE, Grinspoon SK, Klibanski A, Herzog DB: Eating disorders. N Engl J Med 1999; 340:1092–1098

Mehler PS: Bulimia nervosa. N Engl J Med 2003; 349:875–881

Romano SJ, Halmi KA, Sarkar NP, Koke SC, Lee JS: A placebo-controlled study of fluoxetine in continued treatment of bulimia nervosa after successful acute fluoxetine treatment. Am J Psychiatry 2002; 159:96–102

Prozac (fluoxetine) prescribing information (package insert)

Yager J, Devlin MJ, Halmi KA, Herzog DB, Mitchell JE, Powers PS, Zerbe KJ: Eating disorders. FOCUS 2005; 3:503–510 (pp 506–507)

American Psychatric Association: Practice Guideline for the Treatment of Patients With Eating Disorders, 3rd ed. Am J Psychiatry 2006; 163(July suppl):1–54

326

A psychiatrist who is grieving from a recent sudden loss of a spouse shares those feelings with a psychotherapy patient. What is the most ethical interpretation of the psychiatrist's actions?

(A) It may be ethically problematic if the psychiatrist was driven by personal needs rather than by serving the patient's needs.
(B) It is always ethically unacceptable because a psychiatrist should never reveal personal information to a patient.
(C) It is problematic to reveal any information other than the psychiatrist's professional training.
(D) It is not ethically problematic because sharing the psychiatrist's authentic feelings with patients is therapeutic for the patient.

The correct response is option **A**: It may be ethically problematic if the psychiatrist was driven by personal needs rather than by serving the patient's needs

Self-disclosure in psychotherapy need not always be problematic. For instance, a patient has the right to information that is relevant to judge the professional qualifications of the psychiatrist. In the substance abuse treatment arena, self-disclosures are more accepted. Occasional, well-thought-out disclosures for therapeutic effect may also be acceptable in some instances. However, when a psychiatrist discloses information out of personal need rather than for the therapeutic needs of the patient, even if it arises out of deeply felt emotions, the primacy of the patient's best interests is put in jeopardy.

Gabbard GO: Psychodynamic Psychiatry in Clinical Practice: The DSM-IV edition. Washington, DC, American Psychiatric Press, 1994, pp 104–106

Hundert EM, Appelbaum PS: Boundaries in psychotherapy: model guidelines. Psychiatry 1995; 58:345–356

327

Which of the following will cause the greatest increase in serum lithium levels?

(A) Theophylline
(B) Ziprasidone
(C) Hydrochlorothiazide
(D) Celecoxib

The correct response is option **C**: Hydrochlorothiazide

Thiazide diuretics are well established as consistently causing substantial increases in serum lithium levels, sometimes causing lithium intoxication. Theophylline, a xanthine diuretic, increases renal lithium clearance and may lower serum lithium levels. Ziprasidone did not change steady-state levels or renal clearance of lithium (see package insert). In a study of healthy volunteers, celecoxib increased serum lithium levels by a mean of 17%, which does not exclude the possibility of a more clinically meaningful interaction but makes it seem unlikely.

Finley PR, Warner MD, Peabody CA: Clinical relevance of drug interactions with lithium. Clin Pharmacokinet 1995; 29:172–191

Apseloff G, Mullet D, Wilner KD, Anziano RJ, Tensfeldt TG, Pelletier SM, Gerber N: The effects of ziprasidone on steady-state lithium levels and renal clearance of lithium. Br J Clin Pharmacol 2000; 49(suppl 1):61S–64S

328

While reviewing the treatment plan for a patient with methamphetamine dependence, the psychiatrist thinks about how best to help the patient progress from the contemplation phase to the preparation phase. The psychiatrist's approach to treatment in this case is based on the principles of:

(A) 12-step facilitation therapy.
(B) cognitive behavior therapy (CBT).
(C) contingency management therapy.
(D) motivational enhancement therapy (MET).

The correct response is option **D**: Motivational enhancement therapy (MET)

Motivational enhancement therapy (MET) is based on the concept that people move through predictable stages in changing habitual behaviors. As originally described by Prochaska and DiClemente, these stages are precontemplation, contemplation, preparation, action, and maintenance. The treatment goals and, to some extent, therapeutic technique vary according to stage.

DiClemente CC, Velasquez MM: Motivational interviewing and the stages of change, in Motivational Interviewing. Edited by Miller WR, Rollnick S. New York, Guilford Press, 2002, pp 201–216

Nowinski J, Baker S, Carroll KM: Twelve-step Facilitation Therapy Manual. Project MATCH Monograph Series, vol 1. Rockville, MD, National Institute on Alcohol Abuse and Alcoholism, 1995. Available at http://www.commed.uchc.edu/match/pubs/monograph.htm

Kadden R, Carroll KM, Donovan D, Cooney N, Monti P, Abrams D, Litt M, Hester R: Cognitive-Behavioral Coping Skills Therapy Manual. Project MATCH Monograph Series, vol 3. Rockville, MD, National Institute on Alcohol Abuse and Alcoholism, 1995. Available at http://www.commed.uchc.edu/match/pubs/monograph.htm

Miller WR, Zweben A, DiClemente CC, Rychtarik RG: Motivational Enhancement Therapy Manual. Project MATCH Monograph Series, vol 2. Rockville, MD, National Institute on Alcohol Abuse and Alcoholism, 1994. Available at http://www.commed.uchc.edu/match/pubs/monograph.htm

Budney AJ, Higgins ST: A Community Reinforcement Approach: Treating Cocaine Addiction. Therapy manuals for drug addiction, Manual 2. Rockville, MD, National Institute on Drug Abuse, 1998. Available at http://www.drugabuse.gov/TB/Clinical/ClinicalToolbox.html

329

Which of the following is the most effective treatment for catatonic features associated with a manic episode?

(A) Lithium
(B) Electroconvulsive therapy
(C) Divalproex
(D) Clozapine

The correct response is option **B**: Electroconvulsive therapy

Catatonic features may be present in as many as one-third of patients during a manic episode. While the patient may be responsive to benzodiazepines, electroconvulsive therapy is believed to be the most effective treatment for catatonia, "regardless of etiology."

American Psychiatric Association: Practice Guideline for the Treatment of Patients With Bipolar Disorder (Revision). Am J Psychiatry 2002; 159(April suppl). Reprinted in FOCUS 2003; 1:64–110 (p 73)

330

The cornerstone of relapse prevention as a modality of treatment for substance-dependent patients is:

(A) psychodynamic technique.
(B) 12-step group attendance.
(C) motivational enhancement.
(D) skills training.

The correct response is option **D**: Skills training

Relapse prevention is a behavior therapy that combines skill training with cognitive intervention techniques. In this approach, patients are taught behavioral and cognitive skills such as changing thoughts and beliefs, resisting social pressure, increasing assertiveness, and improving interpersonal communication. Relaxation and stress management techniques are also emphasized. The effectiveness of these cognitive behavioral techniques appears to have longer-lasting benefits than some other treatment modalities. They are particularly effective when a co-occurring psychiatric disorder such as anxiety or depression is present.

Marlatt GA, Gordon J (eds): Relapse Prevention: Maintenance Strategies in the Treatment of Addictive Behaviors. New York, Guilford, 1985

Gold PB, Brady KT: Evidence-based treatments for substance use disorders. FOCUS 2003; 1:115–122 (p 116)

Carroll KM, Ball SA, Martino S: Cognitive, behavioral, and motivational therapies, in The American Psychiatric Publishing Textbook of Substance Abuse Treatment, 3rd ed. Edited by Galanter M, Kleber HD. Washington, DC, American Psychiatric Publishing, 2004, pp 369–370

331

Which of the following is the most common sexual disorder in men?

(A) Hypoactive sexual desire disorder
(B) Male erectile disorder
(C) Premature ejaculation
(D) Male orgasmic disorder
(E) Dyspareunia

The correct response is option **C**: Premature ejaculation

Data from the National Health and Social Life Survey showed that almost one-third of men said they had recurring problems with ejaculating too early, making it the most common sexual disorder in men. Premature ejaculation is defined as persistent or recurrent ejaculation with minimal sexual stimulation or before, on, or shortly after penetration and before the person wishes it, resulting in marked distress or interpersonal difficulty.

Laumann EO, Paik A, Rosen RC: Sexual dysfunction in the United States: prevalence and predictors. JAMA 1999; 281:537–544

332

An adult female patient consumes an average of 14 glasses of wine per week, never consuming more than four glasses on any one occasion. Based solely on this drinking pattern, her physician should do which of the following?

(A) Refer her to an addiction specialist for further evaluation.
(B) Recommend that she begin attending AA meetings.
(C) Inform her that she is drinking at a safe level.
(D) Recommend that she reduce her drinking by about 50%.

The correct response is option **D**: Recommend that she reduce her drinking by about 50%

The physician should assess the patient for alcohol-related problems and definitely recommend that the patient decrease her drinking to safer levels. This level of alcohol consumption puts the patient at risk of alcohol-related problems. Nonhazardous drinking for women is seven standard drinks per week, with no more than three per occasion. Without a history of more alcohol-related problems, outside referral is not necessary. The patient will likely respond well to brief office-based intervention.

Fleming MF, Mundt MP, French MT, Manwell LB, Stauffacher EA, Barry KL: Brief physician advice with problem drinkers: long-term efficacy and benefit-cost analysis. Alcohol Clin Exp Res 2002; 26:36–43
Fiellin DA, Reid MC, O'Connor PG: Outpatient management of patients with alcohol problems. Ann Intern Med 2000; 133:815–827

The following four questions (333–336) form a serial vignette.

333

Mr. B, a high school teacher in his mid-30s, was recently separated from his wife and two children. An intelligent and verbally facile man with a particular talent in the arts, Mr. B was plagued by his conviction that he was unacceptable to other people unless he complied with their expectations and gratified their needs. This was a pleasant, agreeable, and compliant facade that hid his feelings of weakness and stupidity. He constantly sought approval from his superiors, but underneath he felt resentment and rebelliousness about others' expecting him to accommodate to their needs and wishes.

Mr. B's mother was an embittered, burdened woman, contemptuous of men and preoccupied with her own needs and interests. His father, while somewhat approachable, had often been away from home trying to make a living to support the family. Mr. B remembered his father as erratic and moody and given to temper outbursts, which, he recalls, would lead to beatings with a leather strap. The middle of three children, the patient felt that his father favored his older sister and that his mother favored his younger brother, and he saw himself as the neglected outsider.

What is the most likely defense mechanism utilized by this patient when first meeting the psychiatrist?

(A) Regression
(B) Altruism
(C) Undoing projection
(D) Intellectualization rationalization
(E) Dissociation

The correct response is option **D**: Intellectualization rationalization

All defense mechanisms, by definition, are outside of the patient's awareness. They function to ward off anxiety and conflict. Rationalization is the use of seemingly logical explanations to make untenable thoughts or feelings more acceptable. In the case of Mr. B, his verbal facility and educational accomplishment make this a likely characteristic of his personality. Regression refers to a partial return to earlier levels of functioning or adaptation in order to avoid painful or conflicted feelings or thoughts.

Altruism is a higher-order defense mechanism. Projection is considered a primitive defense mechanism that is frequently found in patients with significant suspiciousness and that consists of attribution of conflicted feelings, wishes, or thoughts to another person or group. Dissociation is characterized as the splitting off of threatening thoughts or feelings.

Kay J: The essentials of psychodynamic psychotherapy. FOCUS 2006; 4:167–172 (169)

334

Because of an emergency, Mr. B's psychiatrist was 20 minutes late to the second interview. Mr. B makes an offhand and somewhat negative comment about "doctors being too busy these days." In all likelihood, this is an example of:

(A) reaction formation.
(B) transference.
(C) idealization.
(D) splitting.
(E) suppression.

The correct response is option **B**: Transference

A current definition of transference is a combination of a real current relationship and relationships from the patient's past. Reaction formation is the transformation of an unwanted thought or feeling into its opposite. Splitting is the experiencing of others as being all good or all bad (i.e., idealization or deidealization). Suppression is not a defense mechanism since it is the conscious attempt to control unacceptable feelings and wishes. Transference is also outside of the patient's awareness during the initial phase of treatment. Mr. B is offended by the therapist's lateness and expresses his disappointment by characterizing all doctors as being unavailable. There is a likely transference to the patient's father, who was unavailable to the patient during his formative years.

Kay J: The essentials of psychodynamic psychotherapy. FOCUS 2006; 4:167–172 (169)

335

On hearing the irritation in the patient's voice, the clinician begins to explain in detail the reasons for his tardiness and apologizes profusely. He assures the patient that he will not be late for future meetings. This is an example of:

(A) denial.
(B) regression.
(C) countertransference.
(D) deidealization.
(E) dissociation.

The correct response is option **C**: Countertransference

Countertransference is defined broadly as all of the feelings of the therapist evoked by the patient within the therapeutic relationship. Although the term originally referred to a process outside the therapist's awareness and therefore an indication of conflict, it is now used frequently to describe all of the therapist's feelings and behavior stimulated by the patient. Denial is a primitive defense mechanism characterized by a refusal to appreciate information about oneself or the other. Regression refers to a partial return to earlier levels of functioning or adaptation in order to avoid painful or conflicted feelings or thoughts. Deidealization minimizes the other. Dissociation is characterized as the splitting off of threatening thoughts or feelings.

Kay J: The essentials of psychodynamic psychotherapy. FOCUS 2006; 4:167–172 (169)
Inderbitzin LB, Levy ST: Psychoanalytic theories, in Psychiatry. Edited by Tasman A, Kay J, Lieberman JA. Philadelphia, WB Saunders, 1997, pp 443–446

336

In beginning a brief therapy with Mr. B, the most important challenge for this psychiatrist is to:

(A) prescribe an antidepressant.
(B) prescribe an antianxiety agent.
(C) contact the patient's wife for additional history.
(D) establish a therapeutic or working alliance.
(E) set clear limits on the patient's behavior.

The correct response is option **D**: Establish a therapeutic or working alliance

It is true in all types of psychotherapy that the initial task of treatment is to establish a therapeutic or working alliance, without which treatment is unlikely to progress. This alliance represents the willingness of patient and therapist to work collaboratively toward the patient's understanding and changing problematic feelings and behaviors.

It would be premature to prescribe any medication at this point in the treatment relationship because the nature and extent of the patient's symptoms remain unclear. Since Mr. B is seeking treatment, it would be inappropriate to bring another person—his wife, from whom he is separated—into the treatment process. Setting limits on behavior is clearly inappropriate and would undoubtedly establish an adversarial relationship with the patient.

Kay J: The essentials of psychodynamic psychotherapy. FOCUS 2006; 4:167–172 (170)

337

Which of the following psychiatric disorders is considered to be predominantly culture specific?

(A) Bulimia nervosa
(B) Generalized anxiety disorder
(C) Major depressive disorder
(D) Posttraumatic stress disorder
(E) Schizophrenia

The correct response is option **A**: Bulimia nervosa

Bulimia nervosa is considered to be a culture-specific syndrome, occurring predominantly in females in industrialized cultures that value slimness.

Keel PK, Klump KL: Are eating disorders culture-bound syndromes? Implications for conceptualizing their etiology. Psychol Bull 2003; 129:747–769

Sadock BJ, Sadock VA (eds): Kaplan and Sadock's Comprehensive Textbook of Psychiatry, 8th ed. Philadelphia, Lippincott Williams & Wilkins, 2005, p 2007

American Psychatric Association: Practice Guideline for the Treatment of Patients With Eating Disorders, 3rd ed. Am J Psychiatry 2006; 163(July suppl):1–54

338

A 73-year-old man with moderate congestive heart failure and degenerative arthritis in his right knee visits his physician for a scheduled outpatient appointment. Although his physical examination findings from the previous visit are unchanged, the physician notes that the patient appears tired and less interactive than usual. Concerned that the patient may be experiencing a major depressive episode, the physician wishes to gather more information. The presence of which of the following would be most helpful in making a diagnosis of major depressive disorder?

(A) Complaints of pain
(B) Decreased concentration
(C) Loss of appetite
(D) Poor energy
(E) The wish to die

The correct response is option **E**: The wish to die

While anergia, anorexia, somatic complaints, and diminished concentration commonly accompany medical illnesses in older patients, psychological symptoms, including suicidal ideation, decreased self-esteem, and guilt, do not. These symptoms should suggest the diagnosis of depression.

Jacobson SA, Pies RW, Greenblatt DJ: Handbook of Geriatric Psychopharmacology. Washington, DC, American Psychiatric Publishing, 2002, pp 112–113

339

A 46-year-old woman presents to her primary care physician with a 2-month history of low back pain, dull headaches several times a week, insomnia, fatigue, and irritability. She has always been healthy. Findings from her physical examination are all within normal limits, and a review of systems is noncontributory. Routine laboratory tests such as a chemistry panel, CBC, and thyroid function tests are all normal. The most likely diagnosis is:

(A) major depressive disorder.
(B) generalized anxiety disorder.
(C) pain disorder.
(D) hypochondriasis.
(E) somatization disorder.

The correct response is option **A**: Major depressive disorder

In the primary care setting, major depressive disorder most commonly presents with multiple somatic symptoms, with back pain among the most frequent complaints.

Fava M: Somatic symptoms, depression, and anti-depressant treatment. J Clin Psychiatry 2002; 63:305–307

340

A 29-year-old patient with borderline personality disorder is being seen in psychotherapy twice weekly. The psychiatrist realizes that the patient is unconsciously trying to coerce her into acting in a judgmental way. This phenomenon is best described as:

(A) identification with the aggressor.
(B) projection.
(C) projective identification.
(D) regression.
(E) splitting.

The correct response is option **C**: Projective identification

Otto Kernberg described the defense mechanism of projective identification as it occurs in patients with borderline personality disorder. In this primitive defense mechanism, intolerable aspects of the self are projected onto another with the aim of inducing the person to play the projected role, and the two act in unison. It is important that therapists be aware of the process and act neutrally toward such patients.

Sadock BJ, Sadock VA: Kaplan and Sadock's Synopsis of Psychiatry, 9th ed. Philadelphia, Lippincott Williams & Wilkins, 2003, p 809

Gabbard GO: Psychodynamic approaches to personality disorders. FOCUS 2005; 3:363–367

Stern TA, Fricchione GL, Cassem NH, Jellinek MS, Rosenbaum JF (eds): Massachusetts General Hospital Handbook of General Hospital Psychiatry, 5th ed. St Louis, Mosby, 2004, pp 642–643

341

Which of the following is NOT FDA-approved for the treatment of acute mania?

(A) Carbamazepine
(B) Gabapentin
(C) Divalproex
(D) Olanzapine
(E) Risperidone

The correct response is option **B**: Gabapentin

Gabapentin has not been approved by the FDA for treating any aspect of bipolar disorder. Lithium, chlorpromazine, and divalproex were the first agents approved by the FDA for the treatment of acute mania. Since then, five newer antipsychotics—olanzapine, risperidone, quetiapine, ziprasidone, and aripiprazole—have been approved for acute mania. The extended-release formulation of carbamazepine, an anticonvulsant, has also been approved for acute mania.

Tohen M, Baker RW, Altshuler LL, Zarate CA, Suppes T, Ketter TA, Milton DR, Risser R, Gilmore JA, Breier A, Tollefson GA: Olanzapine versus divalproex in the treatment of acute mania. Am J Psychiatry 2002; 159:1011–1017
Ketter TA: Treatment of acute mania in bipolar disorder, in Advances in Treatment of Bipolar Disorder (Review of Psychiatry, vol 24). Washington, DC, American Psychiatric Publishing, 2005

342

The term "four D's of negligence"—duty, dereliction, direct, and damages—refers to:

(A) the questions a defendant physician will be asked at deposition.
(B) what a patient/plaintiff must prove to win a malpractice suit.
(C) the calculation of punitive versus compensatory damages.
(D) the level of care that would be expected of a reasonable physician under similar circumstances.

The correct response is option **B**: What a patient/plaintiff must prove to win a malpractice suit

The four D's of negligence refers to: duty, dereliction, direct, and damages. The physician owes a duty to the patient. When negligence occurs, there is a dereliction of this duty, which directly results in damage to the patient. To win a malpractice suit, a patient/plaintiff must prove by a preponderance of the evidence that the physician owed a *duty* of care to the patient and that negligence (a *dereliction* of this duty) occurred, which *directly* resulted in *damage* to the patient. Option D refers to the standard of care.

Hales RE, Yudofsky SC (eds): The American Psychiatric Publishing Textbook of Clinical Psychiatry, 4th ed. Washington, DC, American Psychiatric Publishing, 2003, p 1586
Simon RI: The law and psychiatry. FOCUS 2003; 1:349–372 (p 350)

343

In a psychotherapy session, a patient reveals that he has been having trouble obtaining an orgasm with his partner. He states that he has always felt aroused when traveling to work on a crowded bus, and he used to think that this enhanced his sexual life. He never thought it was a problem, but now he thinks it is interfering with his relationship. What is the most likely diagnosis?

(A) Exhibitionism
(B) Fetishism
(C) Frotteurism
(D) Pedophilia
(E) Voyeurism

The correct response is option **C**: Frotteurism

This scenario best describes the disorder of frotteurism according to DSM-IV-TR criteria—sexual arousal caused by rubbing up against a nonconsenting person.

American Psychiatric Association: Diagnostic and Statistical Manual of Mental Disorders, Fourth Edition, Text Revision (DSM-IV-TR). Washington, DC, American Psychiatric Association, 2000, p 570
Hales RE, Yudofsky SC (eds): The American Psychiatric Publishing Textbook of Clinical Psychiatry, 4th ed. Washington, DC, American Psychiatric Publishing, 2003, p 758

344

Which of the following comparisons regarding the incidence and prevalence of posttraumatic stress disorder (PTSD) is the most accurate?

(A) The condition is more prevalent in men.
(B) The presence of a psychiatric disorder does not predispose a person to PTSD.
(C) Older individuals have a higher prevalence than younger individuals.
(D) Certain types of trauma are more likely to cause PTSD.

The correct response is option **D**: Certain types of trauma are more likely to cause PTSD

Extreme stressors (such as rape, torture, and combat) significantly increase morbidity of PTSD. When the type of trauma is controlled for, women appear to be at higher risk of developing PTSD compared with men. In one nationwide survey, the highest current (17.8%) and lifetime (38.5%) rates of PTSD were in women who had been exposed to physical assault or rape. PTSD is more common in younger than in older individuals, probably because of the higher incidence of physical violence and accidents in the younger population. Individuals who respond to the initial trauma with high levels of anxiety (e.g., a panic attack), also have a higher risk of developing PTSD after trauma, as are those who perceive an external (vs. internal) locus of control.

Hales RE, Yudofsky SC (eds): The American Psychiatric Publishing Textbook of Clinical Psychiatry, 4th ed. Washington, DC, American Psychiatric Publishing, 2003, p 578

Breslau N, Kessler RC, Chilcoat HD, Schultz LR, Davis GC, Andreski P: Trauma and posttraumatic stress disorder in the community: the 1996 Detroit Area Survey of Trauma. Arch Gen Psychiatry 1998; 55:626–632

Breslau N: The epidemiology of posttraumatic stress disorder: what is the extent of the problem? J Clin Psychiatry 2001; 62(suppl 17):16–22

Resnick HS, Kilpatrick DG, Dansky BS, Saunders BE, Best CL: Prevalence of civilian trauma and posttraumatic stress disorder in a representative national sample of women. J Consult Clin Psychol 1993; 61:984–991

Galea S, Ahern J, Resnick H, Kilpatrick D, Bucuvalas M, Gold J, Vlahov D: Psychological sequelae of the September 11 terrorist attacks in New York City. N Engl J Med 2002; 346:982–987

345

Which of the following statements is correct about the concordance of schizophrenia in the twin of an individual with schizophrenia?

(A) 50% if twin is monozygotic
(B) 75% if twin is monozygotic
(C) Almost 100% if twin is monozygotic
(D) 50% if twin is dizygotic
(E) 75% if twin is dizygotic

The correct response is option **A**: 50% if twin is monozygotic

Between 50% and 60% of monozygotic twin pairs are concordant for schizophrenia. In several studies over recent decades, the concordance in dizygotic twins has ranged from 4% to 15%.

Hales RE, Yudofsky SC (eds): The American Psychiatric Publishing Textbook of Clinical Psychiatry, 4th ed. Washington, DC, American Psychiatric Publishing, 2003, pp 18–19

Sadock BJ, Sadock VA (eds): Kaplan and Sadock's Synopsis of Psychiatry: Behavioral Sciences/Clinical Psychiatry, 9th ed. Philadelphia, Lippincott Williams & Wilkins, 2003, p 465

346

A 33-year-old woman with a diagnosis of borderline personality disorder was recently discharged from medical service after an aspirin overdose. She describes having had thoughts of suicide off and on since early adolescence and has made two previous suicide attempts. In addressing her suicidality in treatment, which of the following approaches would be most appropriate?

(A) Partial hospitalization or brief inpatient hospitalization
(B) Outpatient psychoanalysis
(C) Gabapentin pharmacotherapy
(D) Valproic acid pharmacotherapy

The correct response is option **A**: Partial hospitalization or brief inpatient hospitalization

Of the options listed, long-term partial hospitalization has the most empirical support. Studies of mood stabilizers have been mixed. Although not a listed option, dialectical behavior therapy also has substantial empirical support for the treatment of borderline personality disorder.

Bateman A, Fonagy P: Effectiveness of partial hospitalization in the treatment of borderline personality disorder: a randomized controlled trial. Am J Psychiatry 1999; 156:1563–1569

Bateman A, Fonagy P: Treatment of borderline personality disorder with psychoanalytically oriented partial hospitalization: an 18-month follow-up. Am J Psychiatry 2001; 158:36–42

Lieb K, Zanarini MC, Schmahl C, Linehan MM, Bohus M: Borderline personality disorder. Lancet 2004; 364:453–461

Practice Guideline for the Treatment of Patients With Borderline Personality Disorder (2001), in American Psychiatric Association Practice Guidelines for the Treatment of Psychiatric Disorders, Compendium 2004. Washington, DC, APA, 2004, pp 757–758

347

In addition to a stimulant trial for attention deficit hyperactivity disorder symptoms, the parents of an 8-year-old boy ask what other treatment would be most helpful for managing his refusal to cooperate at home. Which of the following is the best recommendation?

(A) Biofeedback
(B) Behavior therapy
(C) Cognitive behavior therapy
(D) Family therapy
(E) Psychodynamic psychotherapy

The correct response is option **B**: Behavior therapy

Behavior therapy has been documented to be helpful as a component of the treatment of ADHD, especially parent training and classroom behavioral modification approaches.

Sadock BJ, Sadock VA (eds): Kaplan and Sadock's Comprehensive Textbook of Psychiatry, 8th ed. Philadelphia, Lippincott Williams & Wilkins, 2005, pp 2545, 3195

348

A 15-year-old girl is brought in for an emergency evaluation because she has been out all night and refuses to tell her parents where she has been. The parents report that for several months the girl has been irritable and oppositional with severe mood swings. She has been leaving home and school without permission. The girl admits that she has been somewhat moody but insists that her parents are making a big deal about nothing. A preliminary diagnosis of bipolar disorder is made. Which of the following is the most common comorbid condition with bipolar disorder?

(A) Conduct disorder
(B) Generalized anxiety disorder
(C) Oppositional defiant disorder
(D) Posttraumatic stress disorder
(E) Substance use disorder

The correct response is option **E**: Substance use disorder

Substance use or abuse is an important diagnosis to consider in adolescents who present with symptoms consistent with bipolar disorder, both as a possible cause of the symptoms and as an important potential coexisting problem. This diagnosis has significant implications for treatment planning.

Sadock BJ, Sadock VA (eds): Kaplan and Sadock's Comprehensive Textbook of Psychiatry, 8th ed. Philadelphia, Lippincott Williams & Wilkins, 2005, p 3277
Lewis M (ed): Child and Adolescent Psychiatry: A Comprehensive Textbook, 3rd ed. Philadelphia, Lippincott Williams & Wilkins, 2002, pp 783–786

349

A 29-year-old woman is admitted to the hospital with acute herpes simplex encephalitis. Which of the following is the most common residual deficit upon recovery?

(A) Apraxia
(B) Aphasia
(C) Amnesia
(D) Ataxia
(E) Dysarthria

The correct response is option **C**: Amnesia

Acute herpes simplex encephalitis damages the medial, temporal, and orbitofrontal regions of the cortex. Amnesia is the most common residual deficit. The regions of the brain for language, speech, and discrimination of touch are usually not affected.

Wise MG, Rundell JR (eds): The American Psychiatric Publishing Textbook of Consultation-Liaison Psychiatry: Psychiatry in the Medically Ill, 2nd ed. Washington, DC, American Psychiatric Publishing, 2002, pp 86, 688

350

Which of the following is most effective for the psychotherapeutic treatment of obsessive-compulsive disorder?

(A) Biofeedback
(B) Exposure and response prevention
(C) Psychodynamic psychotherapy
(D) Relaxation and visualization
(E) Interpersonal therapy

The correct response is option **B**: Exposure and response prevention

Exposure and response prevention is most effective for the psychotherapeutic treatment of obsessive-compulsive disorder. Relaxation techniques alone are not helpful and are often used as the control in research on obsessive-compulsive disorder.

Practice parameters for the assessment and treatment of children and adolescents with obsessive-compulsive disorder. J Am Acad Child Adolesc Psychiatry 1998; 37(suppl 10):27S–45S
Jenike MA: Clinical practice: obsessive-compulsive disorder. N Engl J Med 2004; 350:259–265
American Psychiatric Association: Practice Guideline for the Treatment of Patients With Obsessive-Compulsive Disorder. Am J Psychiatry, expected 2007

351

Rebound insomnia is most severe after abrupt withdrawal of which of the following medications?

(A) Alprazolam
(B) Clonazepam
(C) Diazepam
(D) Chlordiazepoxide
(E) Quazepam

The correct response is option **A**: Alprazolam

Abrupt withdrawal of any benzodiazepine will cause some degree of rebound anxiety and insomnia. Short-acting compounds have been found to have a greater effect on rebound insomnia on discontinuation. The elimination half-life of alprazolam is intermediate (6 to 20 hours) and is the shortest in comparison to clonazepam, long (>20 hours); diazepam, long (>20 hours); quazepam, long (>20 hours); and chlordiazepoxide, intermediate (6 to 20 hours) but with long (>20 hours) metabolites (demoxepam and nordazepam).

Hales RE, Yudofsky SC (eds): The American Psychiatric Publishing Textbook of Clinical Psychiatry, 4th ed. Washington, DC, American Psychiatric Publishing, 2003, pp 1073–1075
Sadock BJ, Sadock VA: Kaplan and Sadock's Synopsis of Psychiatry, 9th ed. Philadelphia, Lippincott Williams & Wilkins, 2003, p 1025

352

All of the following are symptom clusters of posttraumatic stress disorder (PTSD) EXCEPT:

(A) reexperiencing.
(B) avoidance/numbing.
(C) hyperarousal.
(D) derealization/depersonalization.

The correct response is option **D**: Derealization/depersonalization

Derealization and depersonalization are listed as criteria for acute stress disorder in DSM-IV-TR.

American Psychiatric Association: Diagnostic and Statistical Manual of Mental Disorders, Fourth Edition, Text Revision (DSM-IV-TR). Washington, DC, American Psychiatric Association, 2000, pp 468, 471
American Psychiatric Association: Practice Guideline for the Treatment of Patients With Acute Stress Disorder and Posttraumatic Stress Disorder. Am J Psychiatry 2004; 161(Nov suppl):9

353

In clinical or forensic evaluations when financial compensation or special benefits may be available, a psychiatrist must consider the diagnosis of:

(A) factitious disorder.
(B) malingering.
(C) somatization.
(D) hypochondriasis.

The correct response is option **B**: Malingering

Malingering, the conscious attempt to fake or exaggerate an illness or symptom for personal gain, is the correct answer. Factitious disorder is a self-induced medical problem where the personal goal is not evident. Somatization disorder is a polysymptomatic disorder that begins before age 30, extends over a period of years, and is characterized by a combination of pain and gastrointestinal, sexual, and pseudoneurological symptoms. Hypochondriasis is the fear of having a serious disease based on misinterpretation of somatic signs or symptoms.

American Psychiatric Association: Diagnostic and Statistical Manual of Mental Disorders, Fourth Edition, Text Revision (DSM-IV-TR). Washington, DC, American Psychiatric Association, 2000, pp 485–489, 739, 781–783

354

Avoidance symptoms in posttraumatic stress disorder (PTSD) include which of the following?

(A) Hypervigilance
(B) Intrusive images of the event
(C) Sense of reliving the event or experience
(D) Difficulty recalling important aspects of the event

The correct response is option **D**: Difficulty recalling important aspects of the event

Difficulty recalling is a form of avoidance. In the DSM-IV-TR, posttraumatic stress disorder symptoms are clustered into three categories: reexperiencing, avoidance and numbing, and hyperarousal. Option A is a symptom of hyperarousal, while options B and C are symptoms of reexperiencing the event.

Shalev AY: What is posttraumatic stress disorder? J Clin Psychiatry 2001; 62(suppl 17):4–10
American Psychiatric Association: Diagnostic and Statistical Manual of Mental Disorders, Fourth Edition, Text Revision (DSM-IV-TR). Washington, DC, American Psychiatric Association, 2000, p 468
Davidson JRT: Effective management strategies for posttraumatic stress disorder. FOCUS 2003; 1:239–243

355

Weight gain is LEAST likely to be a side effect of which of the following?

(A) Lithium
(B) Lamotrigine
(C) Divalproex
(D) Olanzapine

The correct response is option **B**: Lamotrigine

When lamotrigine was compared with valproate in a monotherapy study on epilepsy, weight remained stable among patients using the former but not the latter medication (at 32 weeks, mean weight gain was 12.8 pounds on valproate and 1.3 pounds on lamotrigine). Weight gain is a well-established side effect of lithium, divalproex, and olanzapine.

Biton V, Mirza W, Montouris G, Vuong A, Hammer AE, Barrett PS: Weight change associated with valproate and lamotrigine monotherapy in patients with epilepsy. Neurology 2001; 56:172–177

Russell JM, Mackell JA: Body weight gain associated with atypical antipsychotics: epidemiology and therapeutic implications. CNS Drugs 2001; 15:537–551

McIntyre RS, Konarski JZ: Obesity and psychiatric disorders: frequently encountered clinical questions. FOCUS 2005; 3:511–519 (p 516)

356

In Erikson's epigenetic model, each life stage has an identity crisis that must be navigated. Intimacy vs. isolation is the developmental crisis associated with:

(A) school age.
(B) adolescence.
(C) young adulthood.
(D) adulthood.
(E) old age.

The correct response is option **C**: Young adulthood

According to Erikson, the primary task at the life stage of young adulthood, between ages 20 and 40, is to form strong friendships and to achieve a sense of love and companionship or a shared identity with another person. Feelings of loneliness or isolation are likely to result from an inability to form friendships or an intimate relationship.

Erikson EH: The Life Cycle Completed. New York, WW Norton, 1998, pp 56–57

Shaffer DR: Developmental Psychology: Childhood and Adolescence, 5th ed. Pacific Grove, Calif, Brooks/Cole, 1999, pp 45–47

Weiner JM, Dulcan MK: Textbook of Child and Adolescent Psychiatry, 3rd ed. Washington, DC, American Psychiatric Publishing, 2004, p 36

357

Trichotillomania is a difficult symptom to treat with either psychotherapy or medication. Emerging evidence indicates that medication plus which of the following types of psychotherapy is effective?

(A) Exposure
(B) Flooding
(C) Habit reversal
(D) Interpersonal psychotherapy
(E) Psychodynamic psychotherapy

The correct response is option **C**: Habit reversal

Probably the best described and most effective psychotherapeutic technique for the treatment of trichotillomania is habit reversal. The technique has been adapted to both individual and group therapies. Habit reversal includes 13 components, including such things as self-monitoring, relaxation training, habit interruption, overcorrection, and habit inconvenience.

Hales RE, Yudofsky SC (eds): The American Psychiatric Publishing Textbook of Clinical Psychiatry, 4th ed. Washington, DC, American Psychiatric Publishing, 2003, p 796

Hautmann G, Hercogova J, Lotti T: Trichotillomania. J Am Acad Dermatol 2002; 46:807–821

The following vignette applies to questions 358 and 359.

A 19-year-old woman presents to a clinic for treatment of chapped hands. She reports that for several months she has had "this notion in my head" that there are germs everywhere. At first she washed her hands more frequently, but as the thoughts have become more prominent, she now usually wears gloves and washes her hands with diluted bleach several times a day. She says that if she does not complete her cleansing rituals, she cannot stand the anxiety.

The most common comorbid condition with this disorder is:

(A) alcohol abuse.
(B) generalized anxiety disorder.
(C) major depressive disorder.
(D) social phobia.
(E) schizophrenia.

The correct response is option **C**: Major depressive disorder

Two-thirds of patients who have obsessive-compulsive disorder will sometime in their life have an episode of major depression, with about one-third meeting the criteria for current comorbid depression, making it the most common comorbid disorder. All of the other anxiety disorders may be comorbid as well. Finally, obsessive-compulsive disorder can be comorbid with schizophrenia, often making the treatment more difficult.

Kaplan HI, Sadock BJ: Synopsis of Psychiatry. 8th ed. Baltimore, Williams & Wilkins, 1998, pp 610–611
Stein DJ, Hollander E (eds): American Psychiatric Publishing Textbook of Anxiety Disorders. Washington, DC, American Psychiatric Publishing, 2002, pp 183–186

The structural brain abnormality that has been demonstrated most consistently in this disorder is:

(A) asymmetrical septal nuclei.
(B) decreased size of the caudate.
(C) enlarged lateral ventricles.
(D) hypertrophy of the amygdala.
(E) shrinkage of the hippocampus.

The correct response is option **B**: Decreased size of the caudate

This patient is suffering from obsessive-compulsive disorder. Functional brain imaging (e.g., positron emission tomography) has demonstrated increased metabolism and blood flow in the basal ganglia, especially the caudate. Interestingly, structural studies (e.g., computed tomography and magnetic resonance imaging) have found bilaterally smaller caudates in patients with obsessive-compulsive disorder.

Kaplan HI, Sadock BJ: Synopsis of Psychiatry. 8th ed. Baltimore, Williams & Wilkins, 1998, p 610

In which of the following disorders has reduced volume been observed in the prefrontal cortex?

(A) ADHD
(B) Delusional disorder
(C) Obsessive-compulsive disorder
(D) Panic disorder
(E) Schizophrenia

The correct response is option **E**: Schizophrenia

Studies have demonstrated that patients diagnosed with schizophrenia have decreased prefrontal gray matter, decreased prefrontal white matter, and increased ventricle size. The cognitive deficits persist in patients who are not actively psychotic or experiencing negative symptoms.

Hulshoff Pol HE, Schnack HG, Bertens MG, van Haren NE, van der Tweel I, Staal WG, Baare WF, Kahn RS: Volume changes in gray matter in patients with schizophrenia. Am J Psychiatry 2002; 159:244–250

The first step in the evaluation of a patient with male erectile disorder is to:

(A) take a genetic history.
(B) rule out medical problems and substance use.
(C) refer the patient to a sex therapist.
(D) challenge with a test dose of a PDE-5 inhibitor.
(E) order a sleep study.

The correct response is option **B**: Rule out medical problems and substance use

Medical problems and substance use must be considered and carefully assessed during the evaluation of male erectile disorder. From twin studies, the heritability of the risk of dysfunction in having an erection is estimated to be 35%, and of maintaining an erection, 42%. The efficacy of the three available PDE-5 inhibitors (sildenafil, vardenafil, and tadalafil) is approximately 70%, and the three have similar side effect profiles. Caution should be exercised with PDE-5 inhibitors in patients with hypotension and uncontrolled hypertension. The prognosis of male erectile disorder has improved over the years by several groundbreaking treatments: sex therapy, penile prosthesis, intracavernosal injection, and oral PDE-5 inhibitors.

Fischer ME, Vitek ME, Hedeker D, Henderson WG, Jacobsen SJ, Goldberg J: A twin study of erectile dysfunction. Arch Intern Med 2004; 164:165–168
Gresser U, Gleiter CH: Erectile dysfunction: comparison of efficacy and side effects of the PDE-5 inhibitors sildenafil, vardenafil, and tadalafil. Eur J Med Res 2002; 7:435–446
Farre JM, Fora F, Lasheras MG: Specific aspects of erectile dysfunction in psychiatry. Int J Impot Res 2004; 16:546–549

362

A 75-year-old woman with Parkinson's disease develops vivid dreams and night terrors. The most likely explanation for these symptoms is:

(A) the onset of dementia.
(B) a rapid progression of Parkinson's disease.
(C) a normal effect of aging.
(D) an anxiety disorder.
(E) side effects from carbidopa-levodopa.

The correct response is option **E**: Side effects from carbidopa-levodopa

The encephalopathic side effects of carbidopa-levodopa are essentially those of the levodopa. Nearly 30% of patients with Parkinson's disease taking L-dopa have vivid dreams and 7% have night terrors. Delirium occurs in 5%, and a delusional syndrome develops in as many as 3% of patients who take L-dopa for 2 or more years.

Brown TM, Stoudemire GA: Psychiatric Side Effects of Prescription and Over-the-Counter Medications: Recognition and Management. Washington, DC, American Psychiatric Press, 1998, pp 37–38
Krahn LE, Richardson JW: Sleep disorders, in The American Psychiatric Publishing Textbook of Psychosomatic Medicine. Edited by Levenson JL. Washington, DC, American Psychiatric Publishing, 2005, Table 16-10, pp 350–352

363

In which of the following therapies, which has been studied for the treatment of patients with borderline personality disorder, is mindfulness training a central component?

(A) Cognitive behavior therapy
(B) Dynamic psychotherapy
(C) Dialectical behavior therapy
(D) Short-term group psychotherapy
(E) Interpersonal psychotherapy

The correct response is option **C**: Dialectical behavior therapy

Mindfulness is considered a core skill in dialectical behavior therapy, along with tolerance, emotion regulation, and interpersonal effectiveness. Dialectical behavior therapy is well studied and frequently cited as an effective approach to the treatment of patients with borderline personality disorder. Mindfulness training addresses attentional control, described by Linehan as being "in control of attentional processes."

Tasman A, Kay J, Lieberman JA (eds): Psychiatry. Philadelphia, WB Saunders, 1997, p 357

Hales RE, Yudofsky SC (eds): The American Psychiatric Publishing Textbook of Clinical Psychiatry, 4th ed. Washington, DC, American Psychiatric Publishing, 2003, p 1266
Sadock BJ, Sadock VA (eds): Kaplan and Sadock's Comprehensive Textbook of Psychiatry, 8th ed. Philadelphia, Lippincott Williams & Wilkins, 2005, pp 2621–2624

364

Heightened arousal in posttraumatic stress disorder (PTSD) is associated with an increase in which of the following?

(A) Heart rate
(B) Constriction of pupils
(C) Weight
(D) Tidal volume

The correct response is option **A**: Heart rate

The arousal in PTSD is largely due to an increased autonomic response. Therefore, increased heart rate would be a natural occurrence. Constricted pupils, on the other hand, as well as weight gain and an increase in tidal volume would more likely be associated with parasympathetic stimulation. Other physiological findings associated with arousal in PTSD include muscle tension as measured by electromyography and increased sweating.

American Psychiatric Association: Diagnostic and Statistical Manual of Mental Disorders, Fourth Edition, Text Revision (DSM-IV-TR). Washington, DC, American Psychiatric Association, 2000, p 465
Hollander E, Simeon D: Anxiety disorders; in The American Psychiatric Publishing Textbook of Clinical Psychiatry, Fourth Edition. Edited by Hales RE, Yudofsky SC. Washington, DC, American Psychiatric Publishing, 2004, p 600

365

According to DSM-IV-TR, a mixed episode must meet diagnostic criteria for a manic episode and which of the following?

(A) Panic attacks
(B) Rapid cycling
(C) Brief psychotic episode
(D) Major depressive episode

The correct response is option **D**: Major depressive episode

Mixed episodes contain features of both mania and depression. While mixed episodes have been defined by a number of different criteria, DSM-IV-TR requires at least a week during which criteria are met for both a manic episode and a major depressive episode.

McElroy SL, Keck PE Jr, Pope HG Jr, Hudson JI, Faedda GL, Swann AC: Clinical and research implications of the diagnosis of dysphoric or mixed mania or hypomania. Am J Psychiatry 1992; 149:1633–1644

American Psychiatric Association: Diagnostic and Statistical Manual of Mental Disorders, Fourth Edition, Text Revision (DSM-IV-TR). Washington, DC, American Psychiatric Association, 2000, pp 362–363

American Psychiatric Association: Practice Guideline for the Treatment of Patients With Bipolar Disorder (Revision). Am J Psychiatry 2002; 159(April suppl). Reprinted in FOCUS 2003; 1:64–110 (p 81)

366

A psychiatrist is called to see a 78-year-old female patient postoperatively on the surgical service who is said to be "manic." She is hardly sleeping, she is agitated and talking rapidly, and she believes she needs to talk with the President of the United States. Which of the following interventions is most likely to be effective?

(A) Transfer to a psychiatric unit
(B) Divalproex sodium
(C) Haloperidol
(D) ECT
(E) A benzodiazepine

The correct response is option **C**: Haloperidol

An elderly patient who develops acute mental status changes while in the hospital for another problem (this patient is on the surgical service) is most likely suffering from delirium, which is a medical problem (thus options A, B, and D will likely turn out not to be the eventual intervention). Indeed, elderly postsurgical patients are especially at high risk of delirium. Although benzodiazepines can be useful in the management of agitated delirium, the mainstay of delirium management is dopamine blockade with an agent such as haloperidol. Of course, the most important intervention is to identify and treat the cause of the confusional state.

Trzepacz PT: Delirium (confusional states), in The American Psychiatric Publishing Textbook of Consultation-Liaison Psychiatry: Psychiatry in the Medically Ill, 2nd ed. Edited by Wise MG, Rundell JR. Washington, DC, American Psychiatric Publishing, 2002, pp 266–268

Schouten R: Legal aspects of consultation, in Massachusetts General Hospital Handbook of General Hospital Psychiatry, 5th ed. Edited by Stern TA, Fricchione GL, Cassem NH, Jellinek MS, Rosenbaum JF. St Louis, Mosby, 2004, pp 451–452

367

Which of the following variables is most important to take into account when evaluating the score on a Mini-Mental State Exam (MMSE)?

(A) Educational level
(B) Gender
(C) History of alcohol use
(D) Medical history
(E) Past psychiatric history

The correct response is option **A**: Educational level

The formerly used cutoff score of 23 to identify cognitive impairment has been shown to have poor sensitivity for detecting cognitive impairment in better-educated adults. At the same time, individuals with lower educational attainment will be overidentified as cognitively impaired when this cutoff is used. Age- and education-based norms have since been developed for the MMSE.

Spar JE, La Rue A: Concise Guide to Geriatric Psychiatry, 3rd ed. Washington, DC, American Psychiatric Publishing, 2002, pp 158–159

368

The parents of a 5-year-old boy bring their child to a clinic with the complaint that he frequently awakens during the early part of the night screaming; he looks terrified, his pupils are dilated, and he hyperventilates. He is also sweating, agitated, and confused, and he cannot be comforted. When fully awakened, the child has no recall of the event. This presentation is most consistent with:

  (A) narcolepsy.
  (B) nightmare disorder.
  (C) primary insomnia.
  (D) sleep disordered breathing.
  (E) sleep terror disorder.

The correct response is option **E**: Sleep terror disorder

The presentation is most consistent with sleep terror disorder. The most pertinent parts of this vignette are a young child awakening during the early part of sleep in a state of heightened arousal, along with the lack of recall of the event. This would suggest an incident most likely occurring in stages 3–4 of sleep, as this is the most prominent pattern in the early hours. Therefore, consideration would be given to some type of parasomnia associated with deep sleep. The lack of recall for what is happening during the episode suggests that this is not a nightmare. The symptoms are not consistent with the presentation of narcolepsy or a breathing disorder, such as apnea.

Dulcan MK, Martini DR, Lake MB: Concise Guide to Child and Adolescent Psychiatry, 3rd ed. Washington, DC, American Psychiatric Publishing, 2003, pp 165–167

369

A 6-year-old girl is brought to a clinic because of unusual stereotyped hand washing. Pregnancy, labor, and delivery were unremarkable, as were developmental milestones until the age of 8 months, when the child seemed to lose interest in her social environment. Thereafter, significant delays in development were noted. She did not walk until 2 years of age and has had no spoken language. Head growth has stagnated. Recently she has developed breath-holding spells. Examination reveals a small, noncommunicative child who demonstrates truncal ataxia and nonpurposeful hand movements. EEG is abnormal. This presentation is most consistent with:

  (A) Asperger's syndrome.
  (B) autism.
  (C) childhood schizophrenia.
  (D) mild mental retardation.
  (E) Rett's disorder.

The correct response is option **E**: Rett's disorder

In this vignette, development is normal until the age of 8 months and then goes awry, with specific delays and deviance in social, communicative, and cognitive development. Rett's disorder, which occurs only in females, is characterized by an early onset of developmental delays, with deceleration of head growth, loss of purposeful hand movements and stereotypies, and incoordination of gait and trunk movements. The early age at onset suggests the presence of a pervasive developmental disorder rather than schizophrenia, which typically does not present until closer to or during adolescence. In autistic disorder, qualitative impairments are seen in social interaction and communication, along with repetitive and stereotyped patterns of behavior, interest, and activities, but head growth does not decelerate or stagnate, nor is there deterioration in neurological functioning. The same is true for Asperger's syndrome, which presents with many of the signs and symptoms of autistic disorder but without impairments in language or cognitive development. Children with disintegrative disorder develop an autistic-like condition after a longer period (2 or more years) of unequivocally normal development.

Lewis M (ed): Child and Adolescent Psychiatry: A Comprehensive Textbook, 3rd ed. Philadelphia, Lippincott Williams & Wilkins, 2002, pp 587–597

370

Which of the following actions on the part of a psychiatrist constitutes abandonment?

  (A) Failing to show up for a scheduled appointment with a patient
  (B) Referring, with appropriate notification to the patient, an extremely difficult patient to a colleague with more experience in the treatment of the patient's disorder
  (C) Terminating the treating relationship when a patient threatens to sue the psychiatrist
  (D) Prematurely discharging a patient from the hospital

The correct response is option **D**: Prematurely discharging a patient from the hospital

According to Simon (2001), any of the following actions can be construed as abandonment of the patient: failure to inform the patient about medication side effects, failure to admit the patient to the hospital when indicated, not attending (or arranging appropriate attending) to the patient during a hospitalization, prematurely discharging the patient from the hospital, inappropriate or improper referral of the patient, sexual relations with a patient, and termination of the treatment based only on denial of benefits by a third-party payer. Abandonment is a breach of the fiduciary duty of the psychiatrist to act in the patient's best interest. When the therapeutic relationship between the psychiatrist and the patient is "unilaterally and prematurely terminated by the psychiatrist without reasonable notice," abandonment may have occurred. Terminating the treating relationship when a patient threatens to sue may be in the patient's best interest because of the countertransference that almost invariably would occur (it is also difficult to imagine that a patient who has threatened to sue would want to continue in treatment with the same psychiatrist).

Simon RI: A Concise Guide to Psychiatry and Law for Clinicians, 3rd ed. Washington, DC, American Psychiatric Publishing, 2001, p 32–33

371

Common side effects of selective serotonin reuptake inhibitors include:

(A) orthostatic hypotension and dry mouth.
(B) confusion and disorientation.
(C) priapism and arrhythmia.
(D) seizures and hallucinations.
(E) nausea and sexual dysfunction.

The correct response is option **E**: nausea and sexual dysfunction

Common side effects of SSRIs include anxiety, nausea, insomnia, sedation, and sexual dysfunction. Trazodone can cause priapism. Seizures are associated with bupropion. Confusion and disorientation may occur with toxic levels of antidepressants. Orthostatic hypotension and dry mouth occur more commonly with tricyclic antidepressants.

Sadock BJ, Sadock VA (eds): Kaplan and Sadock's Comprehensive Textbook of Psychiatry, 7th ed. Philadelphia, Lippincott Williams & Wilkins, 2000, p 1381

372

Which of the following classes of medications is supported by well-designed studies as the first-line pharmacologic treatment of posttraumatic stress disorder (PTSD)?

(A) Mood stabilizers
(B) Benzodiazepines
(C) Tricyclic antidepressants
(D) Selective serotonin reuptake inhibitors (SSRIs)

The correct response is option **D**: Selective serotonin reuptake inhibitors (SSRIs)

Selective serotonin reuptake inhibitors are recommended as first-line pharmacological treatment for posttraumatic stress disorder. SSRIs have been found to be effective not only in reducing PTSD symptoms but also in treatment of comorbid disorders and associated symptoms. Double-blind placebo-controlled studies support the use of SSRIs as first-line agents for the treatment of PTSD. Sertraline and paroxetine have been approved by the FDA for the treatment of PTSD. Other SSRIs are currently being studied for efficacy. Open-label trials have suggested that nefazodone may be useful for reducing PTSD symptoms. The monoamine oxidase inhibitors and tricyclic antidepressants have been shown in a number of double-blind placebo-controlled studies to be effective, but they are considered second- or third-line agents because of their side effect profiles. Mood stabilizers should be considered, especially when there is accompanying impulsivity or aggressiveness, although further studies are needed to determine the effectiveness of these agents for patients with PTSD.

Hageman I, Andersen HS, Jorgensen MB: Posttraumatic stress disorder: a review of psychobiology and pharmacotherapy. Acta Psychiatr Scand 2001; 104:411–422

Maddux RM, Rapaport MH: Anxiolytic drugs, in Psychiatry, 2nd ed. Edited by Tasman A, Kay J, Lieberman JA. New York, Wiley & Sons, 2003

Hollander E, Simeon D: Concise Guide to Anxiety Disorders. Washington, DC, American Psychiatric Publishing, 2003 p 180

Davidson J, Pearlstein T, Londborg P, Brady KT, Rothbaum B, Bell J, Maddock R, Hegel MT, Farfel G: Efficacy of sertraline in preventing relapse of posttraumatic stress disorder: results of a 28-week double-blind, placebo-controlled study. Am J Psychiatry 2001; 158:1974–1981. Reprinted in FOCUS 2003; 1:273–281

Brady K, Pearlstein T, Asnis GM, Baker D, Rothbaum B, Sikes CR, Farfel GM: Efficacy and safety of sertraline treatment of posttraumatic stress disorder: a randomized controlled trial. JAMA 2000; 283:1837–1844

373

A patient in early recovery from opiate dependence has been maintained on 40 mg/day of oral methadone for the last month. While the patient has not been experiencing any withdrawal symptoms at that dose, the weekly random urine drug tests begin showing a resumption of heroin use. Pharmacologically, the best change to make in medication would be to:

(A) increase the maintenance dose of methadone.
(B) decrease the maintenance dose of methadone.
(C) change the opiate agonist to levo-alpha-acetylmethadol (LAAM).
(D) augment with buprenorphine.

The correct response is option **A**: Increase the maintenance dose of methadone

An oral methadone dose of 40 mg is a low dose. Better outcomes have been achieved with higher doses. There is no reason to change to LAAM at this point. Decreasing or discontinuing treatment would likely lead to even poorer patient outcomes. Buprenorphine may precipitate withdrawal in opioid-dependent patients.

Bickel WK, Amass L: Buprenorphine treatment of opioid dependence: a review. Exp Clin Psychopharmacology 1995; 3:477–489
Preston KL, Umbricht A, Epstein DH: Methadone dose increase and abstinence reinforcement for treatment of continued heroin use during methadone maintenance. Arch Gen Psychiatry 2000; 57:395–404
Strain EC, Bigelow GE, Liebson IA, Stitzer ML: Moderate- vs high-dose methadone in the treatment of opioid dependence. JAMA 1999; 281:1000–1005

374

A 45-year-old man who travels frequently finds that on returning from his most recent trip to a distant city, he has had difficulty maintaining daytime alertness and falls asleep easily and at inappropriate times. Which of the following is the most likely diagnosis?

(A) Circadian rhythm sleep disorder
(B) Dissociative fugue
(C) Dyssomnia
(D) Parasomnia
(E) Narcolepsy

The correct response is option **A**: Circadian rhythm sleep disorder

Circadian rhythm sleep disorder is a persistent pattern of sleep disruption from a mismatch of the patient's endogenous sleep-wake cycle. There are four varieties: delayed sleep-phase type, jet lag type, shift work type, and unspecified type. In jet lag type, the degree of difficulty the patient has is usually related to the number of time zones crossed.

A dissociative fugue is characterized by sudden travel away from one's home with an inability to recall some or all of one's past. A dyssomnia is characterized by a disturbance in the amount, quality, or timing of sleep. A parasomnia is characterized by abnormal behavioral or physiological events occurring in association with sleep or the components of sleep. Narcolepsy is one type of dyssomnia. It involves repeated attacks of refreshing sleep, cataplexy, and recurrent attacks of REM sleep in the form of hypnagogic or hypnopompic hallucinations.

American Psychiatric Association: Diagnostic and Statistical Manual of Mental Disorders, Fourth Edition, Text Revision (DSM-IV-TR). Washington, DC, American Psychiatric Association, 2000, pp 523, 622–629

375

Compared with other dementias, the early presentation in Creutzfeldt-Jakob disease more often includes:

(A) choreoathetosis.
(B) dysarthria.
(C) extrapyramidal symptoms.
(D) frontal release signs.
(E) myoclonus.

The correct response is option **E**: Myoclonus

Myoclonus is a typical manifestation in the early stages of Creutzfeldt-Jakob disease. Extrapyramidal symptoms are found in Parkinson's disease; dysarthria is a sign of head injury; choreoathetosis is a sign of Huntington's disease; and frontal release signs are found in Pick's disease.

Spar JE, La Rue A: Concise Guide to Geriatric Psychiatry, 3rd ed. Washington, DC, American Psychiatric Publishing, 2002, p 217

376

A 27-year-old man has a 4-month history of persecutory delusions about being spied on at work by coworkers. Apart from the delusions, he functions reasonably well, and there is no evidence of medical illness or substance abuse. The most likely diagnosis is:

(A) brief psychotic disorder.
(B) delusional disorder.
(C) major depression with psychotic features.
(D) schizophrenia, paranoid type.
(E) schizophreniform disorder.

The correct response is option **B**: Delusional disorder

According to DSM-IV-TR, nonbizarre delusions in the absence of markedly impaired function and bizarre or odd behavior would qualify for a diagnosis of delusional disorder. Both schizophrenia and schizophreniform disorder are characterized by features such as prominent hallucinations, disorganized speech and behavior, and negative symptoms. An episode of brief psychotic disorder must have a duration of less than 1 month.

American Psychiatric Association: Diagnostic and Statistical Manual of Mental Disorders, Fourth Edition, Text Revision (DSM-IV-TR). Washington, DC, American Psychiatric Association, 2000, pp 323–329

377

Nausea and other gastrointestinal side effects with SSRIs appear to be related to which receptor subtype?

(A) $5\text{-}HT_2$ receptor
(B) DA-2 receptor
(C) DA-4 receptor
(D) H_2 receptor

The correct response is option **A**: $5\text{-}HT_2$ receptor

The short form of the promoter for the serotonin (5-HT) transporter has been reported to predict poor response or intolerance to SSRIs in Caucasians.

Schatzberg AF: Recent studies of the biology and treatment of depression. FOCUS 2005; 3:14–24

378

Which of the following abilities is NOT directly relevant to a person's capacity to make medical decisions?

(A) Communicate or evidence a choice
(B) Understand the facts of the situation
(C) Appreciate how the facts of a situation apply to oneself
(D) Choose an option that reflects what most reasonable persons in that situation would do

The correct response is option **D**: Choose an option that reflects what most reasonable persons in that situation would do

The currently accepted standards relevant to an individual's capacity to make medical decisions do not include whether or not the patient makes the "correct" choice. It is still possible for a fully competent patient to choose an option that few "reasonable" persons would choose. While standards for assessing the capacity to make a decision vary from state to state, the abilities to communicate a choice, to understand, and to appreciate are commonly accepted standards.

Grisso T, Appelbaum PS: Assessing Competence to Consent to Treatment: A Guide for Physicians and Other Health Professionals. New York, Oxford University Press, 1998

379

An 18-year-old woman is starting her freshman year in college. She is living at home with her parents. On campus, she hopes to make friends but usually stays to herself, fearing that she will be rejected by her peers. When called on in class, she avoids eye contact with the professor. Although she almost always knows the answer to questions asked by the professor, she experiences inordinate anxiety that she will make a mistake. In private moments, she refers to herself as "the big nobody." This presentation is most consistent with:

(A) avoidant personality disorder.
(B) dependent personality disorder.
(C) paranoid personality disorder.
(D) schizoid personality disorder.
(E) schizotypal personality disorder.

The correct response is option **A**: Avoidant personality disorder

A number of personality disorders are characterized by a paucity of interpersonal relationships. The cluster A personality disorders (paranoid, schizoid, and schizotypal) are often described as "loners." However, patients with these disorders are not particularly bothered by the lack of relationships. Individuals with an avoidant personality disorder are hypersensitive to rejection by others. Their main personality trait is timidity. Although they desire human companionship, their inordinate fear of rejection prevents them from developing relationships. Their hypervigilance about rejection causes them to lack self-confidence and to speak in a self-effacing manner. In contrast, individuals with dependent personality disorder have a pattern of seeking and maintaining connections to important others rather than avoiding and withdrawing from relationships.

Sadock BJ, Sadock VA: Kaplan and Sadock's Synopsis of Psychiatry, 9th ed. Philadelphia, Lippincott Williams & Wilkins, 2003, pp 812–813
Cloninger CR, Svrakic DM: Personality disorders, in Kaplan and Sadock's Comprehensive Textbook of Psychiatry, 7th ed. Edited by Sadock BJ, Sadock VA. Philadelphia, Lippincott Williams & Wilkins, 2000, pp 1743–1747
American Psychiatric Association: Diagnostic and Statistical Manual of Mental Disorders, Fourth Edition, Text Revision (DSM-IV-TR). Washington, DC, American Psychiatric Association, 2000, p 724

380

The oncology team is concerned because a patient from another culture acts resigned when faced with a diagnosis of terminal cancer. The consulting psychiatrist points out that in the patient's culture illness and death are part of the normal cycle of life. Which of the following best describes the use of culture in this psychiatric formulation?

(A) Interpretive and explanatory tool
(B) Pathogenic and pathoplastic agent
(C) Diagnostic and nosologic factor
(D) Therapeutic and protective element
(E) Management and service instrument

The correct response is option **A**: Interpretive and explanatory tool

There are several ways to look at the function of culture in contemporary psychiatry. Culture as interpretive and explanatory tool allows for describing nonpathologic behaviors within the context of an individual's culture. Culture as pathogenic and pathoplastic agent demonstrates that some psychopathology can result from cultural practices. Culture as diagnostic and nosologic factor frames a specific disease as unique to a culture. Culture can also be therapeutic and protective to one's mental health. Culture as a management and service instrument allows for cultural factors to play a role in the way mental health services are delivered.

Alarcon RD, Westermeyer J, Foulks EF, Ruiz P: Clinical relevance of contemporary cultural psychiatry. J Nerv Ment Dis 1999; 187:465–471

381

According to DSM-IV-TR, which of the following characterizes acute stress disorder (ASD)?

(A) Lasts a maximum of 8 weeks
(B) Does not involve symptoms of hyperarousal
(C) Often occurs as a result of a minor threat
(D) Requires dissociative symptoms for a diagnosis

The correct response is option **D**: Requires dissociative symptoms for a diagnosis

The DSM-IV-TR criteria for the diagnosis of acute stress disorder include the presence of at least three dissociative symptoms (a sense of being in a daze, depersonalization, derealization, a sense of numbing or detachment, or dissociative amnesia). Hyperarousal symptoms are a common feature of both acute stress disorder and PTSD. The duration criteria for acute stress disorder state that the disturbance lasts for a minimum of 2 days and a maximum of 4 weeks and occurs within 4 weeks of the traumatic event. Acute PTSD requires a duration of symptoms less than 3 months, and a diagnosis of chronic PTSD requires that the symptoms have been present for at least 3 months.

American Psychiatric Association: Diagnostic and Statistical Manual Of Mental Disorders, Fourth Edition, Text Revision (DSM-IV-TR). Washington, DC, American Psychiatric Association, 2000, pp 469–472
Kaplan HI, Sadock BJ: Synopsis of Psychiatry: Behavioral Sciences/Clinical Psychiatry, 9th ed. Baltimore, Lippincott Williams & Wilkins, 2003, pp 626–627

382

Olfactory hallucinations are most commonly associated with:

(A) grand mal seizures.
(B) hypoparathyroidism.
(C) parietal tumor.
(D) partial complex seizures.
(E) psychotic depression.

The correct response is option **D**: Partial complex seizures

Olfactory hallucinations are most commonly associated with partial complex seizures, although they can be reported in patients with psychosis or somatization disorders. Olfactory tumors must also be ruled out. Other types of hallucinations, such as taste or kinesthetic hallucinations, may also occur with partial complex seizures. Olfactory hallucinations may also occur in psychotic depression and typically involve odors of decay, rotting, or death.

Sadock BJ, Sadock VA (eds): Kaplan and Sadock's Comprehensive Textbook of Psychiatry, 7th ed, vol 2. Philadelphia, Lippincott Williams & Wilkins, 2000, p 811

383

A new psychologist in town approaches an established psychiatrist and proposes that the psychiatrist refer therapy patients to the psychologist in return for a small percentage of fees collected by the psychologist from treating those patients. This practice is:

(A) not acceptable because it does not put the patients' interests first.

(B) not acceptable because psychiatrists should refer patients to psychiatrist therapists.

(C) acceptable because it provides incentives for all parties to benefit.

(D) acceptable because the psychologist is fairly compensating the psychiatrist.

The correct response is option **A**: Not acceptable because it does not put the patients' interests first

Referrals need to be based on the patients' need, in order to preserve trust in the health care system. The financial arrangement described in this question creates a financial incentive for the psychiatrist that could be in opposition to what is necessary for the welfare of the patient. For instance, there will be situations in which the referral to the therapist may be of financial interest for the psychiatrist but not congruent with the patient's needs. Also, the therapist could try to recoup the costs for referrals by charging more for the services.

Hundert EM, Appelbaum PS: Boundaries in psychotherapy: model guidelines. Psychiatry 1995; 58:345–356
American Psychiatric Association: Principles of Medical Ethics With Annotations Especially Applicable to Psychiatry. Washington, DC, American Psychiatric Press, 2001 (section 2, annotation 7)

384

In order for an individual to recover from PTSD after interpersonal violence, which of the following processes is likely to be most helpful?

(A) Go to court and see the perpetrator brought to justice.

(B) Wait for symptoms to subside with time.

(C) Emotionally engage with the memory of the trauma.

(D) Restore sleep with a benzodiazepine.

(E) Obtain treatment with eye movement desensitization techniques.

The correct response is option **C**: Emotionally engage with the memory of the trauma

For successful processing of traumatic events, three processes must be accomplished: the person must engage emotionally with the memory of the trauma; the trauma story must be organized and articulated in a sequenced and coherent fashion; and the dysfunctional thoughts that commonly occur after trauma must be addressed and corrected.

Davidson JRT: Effective management strategies for posttraumatic stress disorder. FOCUS 2003; 1:239–243

385

A hospital risk manager speaks with you about developing an educational seminar on suicide prevention contracts for emergency department staff. As part of the seminar, which of the following would be a most appropriate point to emphasize?

(A) A patient's willingness to enter into a suicide prevention contract indicates readiness for discharge from an emergency setting.

(B) In emergency settings, suicide prevention contracts are a helpful method for reducing suicide risk but should not be used to determine readiness for discharge.

(C) Using suicide prevention contracts in emergency settings is not recommended.

(D) Suicide prevention contracts can be useful for assessing the physician-patient relationship with individuals who are intoxicated, agitated, or psychotic.

The correct response is option **C**: Using suicide prevention contracts in emergency settings is not recommended

Suicide prevention contracts are only as reliable as the state of the therapeutic alliance. Thus, with a new patient, the psychiatrist may not have had sufficient time to make an adequate assessment or to evaluate the patient's capacity to form a therapeutic alliance, creating little or no basis for relying on a suicide prevention contract. As a result, the use of suicide contracts in emergency settings or with newly admitted and unknown inpatients is not recommended.

Practice Guideline for the Assessment and Treatment of Patients With Suicidal Behaviors (2003), in American Psychiatric Association Practice Guidelines for the Treatment of Psychiatric Disorders, Compendium 2004. Washington, DC, APA, 2004, p 905

386

A middle-aged man consults a psychiatrist at the recommendation of his primary care physician because he has been unable to recover from his deep grief and feelings of abandonment since his divorce 18 months ago. He endorses many symptoms of major depression and has withdrawn from the social activities that he used to enjoy, but he is not suicidal. Of the following things that this patient reports, which would be the most positive indicator that he would be able to benefit from psychodynamic psychotherapy?

(A) He is very angry at his ex-wife.
(B) He has no family history of psychiatric illness.
(C) He has been a successful writer.
(D) He gets significant support from his two best friends.
(E) He is very religious.

The correct response is option **D**: He gets significant support from his two best friends

Option D indicates a capacity for meaningful object relationships, a crucial indicator for psychodynamic psychotherapy. The other items listed are significant to his history but are not as relevant to suitability for psychotherapy. Success at work is a positive indicator to some extent, but it might also indicate that the patient was a workaholic who avoids painful feelings or awareness by plunging himself into his work.

Sadock BJ, Sadock VA (eds): Kaplan and Sadock's Synopsis of Psychiatry: Behavioral Sciences/Clinical Psychiatry, 9th ed. Philadelphia, Lippincott Williams & Wilkins, 2003, pp 923–934

387

Lorazepam may be a better choice of a benzodiazepine than diazepam for an elderly patient because the:

(A) volume of distribution decreases with age.
(B) hepatic oxidation is unaffected by age.
(C) hepatic conjugation is unaffected by age.
(D) glomerular filtration rate is unaffected by age.
(E) hepatic blood flow is unaffected by age.

The correct response is option **C**: Hepatic conjugation is unaffected by age

Lorazepam is primarily metabolized by conjugation, and diazepam by oxidation. Conjugation is unaffected by age, whereas oxidation decreases with age, leading to increases in the half-life of diazepam. Volume of distribution increases with age, whereas glomerular filtration rate and hepatic blood flow decline—all of which would affect both drugs similarly.

Dubovsky SL, Buzan R: Psychopharmacology, in Textbook of Geriatric Neuropsychiatry, 2nd ed. Edited by Coffey CE, Cummings JL. Washington, DC, American Psychiatric Press, 2000, pp 780–781, 796

388

A patient who is an artist is severely depressed and has occasional passive suicidal thoughts. The patient tells the psychiatrist that health insurance benefits have been discontinued and that the patient is no longer able to pay the psychiatric bills. The psychiatrist has decided not to provide free care to this patient. The psychiatrist can avoid abandoning this patient by:

(A) giving the patient a written, 30-day notice of termination and terminating the patient at the end of the 30-day period.
(B) reducing the frequency of the patient's appointments to help make the patient's bill more affordable.
(C) arranging to commission an artwork by the patient in lieu of the professional fees.
(D) continuing to see the patient until acute depression-related crises are resolved and then discharging the patient to the local state-funded community agency clinic.

The correct response is option **D**: Continuing to see the patient until acute depression-related crises are resolved and then discharging the patient to the local state-funded community agency clinic

While an advance notice of termination can sometimes be sufficient, it is inadequate in the case presented in this question, because the patient's condition is severe and may be worsening. Option B will not provide the close monitoring that is necessary for adequate treatment of severe depression with suicidal ideation. Option C describes a bartering arrangement that is highly questionable, as it creates a relationship (artist-patron) that may not always coincide with the goals of the doctor-patient relationship.

American Psychiatric Association: Ethics Primer of the American Psychiatric Association. Washington, DC, American Psychiatric Association, 2001, p 7
Simon RI: A Concise Guide to Psychiatry and Law for Clinicians, 3rd ed. Washington, DC, American Psychiatric Publishing, 2001, pp 32–34
Gutheil TG, Appelbaum PS: Clinical Handbook of Psychiatry and the Law, 3rd ed. Philadelphia, Lippincott Williams & Wilkins, 2000, p 152

389

A primary substance abuse prevention program is being developed for adolescent girls in a large, metropolitan school district in the United States. The school district is diverse, with youths from African, Asian, Caucasian, Middle Eastern, and Native American families. Based on epidemiologic studies, which ethnic group of adolescent girls is at greatest risk of substance use?

(A) African American
(B) Asian American
(C) Caucasian
(D) Middle Eastern
(E) Native American

The correct response is option **E**: Native American

The University of Michigan's annual Monitoring the Future Study (MTF) is a survey of tens of thousands of students in grades 8 through 12. The MTF documents recent trends in substance use, among them a progressively younger age of initiation, particularly for girls. Among girls, drug use is highest in Native Americans and lowest in African Americans and Asian Americans. These differences are thought to be attributable to sociocultural and genetic factors.

Romans SE, Seeman MV: Women's Mental Health: A Life-Cycle Approach. Philadelphia, Lippincott Williams & Wilkins, 2006, pp 133–137
National Institute on Drug Abuse: Gender and ethnic patterns in drug use among high school seniors. NIDA Notes 2004; 18(2). Available at http://www.nida.nih.gov/NIDA_notes/NNVol18N2/tearoff.html

390

Posttraumatic stress disorder (PTSD) is considered to be chronic PTSD after:

(A) 1 month.
(B) 3 months.
(C) 6 months.
(D) 1 year.
(E) 3 years.

The correct response is option **B**: 3 months

Someone who has suffered a life-threatening traumatic event will be diagnosed as having an acute stress disorder in the first month after the trauma. If the duration of the symptoms is less than 3 months, the diagnosis is acute PTSD, and if it is 3 months or more, chronic PTSD.

American Psychiatric Association: Diagnostic and Statistical Manual of Mental Disorders, Fourth Edition, Text Revision (DSM-IV-TR). Washington, DC, American Psychiatric Association, 2000, pp 463–468

391

A 9-year-old boy is seen in the emergency department after attempting to jump out of a moving vehicle. His parents report that he has had a difficult time in the past year. Previously he had done well in school, but now he is struggling academically. He often says he does not want to go to school, "because I am so stupid and ugly." His teacher has contacted his parents and informed them that he is falling asleep in class, seems fatigued, has little to do with his peers, and often does not eat his lunch. The child used to play with friends in the neighborhood, but for the past 2 months has kept to himself, playing alone in his room or just sitting and looking out the window. A few days earlier, he informed his mother of what to do with his most important belongings should he die, but she did not make anything out of it. He has generally seemed very grouchy and "on edge." On questioning, he acknowledges that he was hoping to be killed when he tried to jump out of the car. The most likely diagnosis is:

(A) borderline personality disorder.
(B) major depressive disorder.
(C) oppositional defiant disorder.
(D) separation anxiety disorder.
(E) somatization disorder.

The correct response is option **B**: Major depressive disorder

The diagnostic criteria for major depressive disorder are the same for children and adolescents as adults, except that youths are more likely to present with an irritable mood. This boy exhibits loss of interest in school or play, difficulty sleeping, impaired appetite, fatigue, feelings of worthlessness, and suicidal ideation with an attempt, in the presence of dysphoria and irritability. This is consistent with major depressive disorder.

Dulcan MK, Martini DR, Lake MB: Concise Guide to Child and Adolescent Psychiatry, 3rd ed. Washington, DC, American Psychiatric Publishing, 2003, pp 129–131
Lewis M (ed): Child and Adolescent Psychiatry: A Comprehensive Textbook, 3rd ed. Philadelphia, Lippincott Williams & Wilkins, 2002, pp 768–770

392

The family of a 40-year-old retired police officer reports that in the past year he has been increasingly isolative, withdrawn, and bizarre. He has accused his family of trying to poison him. He put tarps over the windows in his house. He is disheveled and carries a set of torn papers at all times. He has been observed mumbling and talking to himself. He has no history of substance abuse or prior depressive episodes. Which of the following is the most likely diagnosis?

(A) Bipolar disorder
(B) Delusional disorder
(C) Dementia of the Alzheimer's type
(D) Major depression with psychotic features or schizoaffective disorder
(E) Schizophrenia

The correct response is option **E**: Schizophrenia

His diminished social function, evidence of delusional thinking, and behavior related to delusions are indicative of late-onset schizophrenia. Delusional disorder would be the second most likely diagnosis, but patients with this disorder generally do not have hallucinations or such extreme loss of social function.

American Psychiatric Association: Diagnostic and Statistical Manual of Mental Disorders, Fourth Edition, Text Revision (DSM-IV-TR). Washington, DC, American Psychiatric Association, 2000, pp 298–313

393

Clinical signs of major depression may emerge for a patient during bereavement after a parent's death. According to DSM-IV-TR criteria, what is the earliest time interval after the parent's death that this diagnosis is generally made?

(A) 1 month
(B) 2 months
(C) 3 months
(D) 6 months

The correct response is option **B**: 2 months

The diagnosis of major depressive disorder is not usually made until the symptoms of the disorder persist for 2 months after the death. Studies have indicated that if depression is not treated around this time, it is still present 9 months to 1 year after the death.

Zisook S, Shuchter SR, Sledge PA, Paulus M, Judd LL: The spectrum of depressive phenomena after spousal bereavement. J Clin Psychiatry 1994; 55(April suppl):29–36
Zisook S, Shuchter SR: Uncomplicated bereavement. J Clin Psychiatry 1993; 54:365–372

American Psychiatric Association: Diagnostic and Statistical Manual of Mental Disorders, Fourth Edition, Text Revision (DSM-IV-TR). Washington, DC, American Psychiatric Association, 2000, pp 740–741

394

Involuntary hospitalization of a patient with schizophrenia who is hearing voices is justified in which of the following situations?

(A) The patient hears a voice that he cannot resist telling him to kill himself.
(B) Third-party payer deems hospitalization appropriate and will pay.
(C) The patient appears dirty and disheveled.
(D) The patient lacks insight into the nature of his illness.

The correct response is option **A**: The patient hears a voice that he cannot resist telling him to kill himself

If the patient's voices are telling him to kill himself and he feels he must act on these commands, then, although it involves taking away the patient's liberty (or autonomy), the psychiatrist may act in the patient's best interests (beneficence) and hospitalize the patient against the patient's wishes. Involuntary hospitalization of mentally ill individuals brings together the often conflicting ethical principles of autonomy, beneficence, and informed consent, among others. The patient who is hearing voices telling him to kill himself may or may not require involuntary hospitalization. The current standard for involuntary hospitalization in most states is that of dangerousness to self or others. Initially the specified amount of time of hospitalization is determined by the state's law. The psychiatrist's judgment of dangerousness is necessarily dependent on an adequate and appropriate clinical examination, which must be well documented. Whether or not a third-party payer or government agency deems hospitalization the appropriate care, the psychiatrist's ethical obligation is to the patient. Appearing dirty and disheveled does not in and of itself mean that the patient is unable to care for himself. The concept of grave disability, if it is a result of mental illness, can be cause for involuntary hospitalization in some states. Grave disability is usually defined as the inability to provide for one's own food, clothing, or shelter.

American Psychiatric Association: Ethics Primer of the American Psychiatric Association. Washington, DC, American Psychiatric Association, 2001, pp 27–32
Simon RI: The law and psychiatry. FOCUS 2003; 1:349–372 (p 358)

395

Kidney stones are most likely to be a side effect of which of the following?

(A) Gabapentin
(B) Lithium
(C) Lamotrigine
(D) Topiramate

The correct response is option **D**: Topiramate

The package insert for topiramate states that 1.5% of adults exposed to the drug during its development had kidney stones, an incidence two to four times that of the general population. The formation of kidney stones may be related to reduced urinary citrate excretion as a result of carbonic anhydrase inhibition by the drug. The association was noted almost exclusively in patients with epilepsy, although it has also been reported in a patient with bipolar II disorder. Although lithium can adversely affect the kidneys in several ways, the formation of kidney stones is not associated with lithium therapy.

Takhar J, Manchanda R: Nephrolithiasis on topiramate therapy. Can J Psychiatry 2000; 45:491–493
Jones MW: Topiramate: safety and tolerability. Can J Neurol Sci 1998; 25(suppl 3):S13–S15

396

The CEO of a large company is fearful of speaking at a large stockholders' meeting. His fear of public speaking has been a lifelong disability, but he does not have anxiety in other social settings. Which of the following is the most reasonable agent to prescribe?

(A) A benzodiazepine
(B) A beta-blocker
(C) Buspirone
(D) A serotonin norepinephrine reuptake inhibitor (SNRI)
(E) An SSRI

The correct response is option **B**: A beta-blocker

The beta-adrenergic blockers have been used successfully for management of this specific social phobia. Both public speakers and music performers have found them helpful because of the drugs' effectiveness in decreasing manifestations of anxiety in the autonomic nervous system. They have an advantage over benzodiazepines because the beta-blockers do not impair concentration or coordination. The length of time for therapeutic effect of the other agents (SSRIs, SNRIs, and buspirone) makes them impractical for occasional use.

Stein DJ, Hollander E (eds): American Psychiatric Publishing Textbook of Anxiety Disorders. Washington, DC, American Psychiatric Publishing, 2002, p 315

397

A 49-year-old man with schizophrenia taking an antipsychotic asks to change medication because of intolerable side effects. He has had extrapyramidal side effects and has experienced a 24-pound weight gain. His body mass index is now 32.4. His family history is significant for obesity, diabetes, hypercholesterolemia, hypertension, and sudden cardiac death. Of the following medications, which would be the next best one in the management of this patient?

(A) Aripiprazole
(B) Olanzapine
(C) Quetiapine
(D) Risperidone
(E) Ziprasidone

The correct response is option **A**: Aripiprazole

Weight gain and metabolic syndromes are potential side effects of the atypical antipsychotics. Weight gain tends to occur most frequently with olanzapine and clozapine, occurs moderately with quetiapine and risperidone, and is least likely to occur with ziprasidone. Aripiprazole tends to be weight neutral. Of these medications, risperidone is the most likely to cause extrapyramidal side effects. Ziprasidone may cause QTc interval prolongation and should be used with caution in patients with a family history of sudden cardiac death. Because it is weight neutral, aripiprazole is the next drug of choice for treating this patient's schizophrenia.

Schatzberg AF, Cole JO, DeBattista C: Manual of Clinical Psychopharmacology. Washington, DC, American Psychiatric Publishing, 2005, pp 187–206
McIntyre RS, Konarski JZ: Obesity and psychiatric disorders: frequently encountered clinical questions. FOCUS 2005; 3:511–519

398

A 34-year-old man who is comatose, has myoclonic twitching, and has a serum lithium level of 4.2 mEq/L should respond best to which of the following treatments?

(A) Activated charcoal
(B) Hemodialysis
(C) Intravenous sodium chloride
(D) Osmotic diuresis
(E) Plasmapheresis

The correct response is option **B**: Hemodialysis

Severe lithium toxicity, as evidenced in this case by the markedly elevated serum level together with the level of neurologic impairment, is best treated with hemodialysis, which is the most effective way of removing lithium rapidly from the body.

Jefferson JW, Greist JH: Lithium, in Kaplan and Sadock's Comprehensive Textbook of Psychiatry, 8th ed. Edited by Sadock BJ, Sadock VA. Philadelphia, Lippincott Williams & Wilkins, 2005, pp 2839–2851

399

Which of the following is the most common extrapyramidal side effect of antipsychotic medication?

(A) Akathisia
(B) Torticollis
(C) Oculogyric crisis
(D) Neuroleptic malignant syndrome
(E) Tardive myoclonus

The correct response is option **A**: Akathisia

The most common extrapyramidal side effect of antipsychotic medications is acute neuroleptic-induced akathisia, which consists of a subjective feeling of restlessness along with restless movements, usually in the legs or feet. Patients often pace continuously or move their feet. Over a third of patients treated with high-potency dopamine receptor antagonists experience akathisia, particularly when these medications are administered in high doses. Akathisia appears to be less common when lower doses or lower-potency dopamine receptor antagonists are administered and is even more infrequent with atypical antipsychotic agents. Dystonic reactions (including torticollis and oculogyric crises) occur in up to 10% of patients treated with high-potency dopamine receptor antagonists, whereas tardive myoclonus and neuroleptic malignant syndrome are relatively rare.

Sadock BJ, Sadock VA (eds): Kaplan and Sadock's Comprehensive Textbook of Psychiatry, 8th ed. Philadelphia, Lippincott Williams & Wilkins, 2005, p 2829
American Psychiatric Association: Practice Guideline for the Treatment of Patients With Schizophrenia, 2nd ed. Am J Psychiatry 2004; 161(Feb suppl):1–56

400

The best legal protection for a psychiatrist who is accused of malpractice after a patient's suicide is:

(A) the documentation of the patient's risk factors for suicide recorded in the chart.
(B) the patient's documented history of an axis II disorder.
(C) a doctor-patient suicide prevention ("no-harm") contract.
(D) the patient's family having promised to supervise the patient closely.

The correct response is option **A**: The documentation of the patient's risk factors for suicide recorded in the chart

The best legal protection is thorough documentation of a patient's risk factors for suicide. This should include always asking a patient about suicidal ideation and recording chronic and acute risk factors as well as facilitating versus inhibiting factors. It has been noted that as many as 25% of suicidal patients deny having suicidal ideation, so the risk assessment must go beyond simply recording the patient's answer to a question about suicidal thoughts. The psychiatrist should take appropriate steps, if indicated, such as increasing the frequency of visits or even hospitalizing the patient involuntarily. While a comorbid axis II disorder may, especially if it predisposes a patient to impulsivity or uncontrolled rage, represent a chronic risk factor for suicide, documentation of an axis II disorder in and of itself does not protect the psychiatrist from a malpractice allegation. A family's assurance that they will supervise a suicidal patient may be well-intentioned but does not mitigate the psychiatrist's duty to assess thoroughly a patient's risk factors for suicide. Although frequently used in psychiatric and mental health practice, a suicide prevention or "no-harm" contract generally provides minimal legal protection for a psychiatrist accused of malpractice after a patient's suicide.

Simon RI: The suicidal patient, in A Concise Guide to Psychiatry and Law for Clinicians, 3rd ed. Washington, DC, American Psychiatric Publishing, 2001, pp 143–177
Simon RI: The law and psychiatry. FOCUS 2003; 1:349–372 (pp 354–355)

#		#		#		#		#		#		#		#	
1.	E	51.	C	101.	D	151.	E	201.	A	251.	C	301.	D	351.	A
2.	A	52.	B	102.	A	152.	E	202.	C	252.	C	302.	C	352.	D
3.	E	53.	C	103.	D	153.	C	203.	A	253.	A	303.	C	353.	B
4.	B	54.	B	104.	C	154.	C	204.	B	254.	D	304.	A	354.	D
5.	C	55.	C	105.	E	155.	B	205.	B	255.	A	305.	C	355.	B
6.	A	56.	B	106.	D	156.	C	206.	B	256.	D	306.	A	356.	C
7.	C	57.	C	107.	C	157.	A	207.	D	257.	D	307.	A	357.	C
8.	B	58.	E	108.	C	158.	B	208.	E	258.	A	308.	A	358.	C
9.	B	59.	B	109.	D	159.	A	209.	D	259.	D	309.	A	359.	B
10.	B	60.	C	110.	C	160.	D	210.	B	260.	A	310.	C	360.	E
11.	C	61.	A	111.	D	161.	D	211.	A	261.	A	311.	C	361.	B
12.	A	62.	E	112.	A	162.	C	212.	D	262.	E	312.	D	362.	E
13.	C	63.	D	113.	E	163.	B	213.	A	263.	A	313.	D	363.	C
14.	C	64.	A	114.	E	164.	A	214.	E	264.	D	314.	B	364.	A
15.	D	65.	C	115.	D	165.	B	215.	B	265.	B	315.	B	365.	D
16.	C	66.	E	116.	E	166.	D	216.	D	266.	D	316.	A	366.	C
17.	E	67.	E	117.	B	167.	C	217.	A	267.	E	317.	D	367.	A
18.	A	68.	A	118.	D	168.	D	218.	C	268.	B	318.	A	368.	E
19.	A	69.	A	119.	B	169.	B	219.	A	269.	E	319.	E	369.	E
20.	C	70.	A	120.	A	170.	E	220.	C	270.	C	320.	B	370.	D
21.	C	71.	A	121.	D	171.	A	221.	D	271.	E	321.	C	371.	E
22.	C	72.	B	122.	A	172.	C	222.	C	272.	C	322.	A	372.	D
23.	B	73.	E	123.	A	173.	B	223.	B	273.	C	323.	D	373.	A
24.	C	74.	C	124.	A	174.	A	224.	C	274.	C	324.	C	374.	A
25.	E	75.	E	125.	A	175.	C	225.	B	275.	D	325.	D	375.	E
26.	C	76.	D	126.	B	176.	B	226.	A	276.	B	326.	A	376.	B
27.	B	77.	C	127.	B	177.	A	227.	C	277.	A	327.	C	377.	A
28.	B	78.	D	128.	C	178.	B	228.	D	278.	C	328.	D	378.	D
29.	A	79.	C	129.	B	179.	D	229.	B	279.	E	329.	B	379.	A
30.	C	80.	D	130.	E	180.	A	230.	C	280.	E	330.	D	380.	A
31.	B	81.	C	131.	A	181.	D	231.	C	281.	C	331.	C	381.	D
32.	E	82.	E	132.	C	182.	C	232.	C	282.	D	332.	D	382.	D
33.	E	83.	B	133.	D	183.	A	233.	A	283.	B	333.	D	383.	A
34.	B	84.	D	134.	C	184.	A	234.	C	284.	E	334.	B	384.	C
35.	B	85.	B	135.	C	185.	A	235.	C	285.	E	335.	C	385.	C
36.	C	86.	D	136.	B	186.	C	236.	C	286.	B	336.	D	386.	D
37.	B	87.	C	137.	D	187.	D	237.	E	287.	C	337.	A	387.	C
38.	D	88.	E	138.	D	188.	A	238.	B	288.	B	338.	E	388.	D
39.	E	89.	D	139.	A	189.	C	239.	E	289.	C	339.	A	389.	E
40.	A	90.	B	140.	A	190.	B	240.	C	290.	D	340.	C	390.	B
41.	B	91.	D	141.	A	191.	B	241.	D	291.	C	341.	B	391.	B
42.	B	92.	C	142.	D	192.	D	242.	D	292.	C	342.	B	392.	E
43.	C	93.	B	143.	A	193.	E	243.	A	293.	B	343.	C	393.	B
44.	E	94.	E	144.	E	194.	A	244.	C	294.	B	344.	D	394.	A
45.	C	95.	C	145.	A	195.	B	245.	A	295.	D	345.	A	395.	D
46.	B	96.	B	146.	C	196.	B	246.	B	296.	D	346.	A	396.	B
47.	C	97.	B	147.	D	197.	B	247.	C	297.	E	347.	B	397.	A
48.	A	98.	A	148.	E	198.	C	248.	B	298.	C	348.	E	398.	B
49.	D	99.	A	149.	C	199.	A	249.	A	299.	D	349.	C	399.	A
50.	D	100.	B	150.	D	200.	C	250.	C	300.	C	350.	B	400.	A

FOCUS Psychiatry Review: Blank Answer Sheet

1. ___	51. ___	101. ___	151. ___	201. ___	251. ___	301. ___	351. ___
2. ___	52. ___	102. ___	152. ___	202. ___	252. ___	302. ___	352. ___
3. ___	53. ___	103. ___	153. ___	203. ___	253. ___	303. ___	353. ___
4. ___	54. ___	104. ___	154. ___	204. ___	254. ___	304. ___	354. ___
5. ___	55. ___	105. ___	155. ___	205. ___	255. ___	305. ___	355. ___
6. ___	56. ___	106. ___	156. ___	206. ___	256. ___	306. ___	356. ___
7. ___	57. ___	107. ___	157. ___	207. ___	257. ___	307. ___	357. ___
8. ___	58. ___	108. ___	158. ___	208. ___	258. ___	308. ___	358. ___
9. ___	59. ___	109. ___	159. ___	209. ___	259. ___	309. ___	359. ___
10. ___	60. ___	110. ___	160. ___	210. ___	260. ___	310. ___	360. ___
11. ___	61. ___	111. ___	161. ___	211. ___	261. ___	311. ___	361. ___
12. ___	62. ___	112. ___	162. ___	212. ___	262. ___	312. ___	362. ___
13. ___	63. ___	113. ___	163. ___	213. ___	263. ___	313. ___	363. ___
14. ___	64. ___	114. ___	164. ___	214. ___	264. ___	314. ___	364. ___
15. ___	65. ___	115. ___	165. ___	215. ___	265. ___	315. ___	365. ___
16. ___	66. ___	116. ___	166. ___	216. ___	266. ___	316. ___	366. ___
17. ___	67. ___	117. ___	167. ___	217. ___	267. ___	317. ___	367. ___
18. ___	68. ___	118. ___	168. ___	218. ___	268. ___	318. ___	368. ___
19. ___	69. ___	119. ___	169. ___	219. ___	269. ___	319. ___	369. ___
20. ___	70. ___	120. ___	170. ___	220. ___	270. ___	320. ___	370. ___
21. ___	71. ___	121. ___	171. ___	221. ___	271. ___	321. ___	371. ___
22. ___	72. ___	122. ___	172. ___	222. ___	272. ___	322. ___	372. ___
23. ___	73. ___	123. ___	173. ___	223. ___	273. ___	323. ___	373. ___
24. ___	74. ___	124. ___	174. ___	224. ___	274. ___	324. ___	374. ___
25. ___	75. ___	125. ___	175. ___	225. ___	275. ___	325. ___	375. ___
26. ___	76. ___	126. ___	176. ___	226. ___	276. ___	326. ___	376. ___
27. ___	77. ___	127. ___	177. ___	227. ___	277. ___	327. ___	377. ___
28. ___	78. ___	128. ___	178. ___	228. ___	278. ___	328. ___	378. ___
29. ___	79. ___	129. ___	179. ___	229. ___	279. ___	329. ___	379. ___
30. ___	80. ___	130. ___	180. ___	230. ___	280. ___	330. ___	380. ___
31. ___	81. ___	131. ___	181. ___	231. ___	281. ___	331. ___	381. ___
32. ___	82. ___	132. ___	182. ___	232. ___	282. ___	332. ___	382. ___
33. ___	83. ___	133. ___	183. ___	233. ___	283. ___	333. ___	383. ___
34. ___	84. ___	134. ___	184. ___	234. ___	284. ___	334. ___	384. ___
35. ___	85. ___	135. ___	185. ___	235. ___	285. ___	335. ___	385. ___
36. ___	86. ___	136. ___	186. ___	236. ___	286. ___	336. ___	386. ___
37. ___	87. ___	137. ___	187. ___	237. ___	287. ___	337. ___	387. ___
38. ___	88. ___	138. ___	188. ___	238. ___	288. ___	338. ___	388. ___
39. ___	89. ___	139. ___	189. ___	239. ___	289. ___	339. ___	389. ___
40. ___	90. ___	140. ___	190. ___	240. ___	290. ___	340. ___	390. ___
41. ___	91. ___	141. ___	191. ___	241. ___	291. ___	341. ___	391. ___
42. ___	92. ___	142. ___	192. ___	242. ___	292. ___	342. ___	392. ___
43. ___	93. ___	143. ___	193. ___	243. ___	293. ___	343. ___	393. ___
44. ___	94. ___	144. ___	194. ___	244. ___	294. ___	344. ___	394. ___
45. ___	95. ___	145. ___	195. ___	245. ___	295. ___	345. ___	395. ___
46. ___	96. ___	146. ___	196. ___	246. ___	296. ___	346. ___	396. ___
47. ___	97. ___	147. ___	197. ___	247. ___	297. ___	347. ___	397. ___
48. ___	98. ___	148. ___	198. ___	248. ___	298. ___	348. ___	398. ___
49. ___	99. ___	149. ___	199. ___	249. ___	299. ___	349. ___	399. ___
50. ___	100. ___	150. ___	200. ___	250. ___	300. ___	350. ___	400. ___

Jerald Kay, M.D., Professor and Chair, Department of Psychiatry, Wright State University School of Medicine, Dayton, Ohio
No financial affiliations with commercial organizations.

Scott Y.H. Kim, M.D., Assistant Professor, Department of Psychiatry, Bioethics Program, and Center for Behavioral and Decision Sciences in Medicine, University of Michigan Medical School, Ann Arbor, Michigan
No financial affiliations with commercial organizations.

Joan A. Lang, M.D., Professor and Chair, Department of Psychiatry, Saint Louis University, St. Louis, Missouri
No financial affiliations with commercial organizations.

Martin H. Leamon, M.D., Associate Professor of Clinical Psychiatry, University of California–Davis, Sacramento
No financial affiliations with commercial organizations.

Alan K. Louie, M.D., Director, San Mateo County Mental Health Services, Psychiatry Residency Training Program, San Mateo, California
Consultant or Speaker: Abbott Laboratories; Bristol-Myers Squibb; Cephalon; Ciba-Geigy; Lilly; Forest; Glaxo Wellcome; Janssen; Parke Davis; Sandoz; SmithKline Beecham; Wyeth Ayerst.

Annette M. Matthews, M.D., Psychiatrist, Portland Veterans Affairs Medical Center, Portland, Oregon; Assistant Professor of Psychiatry, Oregon Health and Science University, Portland, Oregon; American Psychiatric Association/Bristol-Myers Squibb Fellow in Public and Community Psychiatry
Other Financial or Material Support: APA/Bristol-Myers Squibb fellowship.

Patricia I. Ordorica, M.D., Associate Chief of Staff for Mental Health and Behavioral Sciences, James A. Haley VA Hospital; Clinical Director, Counterdrug Technology Assessment Center (CTAC) Drug Addiction Study; Director, Addictive Disorders, and Associate Professor of Psychiatry, University of South Florida, Tampa
Consultant/Speaker: Bristol-Meyers Squibb; Pfizer, Inc.

David W. Preven, M.D., Clinical Professor in the Department of Behavioral Sciences and Psychiatry, Albert Einstein College of Medicine, Montefiore Medical Center, Bronx, New York
Speaker: Pfizer, Inc.; Forest.

Rima Styra, M.D., Toronto General Hospital, University Health Network, Department of Psychiatry, Toronto, Ontario, Canada
No financial affiliations with commercial organizations.

Christiane Tellefsen, M.D., Clinical Assistant Professor, University of Maryland School of Medicine and Johns Hopkins University School of Medicine, Baltimore, Maryland
No financial affiliations with commercial organizations.

Eric R. Williams, M.D., Child and Adolescent Psychiatrist, Raleigh, North Carolina
No financial affiliations with commercial organizations.

Isaac Wood, M.D., Associate Professor of Psychiatry and Pediatrics; Associate Dean of Student Activities; Director of Medical Student Education in Psychiatry, Virginia Commonwealth University School of Medicine, Richmond, Virginia
No financial affiliations with commercial organizations.

Disclosure of Unapproved or Investigational Use of a Product

FOCUS examination questions may contain information on off-label uses of particular medications. Off-label use of medications by individual physicians is permitted and common. Decisions about off-label use can be guided by the evidence provided in the scientific literature and by clinical experience.

Index of Questions by Topic

This index provides a guide for review of questions by topic area. Many questions apply to more than one topic area but are indexed by a single topic.